Natural Health

Pain Management For The 21st Century

Bruce R. Hocking, D.A.c, *Acupuncturist*, M.D.M.A.

ISBN 0-9681714-0-0

Table of Contents

ETPS Therapy Introduction .... 1 - 15

Quick Reference Guide .... 16 - 17

Dermatome Chart 18

Finger Measurements (point location) 19

ETPS Pain Therapy Introduction .... 20 - 49

Parasympathetic Points .... 21 - 22

Standard Protocol Back .... 23 - 27

Standard Protocol Neck .... 28 - 30

General Pain Disorders .... 31 -154

World Health Organization (WHO) 155

Index .... 156 -158

Special Thanks To:

Kimberly, Orion & the ETPS Group
also,
In memory my loving Father
Reginald Hocking

Important reminder:

The points recommended for treatment in this book are suggested only and are in no way guaranteed to assist in any condition. While the suggested points have proven helpful to some, the author in no way takes responsibility for the outcome of any Acutherapy treatment. It is recommended you receive a Medical Doctor's diagnosis for your condition prior to starting any ETPS Therapy program.

THE OPEN INTERNATIONAL UNIVERSITY
FOR
COMPLEMENTARY MEDICINES

Reply to:
28, International Buddhist
Centre Road,
Colombo 6, Sri Lanka.

CHARTER OF MEDICINA ALTERNATIVA
(ALMA ATA DECLARATION 1962)

Ref. No. MA/20
Date 5.2.2000

I wish to congratulate Dr. Bruce Hocking on his development of ETPS (Electro Therapeutic Point Stimulation) Therapy and the writing of this book.

Bruce has cleverly combined acupuncture with segmental and dermal therapy to produce ETPS. The integration of these therapies permits the treatment of many chronic pain syndromes.

I have assessed the efficacy of this therapy on many chronic pain patients at our hospital. I am most certainly impressed with the results obtained with ETPS.

While wishing him the best for the future, I wish to nominate him for the accolade Physician of the Year 2000 A.D. which will be conferred on him at the next World Congress in Colombo, Sri Lanka.

Lord Pandit Prof. Dr. Sir Anton Jayasuriya
Consultant Rheumatologist & Acupuncturist
Colombo South Government General Hospital
Kalubowila, Sri Lanka.

ETPS Therapy Overview:

A New Modality for the Treatment of Chronic Pain*

***Abstract: AAPM's 6th Edition of Pain Management: A Practical Guide for Physicians, 2001**

Pain, especially chronic pain, is a debilitating disease. It is one of the most unpleasant experiences for any human being to endure. Pain is the major reason why most people seek the attention of a physician or therapist.

Despite major advances in science and medicine with regard to drugs and surgery, eliminating or even reducing chronic soft tissue pain has been an elusive task for western medicine. Despite years of education, there are no courses titled Pain 101 in medical or therapy schools. Therefore, the current treatment approaches for pain, in most cases, provide unsatisfactory outcomes to suffering patients.

Finally, Relief from Pain:

Now there is relief for the suffering patient! ETPS Therapy is the world's first hybrid modality specifically designed for the treatment of chronic/acute soft tissue pain. ETPS Therapy applies brief, concentrated DC micro-stimulation to acupuncture points that relate to specific muscles, tissues and nerves that isolate and then treat, root causes of pain.

The theoretical underpinnings of ETPS are based on the integration of acupuncture, osteopathy, trigger point, neuromuscular and neural therapies. Its unique contribution to pain relief comes from the synthesis of these different approaches, combining the therapeutic 'pearls' of different modalities into simple, easy-to-use and highly effective series of protocols. The following manual provides the ultimate integrative pain "cookbook" for the treatment of pain.

ETPS is based on the theories that:

- Pain disorders are controlled by the autonomic nervous system (ANS).
- When the ANS becomes heightened or upregulated, the pain cycle is triggered, and will continue to be triggered until the pathology(s) causing un-regulation is eliminated. In many cases of pain, there is also **hypersensitivity** of the ANS called "**Denervation Supersensitivity**".
- This causes an amplification of the perception **of all senses**, such as heat, pressure & of course pain. This hypersensitivity is often seen in Fibromyalgia (2,4*).

ETPS theorizes that the chronic pain cycle is controlled by:

- Structural changes in the jaw, neck & sacrum that jam the nervous system
- Nerve root entrapment (called radiculopathy) which affect the limbs/ organs by reducing motor impulses & chemically changing nerve pathways
- Emotional blockages from past trauma - limbic system
- Physical scars left behind from injuries or surgeries - neural therapy
- Energetic imbalances in the organ system - traditional acupuncture
- **Postural Stress Syndromes (PSS), a bi-product of the above**, where asymmetrical movements of the body inhibit *(shut down)* muscles and transfer the task to compensating muscles which are not accustomed to such work. PPS is the basis of repetitive stress injuries. PPS increases wear & tear on the body and accelerates joint degeneration (arthritis).

ETPS is applied to both acupuncture and trigger points. The main difference between the treatment of acupuncture points and trigger points is their location, and with 93% of trigger points correlating to acupuncture points (6*). Acupuncture points are usually treated far removed from the injury or pain site, and trigger points are treated for local pathology.

NOTE: As a rule of thumb, acupuncture points located furthest from the pain site are usually the most powerful in providing pain relief.

The ETPS pain protocols presented in this manual are formulated using acupuncture & trigger points to isolate specific muscles, nerves and spinal segments that are believed to be primary cause(s) of the pain condition. One reason for the success of ETPS Pain Therapy is that it treats the patient as a whole, not just the local symptomology.

Why is ETPS stimulation optimal for pain relief?

Because it works on the same frequency as your nervous system! ETPS is applied non-invasively to acupuncture points using concentrated, low frequency Direct Current Microstimulation. The Biomedical Engineering Handbooks states "DC current heals, AC current kills".

Since the human body's nervous system "runs" on a low-frequency Direct Current (DC) impulse, this stimulation allows altered nerve function to be restored to normal & significantly accelerate tissue repair. By duplicating the same frequency of the human nervous system, ETPS can relax muscles and provide a significant calming response. **AC "TENS" and ultrasound cannot do this.**

Dr Robert Becker, Orthopedic surgeon, researcher and the father of osteogenesis (microcurrent therapy) documented in his book, **The Body Electric,** "the perineural cells or nerve sheaths carry a direct current of electricity, prompting the body to grow, heal, regenerate and repair itself. **No subsequent healing of any injury may occur without DC stimulation"(7*).**

Dr Bruce Pomeranz, the scientist who discovered endorphins (the body's natural opiates) through acupuncture, found that non-invasive, low frequency, DC stimulation (ETPS) can produce the same endorphin releasing affects as traditional needling. This led to the ability of non-acupuncturists, such as laypeople and pain sufferers, to easily apply non-invasive acupuncture (ETPS) at home or clinically.

Conclusion: in order to provide tissue change and long-term relief from pain, DC micro-stim (ETPS) must be applied to the patient

Why ETPS applied to acupuncture points?

For over 5000 years mankind has turned to acupuncture for pain relief. It is man's oldest known form of medicine, and has changed little in its approach over time. Research proves it works, with millions of people each year turning to acupuncture and electro-acupuncture for the management of their pain.

The ETPS device locates & treats acupuncture points with the optimal therapeutic stimulation, providing a non-invasive alternative to acupuncture or trigger point needling. When combined with the protocols outlined in this manual it provides a powerful tool in the fight against pain.

Conclusion:

ETPS is a gift to all suffering pain patients. ETPS can manage chronic pain, improve the quality of life and provide pain sufferers a means of self control. ETPS provides a simple easy-to-apply tool where patient treatment can continue on an as-needed basis in the home setting.

ETPS device is FDA approved & ETPS Therapy is CPT reimbursable. For additional information on upcoming ETPS CE Pain seminars in your area, contact **1-800-567-PAIN (7246), or visit www.acumedmedical.ca**

ETPS Pain Therapy

Acupuncture

Classical acupuncture therapy is a vast body of ancient knowledge collected and compiled over many centuries by the Chinese. Since acupuncture therapy is said to influence the entire body, the diagnosis of a disease is often very different from a diagnosis with western medicine. Western medicine often looks for an external cause or agent to explain the disease. Eastern medicine, on the other hand, looks at the body as a whole in which health is considered to be a state of total harmony between the physical, emotional and spiritual states of the individual. In eastern medicine, symptoms like pain are often considered unimportant. Such symptoms are seen as merely part of the energetic, chemical and structural disharmonies throughout the body.

Each traditional acupuncture point has a specific anatomical location. Each point individually or collectively exerts an influence on specific muscles, tissues, segments, emotions & sometimes entire systems (i.e. circulatory).

All **acupuncture points display a lowered electrical resistance in relation to their surrounding skin. Therefore these points may be** precisely detected on the skin's surface using an electrical point finder that can measure variances in skin resistance (ohms).ETPS has a highly accurate built-in point finder. **This enables non-acupuncturists to accurately locate and treat acupuncture points without formal medical training.**

Acupuncture & Pain Relief

In the mid 1970s, it was scientifically discovered that naturally occurring pain relieving opiates, **called endorphins,** could be released with acupuncture needling and DC electro-stimulation of acupuncture points (ETPS)(1*). These natural pain relievers circulate throughout the body and assist in relieving pain and speeding up the soft tissue healing process. **This "endorphin" discovery greatly increased the acceptance of Acupuncture into the West by providing a scientific model as to why and how it actually works for pain relief.**

ETPS Muscle Relaxing

Although the endorphin theory offers to the west one of the most concrete explanations as to why Acupuncture works, it does not account for why Acupuncture or ETPS works so quickly with soft tissue pain. Scientifically, endorphins take many hours to fully secreted into the circulatory system. The endorphin theory offers no reasons as to why Acupuncture or ETPS offer such an immediate and dramatic pain relieving responses with some patients.

Another theory that supports the immediate pain relief of ETPS is the theory of **"contracted or shortened muscles"**. This theory suggests that tightened or contracted muscles not only place strain on the body's mechanics, but they also place the nerves in a hypersensitive state, causing an amplification of pain for the suffering person, (called hypersensitivity or 'dennervation supersensitivity"). The belief is this amplification of the ANS is the basis of most chronic pain syndromes.

By releasing these tightened or contracted muscles, you may reinnervate the neural pathways and allow the suffering person to return to normal levels of pain tolerance. By releasing and relaxing the muscles, you permit the pain sufferer to achieve a more relaxed state, greater range of motion, and less pressure on the nerves. This will reduce the amplification (patient's perception) of their own pain levels.

By keeping the muscles soft and supple, you guard against further injury, and permit the natural healing forces of the body to take place. This is one of the most viable rationalizations as to this speedy and dramatic pain relieving response of ETPS and is supported by EMG findings.

Often with this theory, you stimulate acupuncture points far removed from the areas of symptomology, and treat the actual source of pain. For example, the carpal tunnel sufferer would treat the lower back, then neck, and then if necessary, forearm muscles to relieve pain in the wrist region. This is because the tendons, which are inflamed, are attached to muscles which are tightened, & are controlled by nerves emanating from the spine. Theory: by relaxing muscles, you relieve the stress on the tendons, joints and nerve roots directly involved with that muscle.

The benefits of ETPS are similiar to receiving a "super" massage from the inside out! This theory may seem simple, but this approach works because lasting results are often obtained within minutes, of ETPS treatment, not days or weeks after multiple therapy sessions.

Many back pains, whiplash, migraines, repetitve strain injuries, tension headaches, fibromyalgia and carpal tunnel pain syndromes, etc. respond wonderfully to this type of pain management technique. Together, these three theories offer a good explanation as to why ETPS Therapy is so successful with many hard to manage chronic pain disorders.

ETPS Therapy Research - Evidence Based Medicine (EBM)

An independent Florida Hospital study, comparing 2 standardized patient groups (n=86), one group applying TENS (AC stim with pads) and the other Physical Therapy group with ETPS (DC stim applied to acupuncture points) **produced some surprising results:**

Conclusion: The ETPS Therapy group had significantly greater reduction in pain **(83% vs 48%)** than the traditional TENS modality group. "ETPS is a highly effective modality when combined with traditional physical therapy", says Mitch Fried, M.D., Director of Rehab. (8*)

One of the most striking aspects of ETPS Therapy is the almost complete lack of adverse side effects and complications resulting from its use. This fact, coupled with ETPS's impressive track record for treating a wide variety of painful disorders, makes ETPS a desirable treatment for any suffering pain patient or clinician treating pain.

References:

(*1) Cheung R., McKibbon L., Roy B., Pomeranz B. Electroacupuncture elevates blood cortisol levels in horses: sham treatment has no effect. International Journal of Neuroscience. 10(2-3):95-7, 1980.

Voll R. Twenty Years of Electroacupuncture therapy using low frequency current impulses. Am J Acupuncture 1975;3:291 314

Engel J. Acupuncture biological basis: tracking an internal analgesic. Sci Demension 1982; 3: 4-8

(*2) Gunn, C.C., Milbrandt, W.E.: Tenderness at motor points - A Diagnostic and prognostic aid for low back injury. Bone and Joint Surg 58A (6): 815-825, 1976

(*3) Bradley, W.G., Disorders of Peripheral Nerves. Blackwell Scientific Publications, Oxford (1974)

(*4) Cannon, W.B., Rosenbleuth A.: The Supersensitivity of Denervated Structures. New York, MacMillan, PP 1-22, 185,1949.

(*5) Gunn, C.C., Milbrandt, W.E., Dry Needling of muscle motor points for chronic low-back pain; a randomized clinical trial with long term follow-up. Spine, 5:3 (1980) 279-291

Ochoa, J.L., Torebjork, E., Marchettini, P., Sivak, M., Mechanisisms of neuropathic pain: cumulative observations, new experiments and further speculation. In: H.L. Fields, R.Dubner, F. Cervero (Eds.), Advances in pain Research and Therapy, Vol 9. Raven Press, New York (1985).

Thomas, P.K., Symptomatology and differential diagnosis of peripheral neuropathy: clinical features and differential diagnosis. In: P.J. Dyck, P.K. Thomas, E.H. Lambert, R. Bunge,(Eds.), Peripheral Neuropathy, Vol II. W.B. Saunders, Philadelphia (1984) 1169-1190.

(6) Trigger Points and Classical Acupuncture Points: Part 1: Qualitative and Quantitative Anatomic Correspondences- PT Dorsher MD, Department of Physical Medicine and Rehabilitation, Mayo Clinic, Jacksonville, FL

(7*) R. Becker, The Body Electric 1985, (page 106, 183).

(8*) Rehab Report Volume 2, Issue 2, Summer 2005: An independent non-published internal study

ETPS Pain Therapy

This is a brief introduction to pain management with the revolutionary ***Electro Therapeutic Point Stimulation (ETPS)*** therapy approach. We hope this book will provide the reader with an excellent foundation into point therapy and will be used successfully by both pain sufferers and therapists who treat painful conditions.

Relieving Chronic Pain with ETPS

Pain has been around since the beginning of humanity. Pain has served a useful purpose by providing a first line of defence for our bodies. Pain allows us to adapt our lifestyle for survival.

Unfortunately, many of us suffer from long lasting, crippling pain called ***chronic pain.*** Chronic pain is classified as pain lasting for 3 - 6 months or longer. At the source, all chronic pains seem to be caused by some dysfunction of the nervous system, called neuropathic pain or neuropathy. Neuropathy is defined as ***"functional alterations of the nervous system"***, *which simply means:* ***when a nerve is not functioning properly it becomes supersensitive and behaves abnormally.***

Neuropathic pain conditions include many repetitive strain injuries (RSI's), whiplash, back pains, headaches, migraines, carpal tunnel syndrome and fibromyalgia. These "lifestyle" conditions may display different symptoms, but their origins all lie within neuropathy.

Chronic neuropathic pain requires a physical input (such as acutherapy needling or concentrated ***ETPS*** stimulation), in order to release contracted muscles. Releasing muscles helps to break the pain cycle and provide lasting pain relief to the sufferer.

Medication and surgery have a poor track record in treating these long-term chronic conditions. It is documented that properly applied ***ETPS*** stimulation will relieve chronic neuropathic pain in several ways:

1. Relaxing muscle spasm and releasing contracted muscles
2. Reducing heightened sensitivity of neural pathways
3. Releasing natural pain relievers called endorphins and thus providing a natural, non-toxic form of pain relief.

Pain Management with ETPS

The keys to successful pain management using ***ETPS*** include the following elements:

1. A thorough medical diagnosis
2. Proper point selection for your condition
3. Locating these points precisely and accurately
4. Stimulating these points for a therapeutic response
5. Safely and conveniently performing the above as needed

A Thorough Medical Diagnosis

It is imperative that as a chronic pain sufferer you receive a thorough medical examination and diagnosis **before** attempting ***ETPS*** techniques of pain management. The reason for this, is that you must determine the root cause of your pain. Once properly diagnosed, refer to the section of the book relating to your pain and stimulate the recommended points with the intent of eliminating or reducing the cause of your pain.

The most important step to a pain free existence is a proper medical diagnosis of your condition.

Locating Points with Manual & ETPS device

Historically, the location of acutherapy points was determined by a combination of ***finger measurement and skilled hands***. Today it has been established that *acupuncture, motor and trigger points* may all be located on the skin surface using a non-invasive electronic point finder, which the ETPS device has built-in. Science has discovered that these points display a lowered electrical resistance in relation to the surrounding skin. **Electrical point finders simply locate these points by measuring differences in this resistance. Proper and accurate point location requires the following:**

1. **Use finger measurements to locate general area**
2. **Use Finger pressure (palpation) to identify local tenderness**
3. **Use ETPS Point finder to "zero" in on the point**

ETPS Point location:

First step- finger measurements

refer to the manual and read the description on how to locate the desired point. It will usually describe a finger measurement (page 16) in relation to a specific body location. Next to each description is a diagram of the acupoint, which is used as a visual reference to approximate the location of a treatment point.

Second step-papate for local tenderness:

after locating the point with a finger measurement and diagram, press and rotate ***(palpate)*** your index finger or thumb in the vicinity of the illustrated point searching for a sharp tenderness in the muscle tissue. A skilled pair of hands may *"**sense**"* the point, which sometimes feels like a small marble or ball bearing when pressed. A greater pressure may have to be applied for some points that are located deeper in the tissue.

Third step-Use point finder:

place the tip of the unit in the general vicinity of the tender acupuncture point and slowly roam the tip around the skin surface until the light flickers off and the audible tone rises sharply. When the light is off and the tone is high, you have successfully located a treatment point.

How to use the Sensitivity Control to locate points:

To adjust for different skin types, units have a built-in sensitivity control. People with wet skin will find point location too easy, conversely, people with dry skin, will find point location more difficult. For those with dry skin, adjust the setting towards *"**DRY**"*. For those with wet skin, adjust

Trouble Shooting for Point Location

If you are ***locating too many points in a region,*** it may be because you are applying too much pressure with the unit or your skin is too moist. First lighten your touch. If this does not help, it may be that your ***skin is too moist.*** Use your sensitivity adjustment to correct this problem by adjusting towards "wet". Alternatively, ***if you have difficulty finding the point,*** your ***skin may be too dry.*** Adjust the sensitivity dial towards "dry" and apply more pressure for point location.

When Treating Another Person

In order to establish a circuit, when treating another person ***you must touch their skin with the palm of your hand.*** Use the palm of your free hand ***(the one not holding the unit).***

IMPORTANT: SLOW DOWN & FEEL THE TREATMENT

With a point finder, it is important that you GO SLOWLY when searching for points. It takes a millisecond for the unit to register the changes in skin resistance, and moving too quickly does not allow the unit a chance to positively identify a minute area of low skin resistance. **The audible tone will also assist you when searching for a point.** The higher the pitch, the more "active" the point. In summary, the higher the pitch, the lower the resistance, the stronger the stimulation. **Pain relief does not depend on strength of stimulation.** Using the ETPS unit on high or low intensity often produces the same results. One keys to provide effective pain relief is to actively select and stimulate the most tender treatment points relating to your injury. These points *(called "Ah Shi")* are always most active (or tender) during the first treatment. Often after a single application, the tenderness will decrease significantly.

ETPS Therapy at Home

Today's portable units are specifically designed for safe, easy, home use. They are designed to provide an inexpensive tool for the average pain sufferer to effectively manage pain without the ***overuse of medication or the reliance on frequent professional therapy sessions.***

ETPS protocols presented in this manual will illustrate and describe the series of points to treat for a wide variety of pain conditions. Beside each point in the manual will be the polarity setting, either ***tonify (+) or sedate (-)***. Selecting the correct polarity for your condition is as easy as flicking a switch on your unit. **The polarity changes the direction of current flow, creating reducing (ice) effect on negative and strengthening (heat) effect on positive polarity.**

The hand-held unit will electrically locate and stimulate individual points. **Stimulation of a point is initiated with a push of the treatment button. The recommended treatment time <u>per point</u> is 15 - 30 seconds (approximately 25-50 "beeps").**

ETPS provides a physical form of stimulation that can actually change the physiology of the injury. Relaxing the muscle & connective tissues goes beyond masking the pain, and will provide immediate and often long lasting pain relief as well as greater functional mobility to pain sufferers.

The portable kit allows for readily available pain relief both in the privacy of your own home or on the road, whenever or wherever you need it, without relying on medication. Instructional support is available through a toll free support line ***1-800-567-PAIN.***

Medical Treatment

Do not discontinue any medical treatment you may be having without consulting your medical adviser. If your problem persists despite the use of point stimulation, seek medical advice to investigate more serious causes to your conditions.

What You Should Feel applying ETPS

The sensation you feel will vary considerably from point to point. With most points you will feel a tingle sensation and with active or tender points you may feel a ***"hot needle" or biting sensation***. **This will all vary due to the skin resistance relating to the tenderness of the point. The more tender the point, the lower the resistance and stronger the sensation.** The treatment of some tender points may even be uncomfortable. You may need to stimulate these points in short bursts until the treatment becomes more tolerable.

When to Expect Results

In some cases the conditions you are treating may be chronic and may have been present for some time. As these cases will generally take longer to respond, look for increased improvement in your condition after each treatment. Recent or acute conditions will improve more rapidly, usually within 1-3 applications.

Frequency of Treatment

In the first week, stimulate once or twice per day. During the second week, you can reduce this to once every day or two. In the third week, begin to space your treatments to every 2 - 3 days. ***ETPS*** has a cumulative therapeutic effect and as time goes by you should require fewer treatments. For many chronic conditions that cannot be cured, applying 2 - 3 times per week on a preventative basis may be best suited. You will find your own comfort zone after several weeks.

Be patient

Patience may be required for the novice. If you experience difficulties, ***relax*** and let the application flow. The unit will do all the work for you, and the harder you try the more difficult it will seem. ***Relax and enjoy*** the treatment. Remember to call our toll-free number should you have any further questions. **Toll-free support line: 1-800-567-7246.**

Important Reminders

1. **Following the first treatment,** it is not uncommon to experience a **temporary "stirring up", or worsening, of the condition.** This is a common reaction following traditional therapy treatments and is usually a promising sign. If stirring up occurs for more than 2 applications, **switch the polarity setting and immediately stimulate again. This should reduce your pain quickly.**

2. Some people find that **better results are obtained by stimulating in several short sessions rather than 1 long session,** even if they are only a few hours apart.

3. As a general rule of thumb, treat the neck for all upper limb disorders **first**, and treat the lower back for all painful disorders of the lower limbs **first.**

4. For further suggestions or other helpful application tips **call 1-800-567- PAIN (7246), and ask for the therapist.**

5. Apply stimulation to all points listed in manual during the initial session. Subsequently, stimulate ONLY the points which display the greatest tenderness.

NOTE:

If the stimulation on negative is too STRONG even on low intensity, this is your body's way of telling you that the stimulation should be applied on POSITIVE.

Getting Started - Quick Reference

Here are a few commonly asked questions when patients begin to do self-treatments at home.

Q How do I hold the ETPS unit?

A It is most comfortable to hold the ETPS like a pen or big pencil. Position the unit so that the buttons and dials face DOWN at about a 45 degree angle and so that the middle finger may comfortably press the center button, *(your index finger works hard enough already)*.

Q Where do I set the dial that reads "wet/dry" 1-9?

A This dial is simply a sensitivity meter that can be adjusted according to the skin surface in which you are working. For example, if the skin you are treating is dry, place the dial on a higher number to achieve maximum point location.

If you are working on oily or sweaty skin, you will need to turn the dial to a lower number in order to properly locate points. *(This dial does not change the intensity of the unit in any way)*.

Q If I am applying the ETPS device to someone else, which person should be grounding the unit?

A The person using the ETPS is usually the person who touches the metal plate or wears the wrist band. To achieve maximum results, make sure to keep your thumb on the metal ground plate (for the Canadian ETPS device) or position the metal plate of the wrist band against the inside portion of your wrist (for the USA ETPS device).

Q How do I find the points to treat and how long do I stimulate each point?

A This unit is designed to help you find optimal points to treat. Turn to the page in the ETPS manual that refers to your condition. The points are listed in order of therapeutic importance. Refer to the manual and read the description of point location. Use finger measurments to determine general area of point location. Plapate the area for tenderness, as many of ther listed points are tender and easy to located through touch.

ETPS unit has both visual and audible point locators. With the unit turned on, guide the tip around the area you have palpated and selected for treatment. The device will emit a high pitched sound which will vary depending on the close your are to the point. Roam the tip of the unit around until the hear a very high pitch and the indicator light flicker "off". (light is located next to the ground plate). With a high pitch and the light off you have correctly located a trigger or acupuncture point. To initiate stimulation, simply push down and hold the gray “treatment ” button for approximately 10 -30 beeps *(depending on sensitivity)* for each point. Treamnet button is located on opposite side of unit to ground plate.

Q Some points are very tender when I stimulate them. Can I skip these points?

A If a point is too painful to simulate on high, then turn the intensity dial down to low (located beside treatment button). After you have done that, you should be able to stimulate the tender point again without nearly as much discomfort. The increased tenderness in that area is an indication of strong relationship that point has with muscle/nerve damage and it should not be skipped over and ignored. Tender points usually provide optimal relief to patients.

Dermatome Chart

The Nerve Pain Pathways

If your pain is following any of these nerve pathways, treat at the nerve root with ETPS for exceptional relief

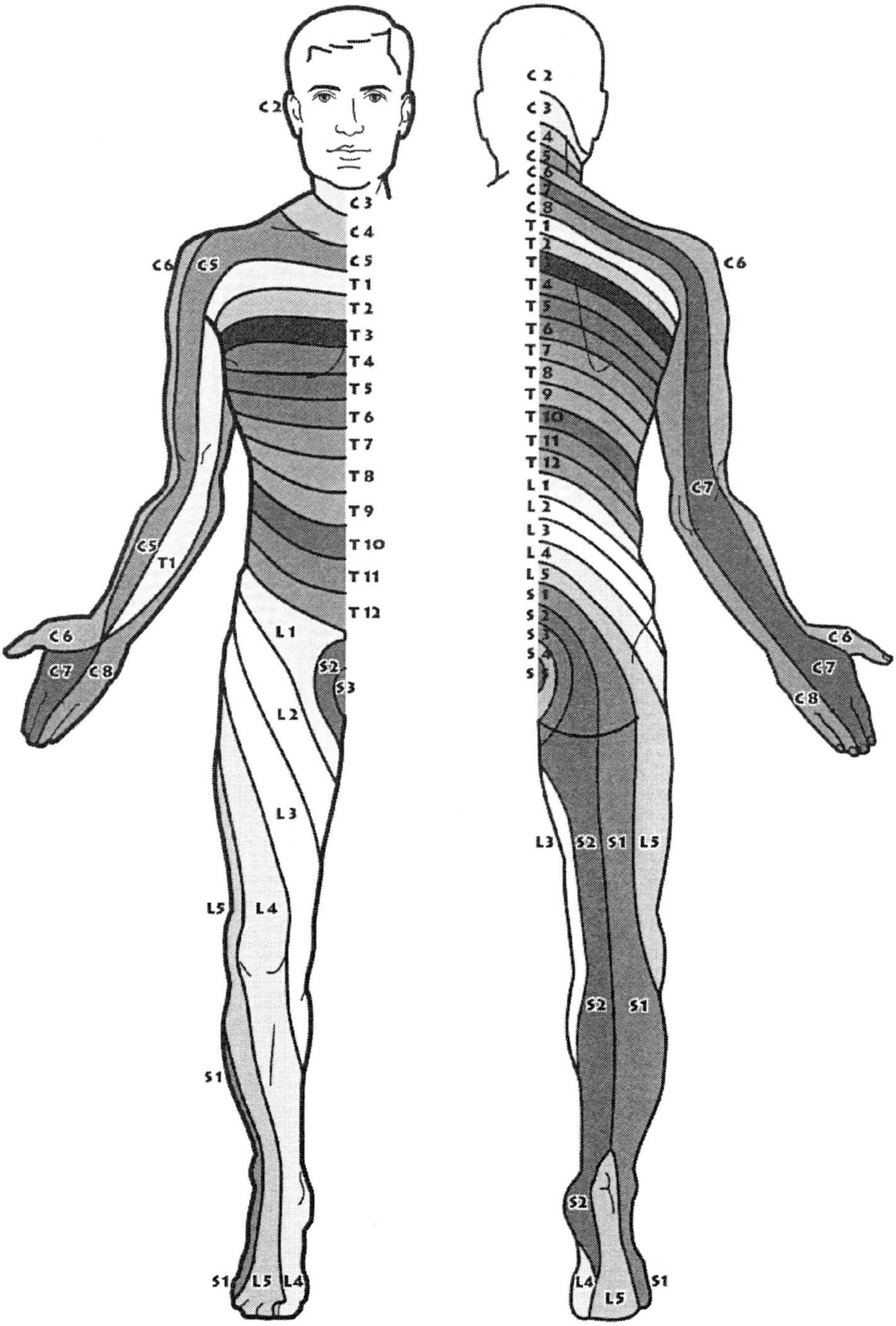

Finger Measurements for Point Location

The following illustrations show the common finger measurements used to locate meridian points. In this manual, "cun" measurement has been replaced with finger measurement for simplicity and ease of use. For accuracy, use the 1st knuckle on the thumb and the 2nd knuckle on the fingers for measurement purposes.

Here are the three most common measurements for point location throughout this book. After finger measuring, press and rotate for tenderness, then use the point locator to search for optimal application site.

1 Thumbs width = 1 "cun"

Use first knuckle for measurement

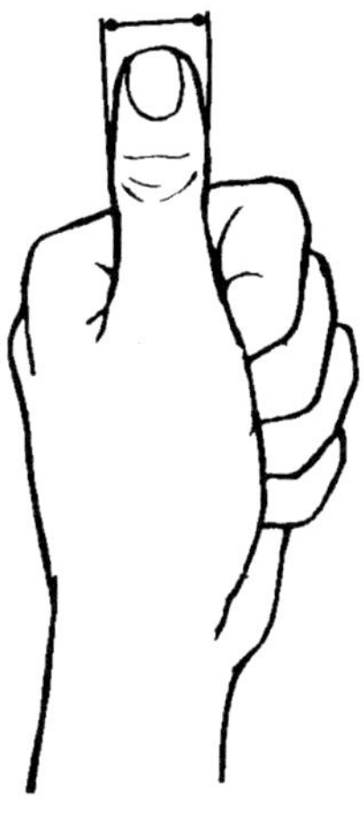

2 Fingers width = 1.5 "cun"

Use 2nd knuckle for measurement

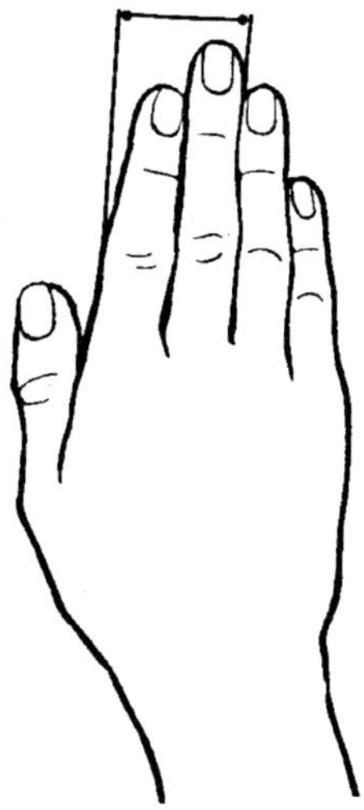

4 Fingers width = 3 "cun"

Use 2nd knuckle for measurement

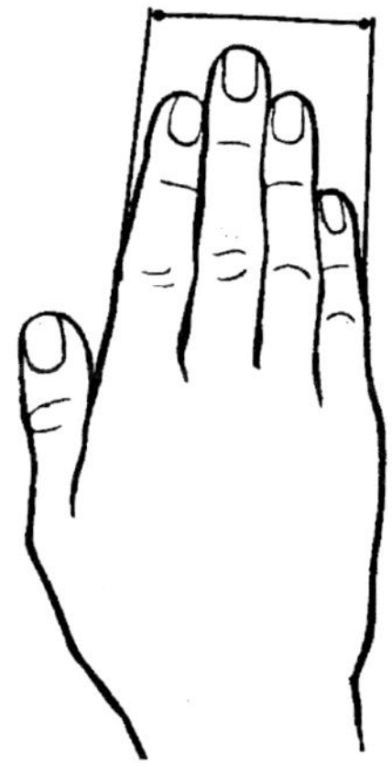

Treating Chronic Pain

Treating Pain

Step 1 : Parasympathetic (calming) Points

Step 2: Standard Protocol - Back

Step 3: Standard Protocol - Neck

Parasympathetic (Calming) Points

Parasymapthetic points may be used to calm a distressed or hypersensitive patients prior to initiating a treatment. They may also be used very successfully as treating these points will relax the nervous system, often releasing any shortened (tightened) muscles involved with the pain condition.

Golden Triangle

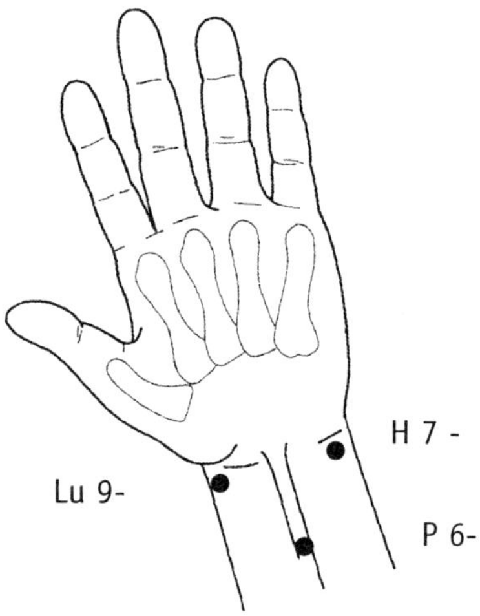

Lu 9 In the groove at the thumb side of the wrist crease, and inside of the tendon.

H 7 On the little finger side of the wrist crease, to the inside of the tendon.

NOTE: The therapeutic wrist crease where H7 and Lu 9 are found is located 1/4 inch proximal from the most distal wrist crease OR 2 thumbs width distal from (away from) P6. For further instructions on point location, please call 1-800-567-7246 (PAIN).

P 6 3 fingers width from the most distal wrist crease, in between the tendons.

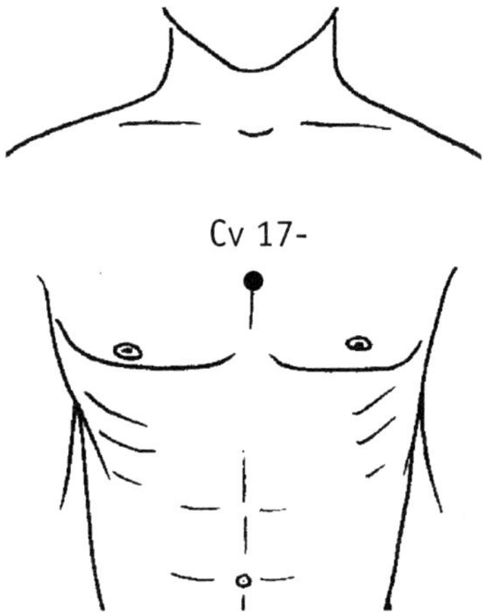

Cv 17 On the breast bone at the heart level or the 4th rib space. Tender when pressed.

Parasympathetic (Calming) Points

Sp 6 3 fingers width above the inner ankle and just behind the prominent shin bone.

K 3 Halfway between the Achilles tendon and the inner ankle bone.

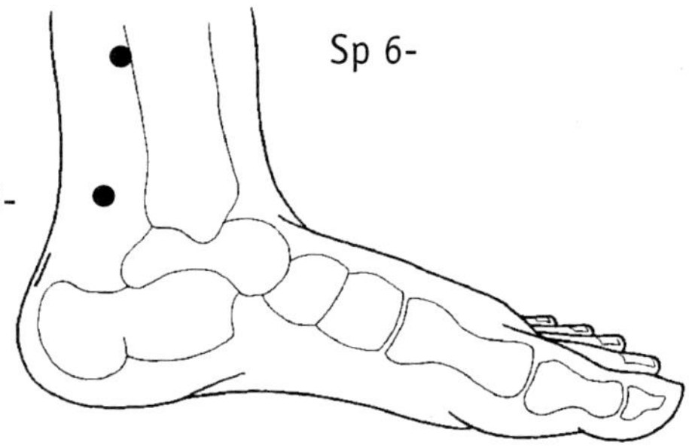

B 62 In the depression half a finger below the outer ankle bone.

Gv 20 On the midline of the top of the head, halfway between the ears.

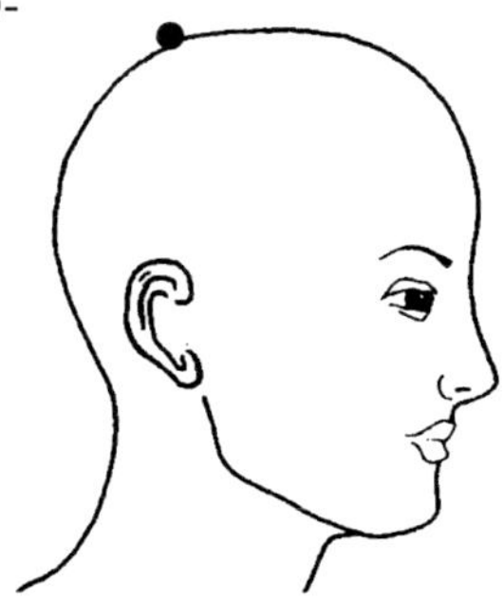

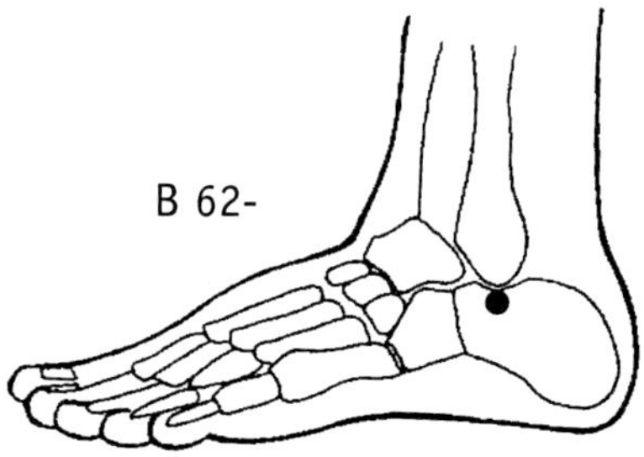

Standard Protocol - Core Therapy

The following Standard Protocol is the second step to treating any pain condition and we recommend that it be applied regardless of the type of pain diagnosis.

Step 1: Standard Protocol

Back Shu Points

Located 2 fingers width to each side of the spine below the spinal bone.

Treat segment by segment bilaterally using 2 ETPS units simultaneously, or using a single ETPS unit, treat alternating sides in a "zig zag" pattern.

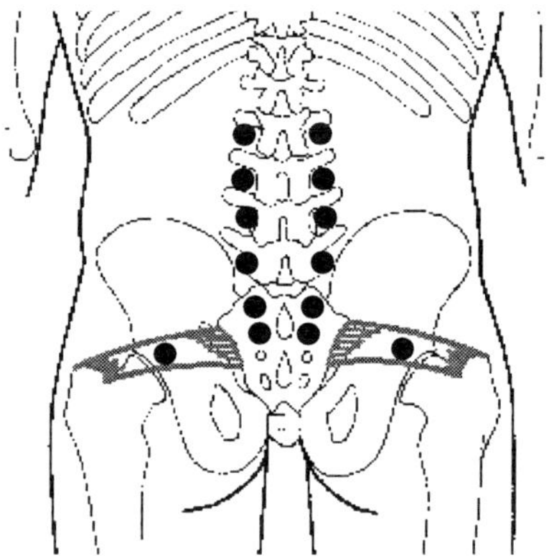

Piriformis Trigger Point

This tender point is located approximately half way between the sacrum (the trianglar bone at the base of the spine) and the hip joint. Press and rub (palpate) the general area until a tender point is located.

Gb 31 This point is located at the end of the middle finger, with your hand lying flat at the side of your thigh.

Gb 34 4 fingers width below the outside of the knee and just in front of and below the knobby head of the fibula bone.

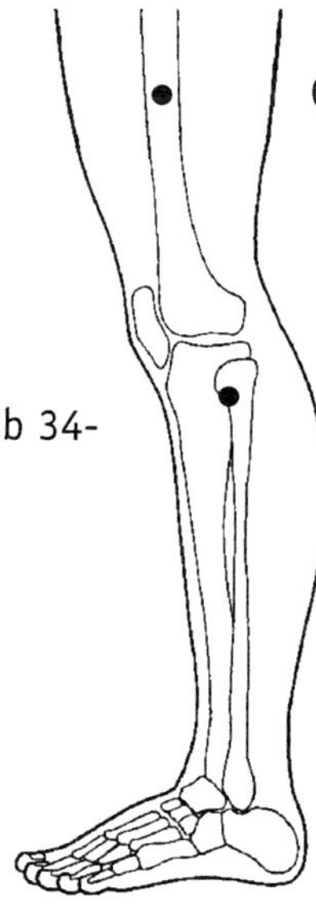

Standard Protocol - Core Therapy

If you are experiencing back pain that is stiff and more severe in the morning as you wake up, or if it feels worse towards the end of the day it will be beneficial for you to follow the steps below.

Step 2: Neural Points

B 40 On the middle of the crease behind the knee.

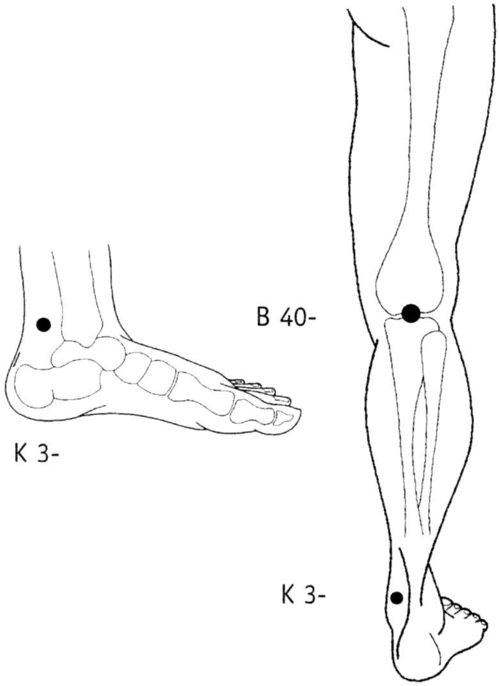

For back pain that's more severe in the morning:

K 3 In the hollow midway between the tip of the inner ankle bone and the Achilles tendon.

For back pain that's more severe in the evening:

B 60 In the hollow midway between the tip of the outer ankle bone and the Achilles tendon.

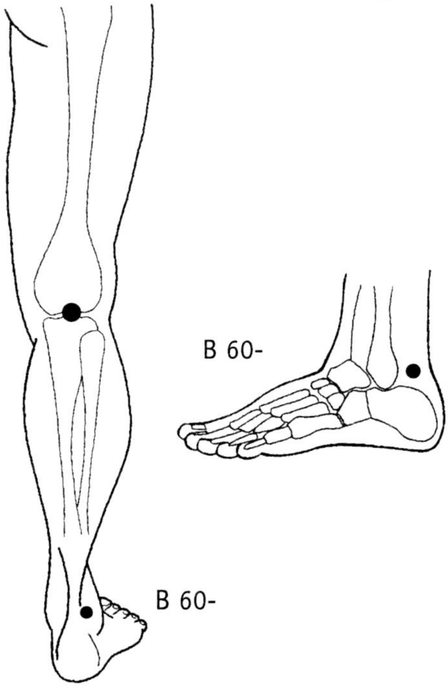

Standard Protocol - Core Therapy

Step 3: Sacral Triangle

The following points should release the hips and paraspinal muscles. Sedate them if you require additional relief.

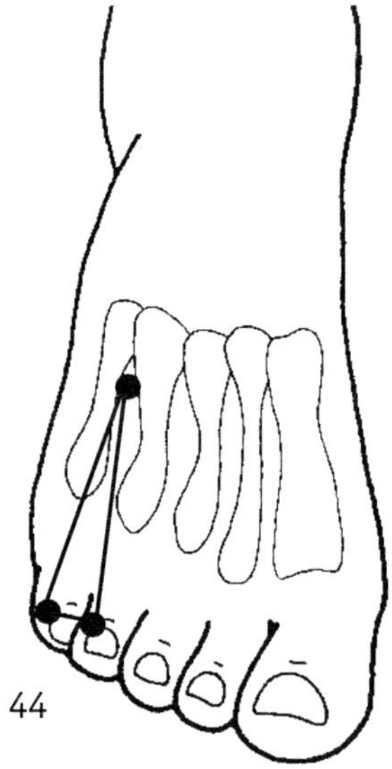

Gb 41 In the depression where the 4th and 5th toe bones meet.

Gb 44 At the base of the outer side of the 4th toe nail.

B 67 At the base of the outer side of the 5th toe nail.

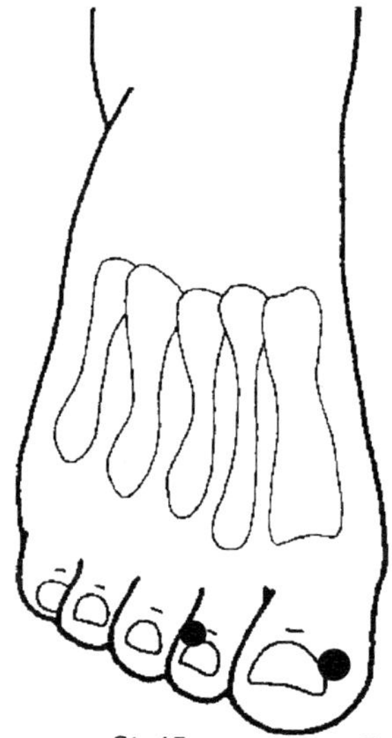

Step 4: Psoas Release

St 45 At the base of the outer side of the 2th toe nail.

Sp 1 At the base of the inner side of the big toe nail.

Core Therapy - Gluteal Release

If you require additional relief (after applying stimulation to steps 1-4) for your back condition, apply to the following points.

Step 5: Gluteal Release

Gluteal release

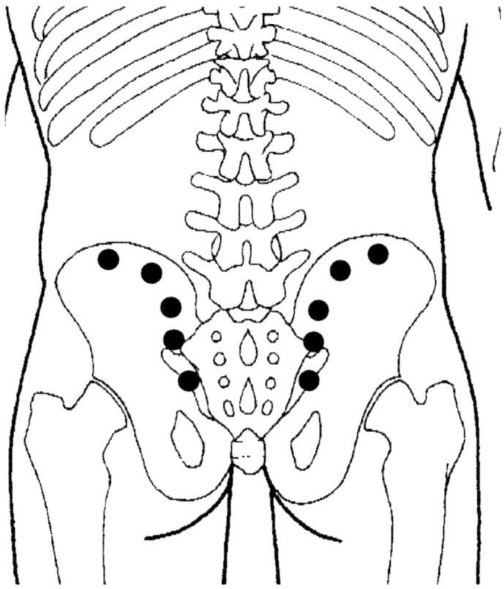

Locate these points on the lower border of the PSIS (posterior superior iliac spine). It is the bone at the top of the buttocks, running from the hips
to the sacrum.

Treat every tender point located on the lower border for powerful relief of back pain.

Protocol: Neck & Upper Limbs

Usually caused by soft tissue muscle strain due to work, sport related overuse or just poor posture. Symptoms include pain, tenderness with muscle spasms and inflammation evident upon palpation.

Step 1: Standard Protocol

To treat the neck, begin with Standard Protocol for Back Pain. Then continue to treat the neck with the points listed on next page (pg. 29).

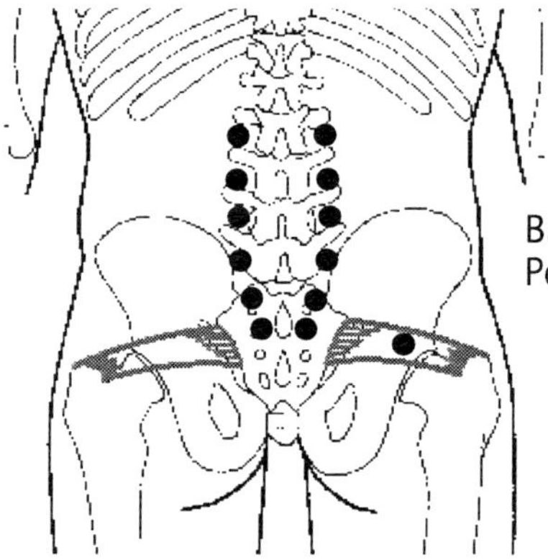

Back Shu Points

Located 2 fingers width to either side of the spine below each spinal bone.

Piriformis Trigger Point

Approximately half way between the sacrum *(the trianglar bone at the base of the spine)* and the hip joint. Palpate the general area until a tender point is located.

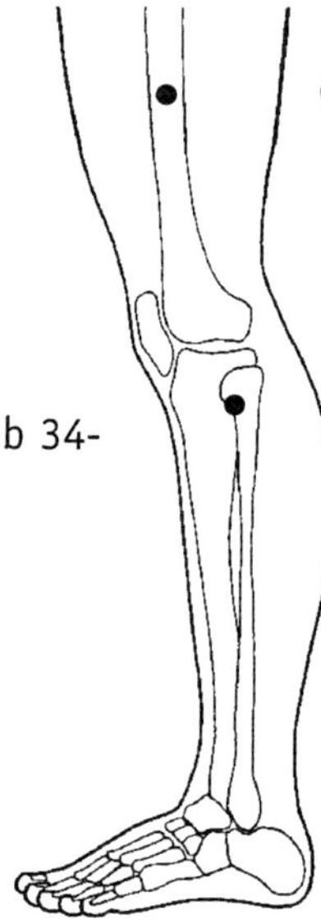

Gb 31 This point is located at the end of the middle finger, with your hand lying flat at the side of your thigh.

Gb 34 4 fingers width below the outside of the knee and just in front of and below the knobby head of the fibula bone.

Protocol: Neck & Upper Limb Pain

For all disorders involving the upper limbs & neck, the following procedure called the paraspinal release, should be performed. Treating these points will release any shortened muscles involved with radiculopathy (nerve root entrapment), which influence pain along the upper extremities.

Step 2: Posterior Neck & Trapezius release

Gb 20 Below the base of the skull, in the hollow just outside the main spinal muscles of the neck.

B 10 Located 2 fingers width from the middle of the spine, at the middle of the natural hair line at the back of the neck.

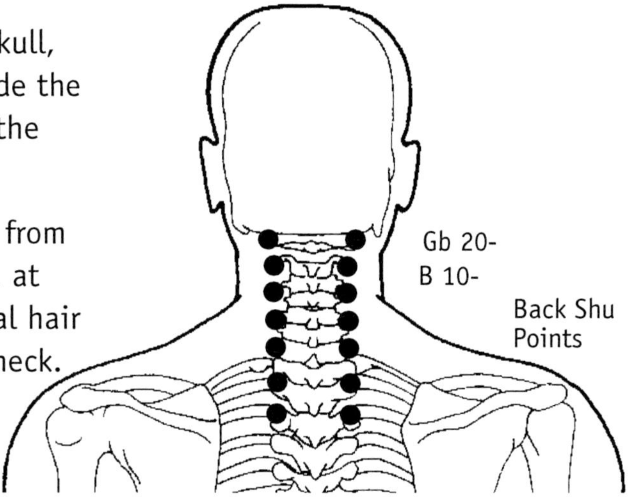

Back Shu Points
Located 2 fingers width to either side of the spine below each spinal bone.

Gb 21 Halfway between the prominent bone at the bottom of the neck and the outer tip of the shoulder.

Tw 15 1 thumbs width below GB 21.

Si 13 4 fingers width below GB 21, just on top of the spine of the shoulder blade

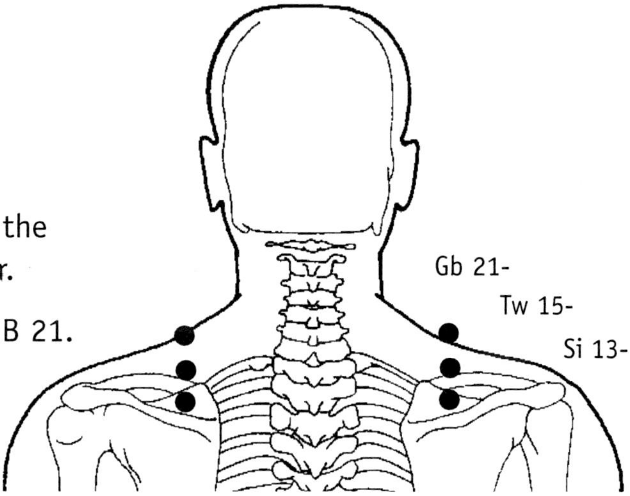

Protocol: Neck & Upper Limbs Pain

Step 3: Lateral Neck Release

Gb 20 Below the base of the skull, in the hollow just outside the main spinal muscles of the neck.

B 10 Located 2 fingers width from the middle of the spine, at the middle of the natural hair line at the back of the neck.

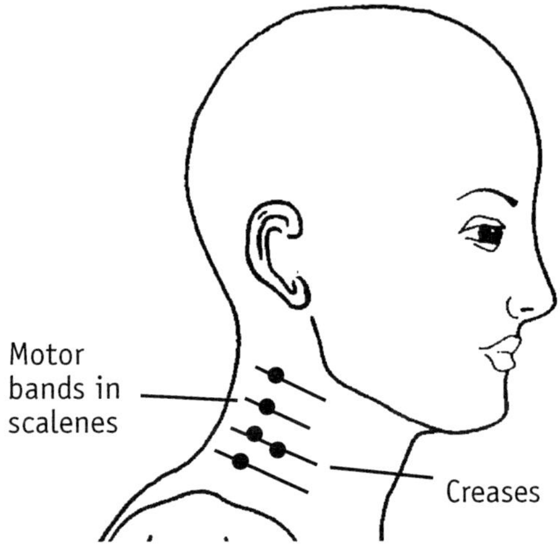

Step 4: Distal Acupoints for the Neck Release

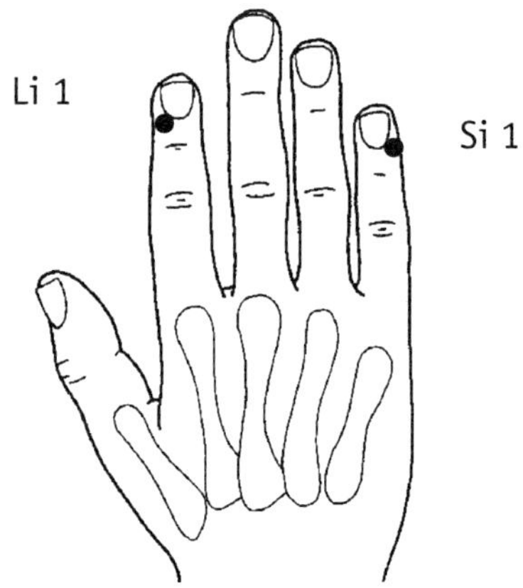

Li 1 At the inner base of the index finger nail

Si 1 At the outer base of the little finger nail.

Si 3 With the hand in a loose fist, this point is located at the end of the main transverse hand crease.

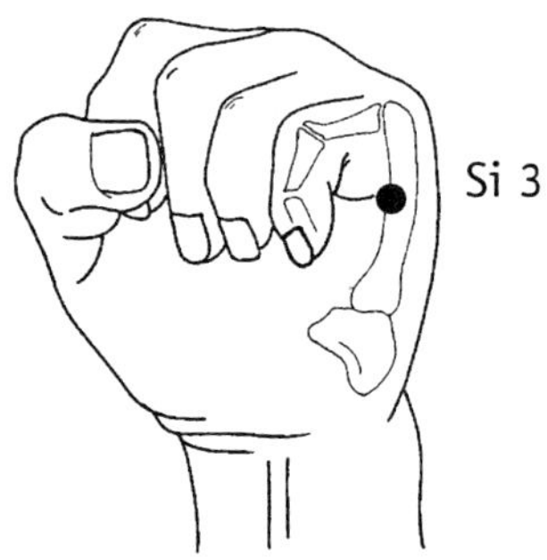

Pain Disorders

"If you cannot be king
be a healer"

(Ancient Sinhala quote from
a manuscript dated 500 B.C.)

Abdominal Pain

Consult a Doctor before treating any points. Once diagnosed, stimulate the distal points before local points. If pain is of muscle or neural origin, the following points should be sedated for relief.

Cv 12 In the midline, midway between the umbilicus and the lower end of the breast bone. *Fig. 1*

St 25 2 thumbs width ***to each side*** of the belly button. *Fig. 1*

Cv 6 In the midline, 2 fingers width ***directly below*** the belly button. *Fig. 1*

St 36 4 fingers width below the kneecap, and 1 fingers width to the outside of the shinbone. *Fig. 2*

Gb 34 4 fingers width below the outside of the knee and just in front of and below the knobby head of the fibula bone. *Fig. 3*

Liv 3 On the top of the foot in the hollow between the 1st and 2nd toes, where the bones meet. *Fig. 4*

St 44 At meeting of the base of 2nd and 3rd toes in the web. *Fig. 4*

Jing Well Points
At the outer base of the toe nails. *Fig. 4*

Fig. 1

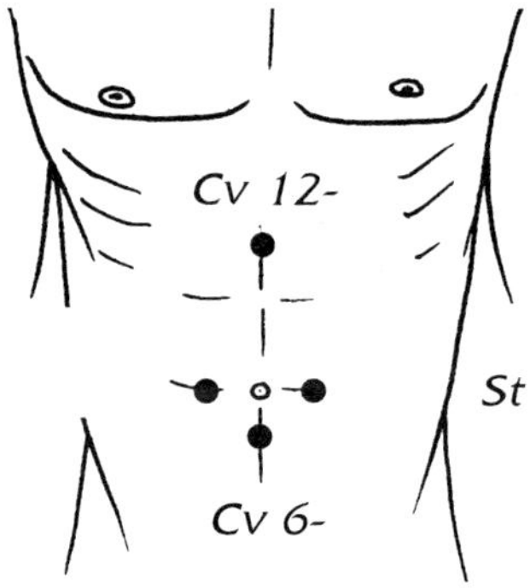

Fig. 2

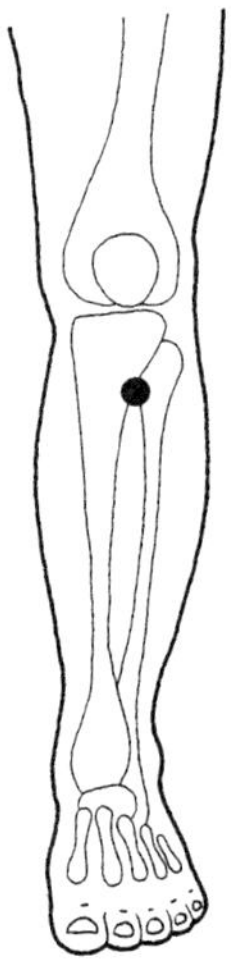

Fig. 3

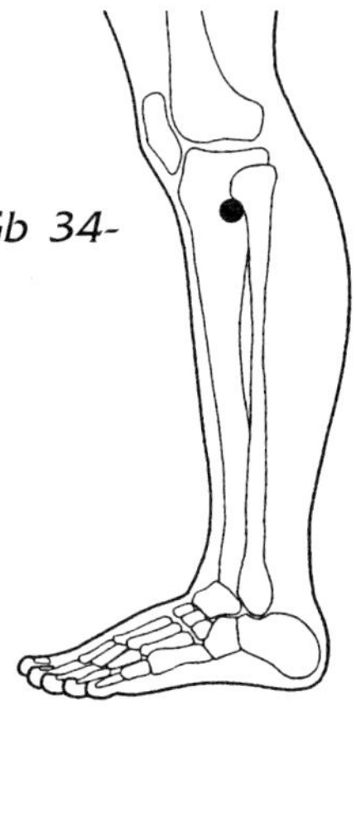

Fig. 4

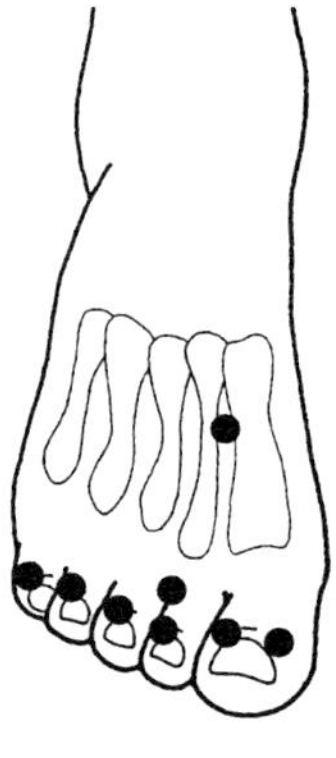

Achilles Tendonitis

***A** common sports injury where the tendon at the back of the heel becomes very tender and painful, usually due to overuse or a traumatic injury. Start with the Lower Back and Hips, then release any tight calf muscles.*

Back Shu Points:
Located 2 fingers width to each side of the spinal bones. ***Sedate these points from the lower back to the sacrum. Above points innervate the affected region(s) and often provide substantial relief to the patient.*** *Fig. 1*

Fig. 1

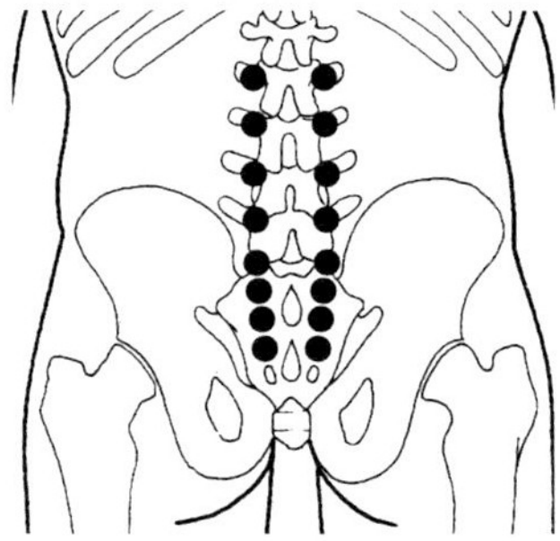

Piriformis Trigger Points:
Approximately half way between the sacrum (the triangular bone at the base of the spine) and the hip joint, or one hands width above GB 30. *Fig. 2*

Fig. 2

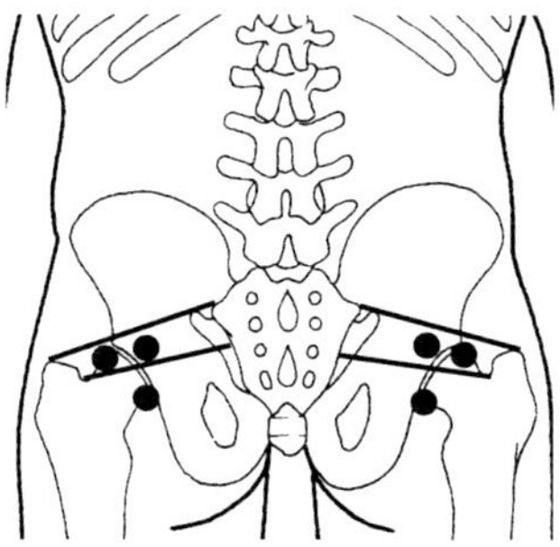

Gb 30 This point is directly in the middle of each "cheek", equal distance from all sides. *Fig. 2*

Gb 31 Standing erect with your hands laying the side of the thigh. This point is at the ***tip of the middle finger***. *Fig. 3*

Fig. 3

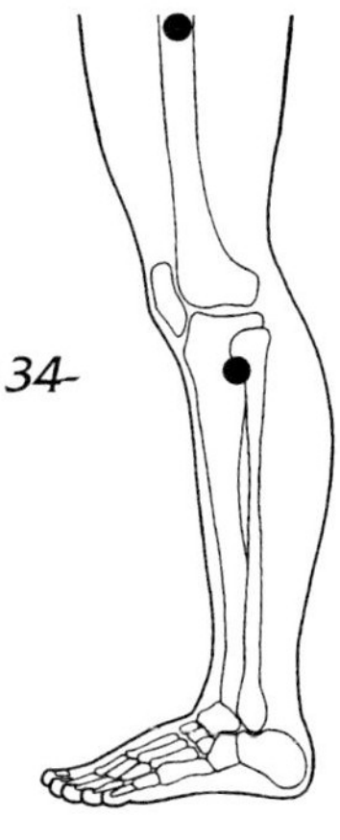

Gb 34 4 fingers width below the outside of the kneecap, and just in front of and below the knobby head of the fibula bone. *Fig. 3*

Fig. 4

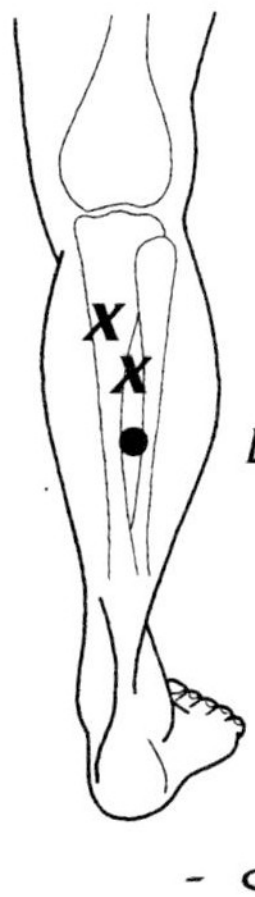

B 57 At the mid point of the calf where the calf muscle narrows to form the tendon, between the 2 calf muscles. *Fig. 4*

- continued next page

Achilles Tendonitis

If additional relief is required, sedate the following points in the order illustrated.

Gb 34 In front of and below the head of the fibula bone, located 4 fingers width below the outside of the kneecap. *Fig. 1*

B 60 In the hollow midway between the tip of the outer ankle bone and the Achilles tendon. *Fig. 1*

St 41 On the front of the ankle, on the crease in between the 2 ankle tendons. *Fig. 2*

Liv 3 On top of the foot, in the hollow where the 1st and 2nd toe bones meet. *Fig. 2*

St 44 At meeting of the base of the 2nd and 3rd toes, in the web. *Fig. 2*

Sp 6 3 fingers width above the inner ankle bone and behind the prominent shin bone. *Fig. 3*

K 3 In the hollow, midway between the tip of the inner ankle bone and the Achilles tendon. *Fig. 3*

Sp 5 Below and in front of the tip of the inner ankle bone, in the depression. *Fig. 3*

Sp 3 Just above the "Bunion" bone at the base of the big toe, ***at the junction of the red and white skin***. *Fig. 3*

Fig. 1

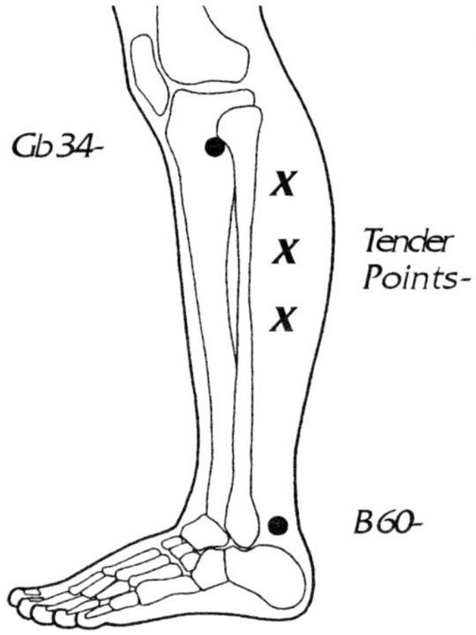

Fig. 2

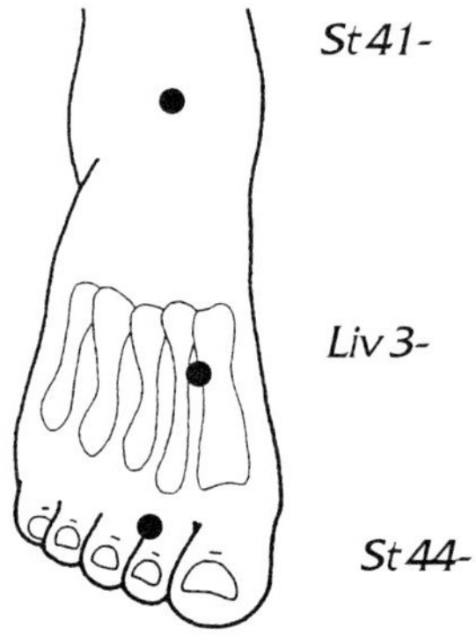

Fig. 3

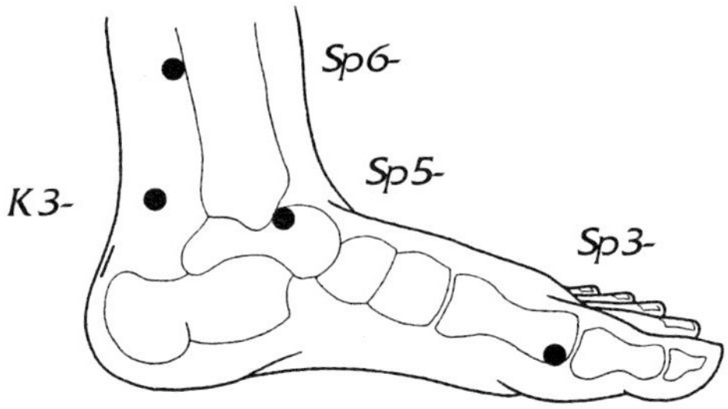

Ankle Sprain & Pain

Consult a Doctor before treating any points. For chronic conditions, stimulate at the points on this page first. The distal and local points on the following page may be used after the below points. Sedate points for maximum relief.

Back Shu Points:

Located 2 fingers width to each side of the spinal bones. ***Sedate these points from the middle to the lower back. Above points innervate the affected region and often provide substantial relief.*** *Fig. 1*

Piriformis Trigger Points:

Approximately half way between the sacrum (the triangular bone at the base of the spine) and the outside hip joint. Or, one hands width above GB 30. Press and rub (palpate) the general area until tenderness is detected. *Fig. 2*

Gb 30 This point is directly in the middle of each "cheek", equal distance from all sides. *Fig. 2*

Gb 31 Stand erect, hands flat along the side of the thigh. This point is at the ***tip of the middle finger***. *Fig. 3*

Gb 34 4 fingers width below the outside of the kneecap, and just in front of and below the knobby head of the fibula bone. *Fig. 3*

Fig. 1

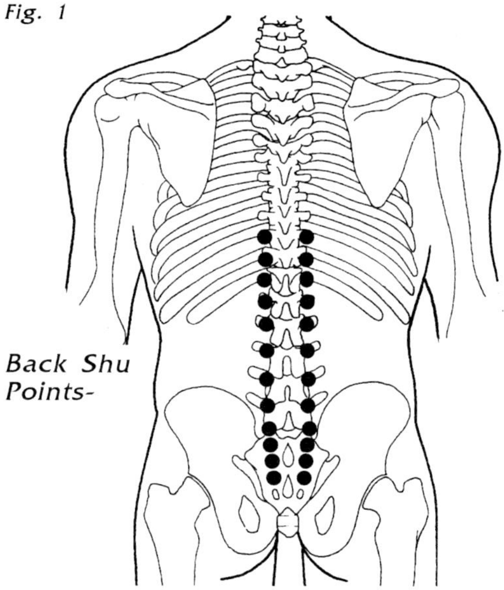

Fig. 2

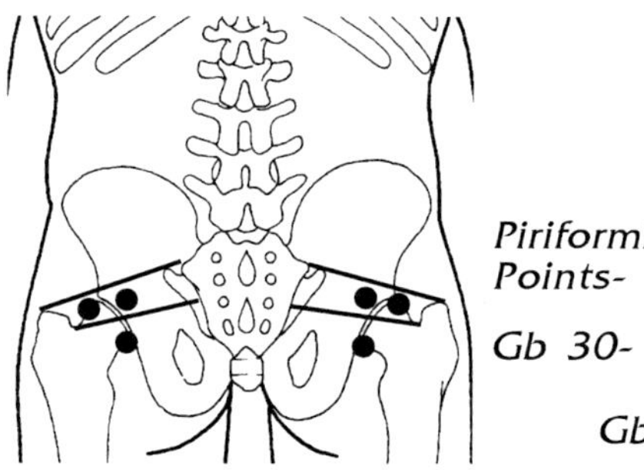

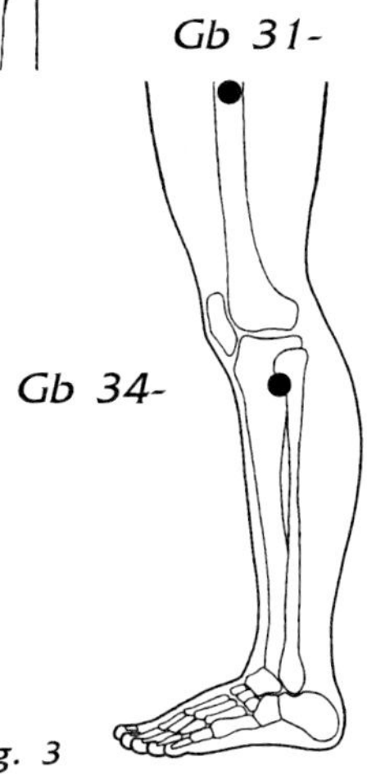

Fig. 3

Ankle Sprain & Pain

***A**fter treating the lower back and buttocks on the previous page, sedate the following points (on both feet) daily until the pain & swelling subsides.*

B60 This lies in the hollow midway between the tip of the outer ankle bone and the Achilles tendon. *Fig. 1*

Gb 40 In the hollow just in front of the outer ankle bone. *Fig. 1*

B 62 In the depression half a finger below the outer ankle bone. *Fig. 1*

St 41 On the front of the ankle, in the crease in between the 2 ankle tendons. *Fig. 2*

Liv 3 On the top of the foot, in the hollow between the 1st and 2nd toes, where the bones meet. *Fig.2*

Sp 6 3 fingers width above the inner ankle and just behind the prominent shin bone. *Fig. 3*

K 3 Halfway between the Achilles tendon and the inner ankle bone. *Fig. 3*

K 5 1 thumbs width below the inner ankle bone. *Fig. 3*

K 6 Below and in front of the tip of the inner ankle bone, in a depression. *Fig. 3*

Sp 3 Just proximal to the "Bunion" bone at the base of the big toe, ***at the junction of the red and white skin.*** *Fig. 3*

Fig. 1

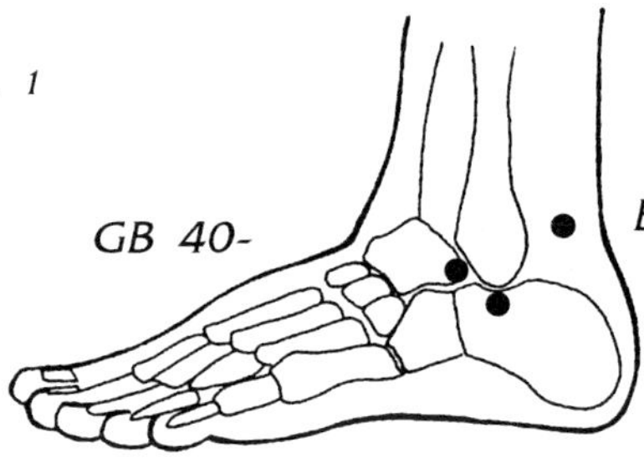

Fig. 2

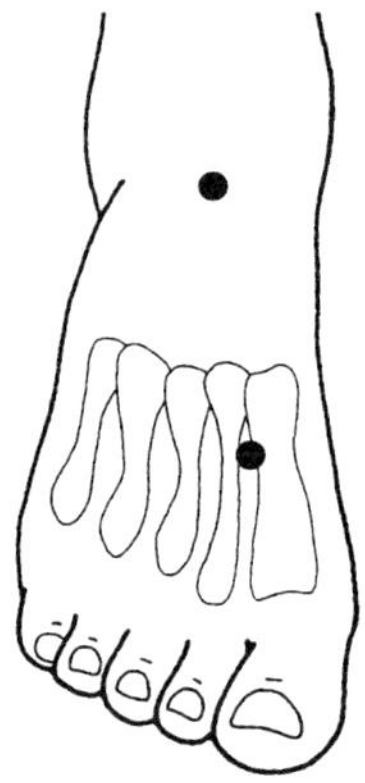

Fig. 3

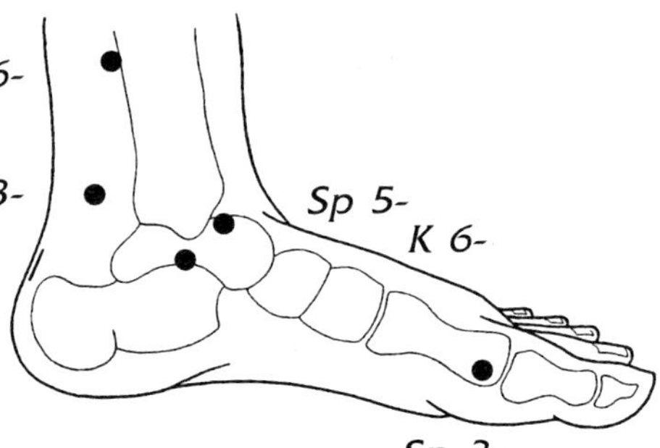

Ankylosing Spondylitis

For chronic conditions, sedate the following parasympathetic points in order to decrease the sensitivity of the spine. For additional relief, sedate the local points on the following page.

Lu 9 In the groove at the thumb side of the wrist crease, and inside of the tendon. *Fig. 1*

H 7 On the little finger side of the wrist crease, to the inside of the tendon. *Fig. 1*

P 6 3 fingers width from the most distal wrist crease, in between the tendons. *Fig. 1*

Sp 6 3 fingers width above the inner ankle and just behind the prominent shin bone. *Fig. 2*

K 3 Halfway between the Achilles tendon and the inner ankle bone. *Fig. 2*

B 62 In the depression half a finger below the outer ankle bone. *Fig. 3*

Cv 17 On the breast bone at the heart level or the 4th rib space. Tender when pressed. *Fig. 4*

Fig. 1

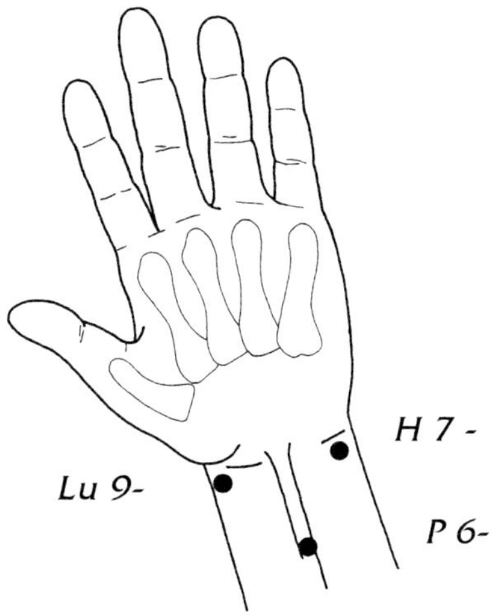

Fig. 2

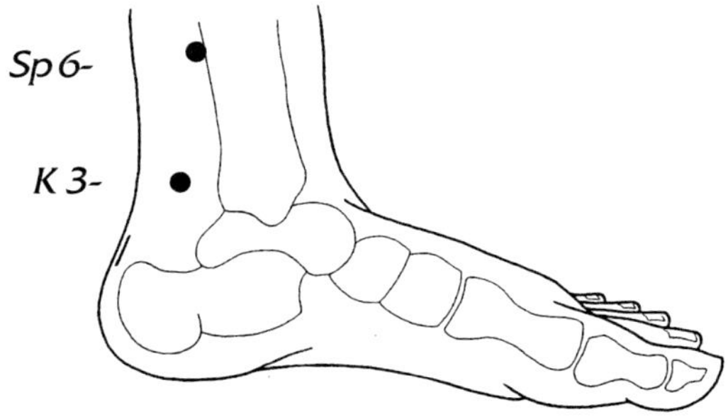

Fig. 4

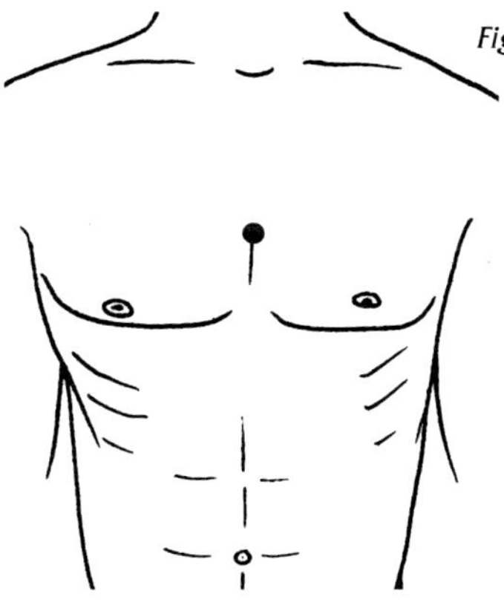

Fig. 3

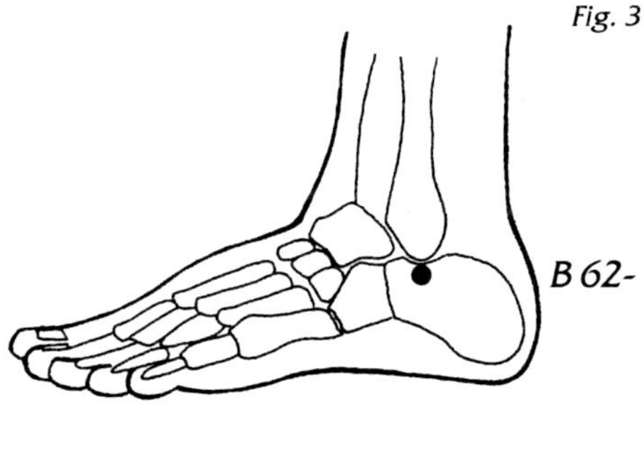

- continued next page

Ankylosing Spondylitis

A *chronic and progressive inflammatory arthritic disease affecting the spinal joints and adjacent connective tissues. Symptoms include back pain, stiffness on awakening and nocturnal pain and stiffness causing insomnia. Sedate the following points to help relax paraspinal muscles (loosen connective tissue) to help relieve discomfort and pain. Apply frequently to entire length of spine.*

Fig. 1

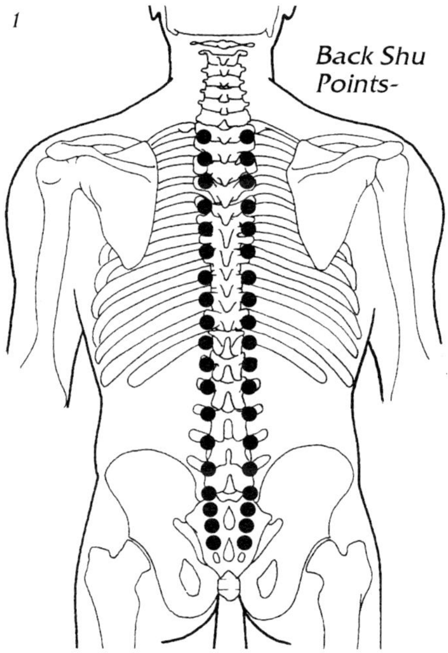

Stimulate in the affected region

Back Shu Points

2 fingers width to each side of the spine, ***at the level of the lower border of the spinal bumps. Stimulate in the area(s) of problems. Neck, mid, lower or all of the back region may be stimulated for relief.*** *Fig. 1*

B 40 On the middle of the crease behind the knee. *Fig. 2*

B 60 This lies in the hollow midway between the tip of the outer ankle bone and the Achilles tendon. *Fig. 2*

Li 4 In the fleshy mass between the thumb and index finger. *Fig. 3*

Tw 5 2 thumbs width above the middle of the wrist crease, between the 2 forearm bones. *Fig. 3*

Fig. 2

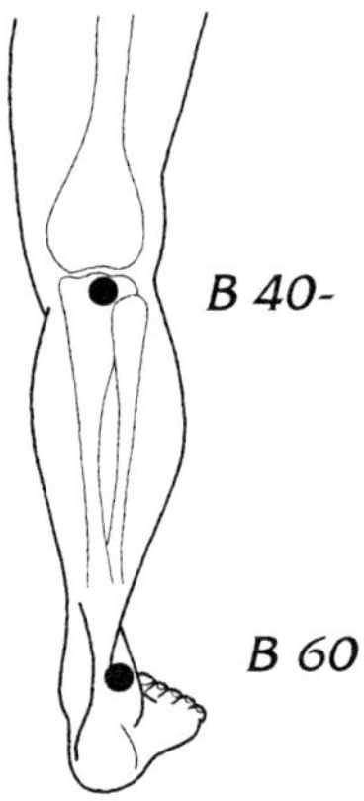

Fig. 3

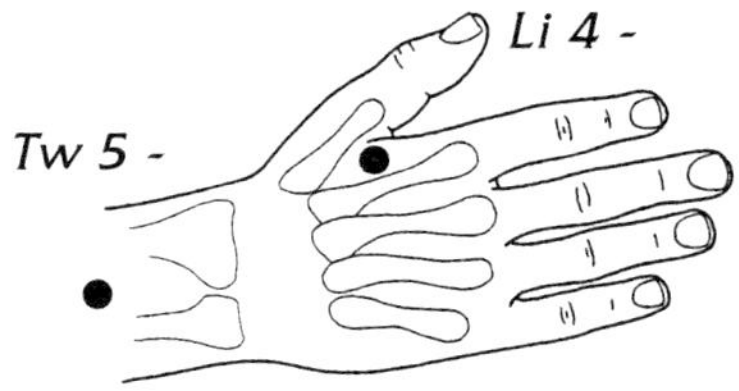

Back Pain - Chronic

For chronic conditions, sedate the following parasympathetic points in order to decrease the sensitivity of the spine. For additional relief, sedate the local points on the following page.

Lu 9 In the groove at the thumb side of the wrist crease, and inside of the tendon. *Fig. 1*

H 7 On the little finger side of the wrist crease, to the inside of the tendon. *Fig. 1**

P 6 3 fingers width from the most distal wrist crease, in between the tendons. *Fig. 1*

Sp 6 3 fingers width above the inner ankle and just behind the prominent shin bone. *Fig. 2*

K 3 Halfway between the Achilles tendon and the inner ankle bone. *Fig. 2*

B 62 In the depression half a finger below the outer ankle bone. *Fig. 3*

Cv 17 On the breast bone at the heart level or the 4th rib space. Tender when pressed. *Fig. 4*

Fig. 1

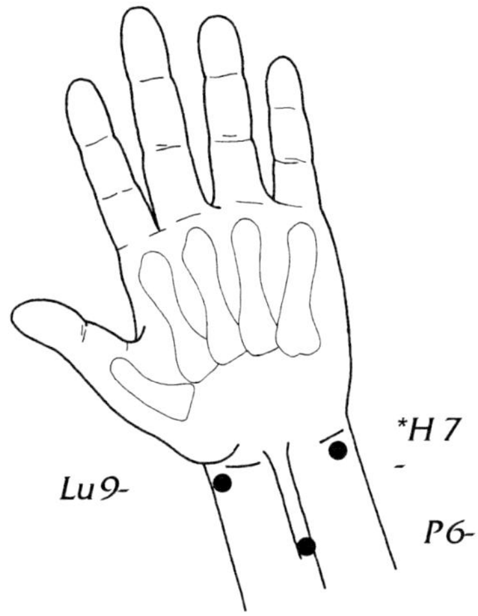

Fig. 2

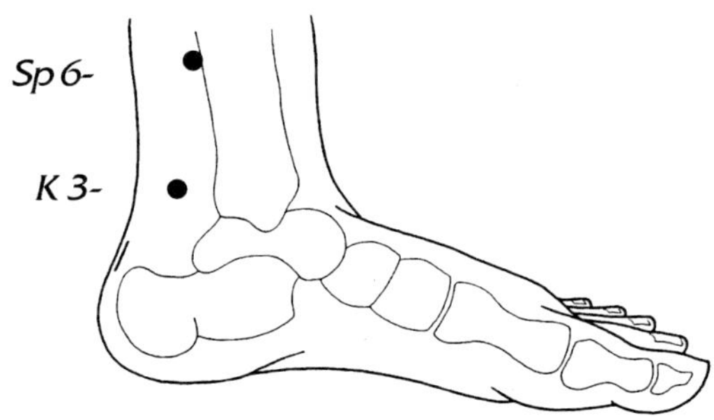

Fig. 4

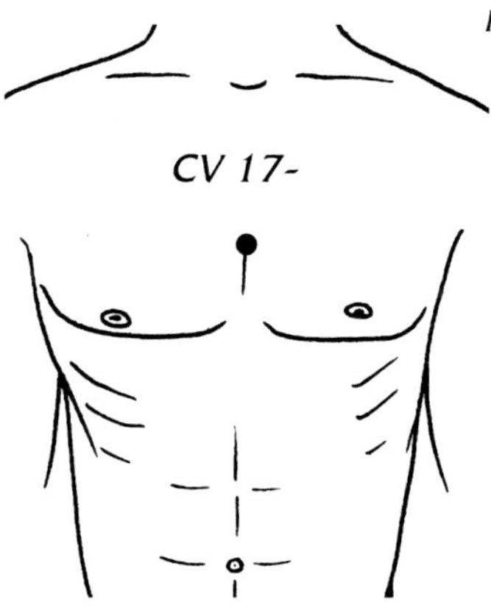

Fig. 3

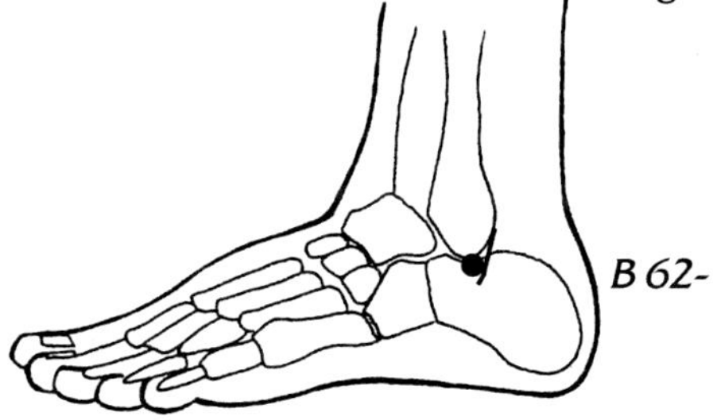

Back Pain - Lower

***U**sually caused by soft tissue muscle strain due to repetitive overuse, postural imbalances or just poor lifestyle. For relief, sedate the following points to relax muscles and calm the nervous system.*

Back Shu Points:
Located 2 fingers width to each side of the spinal bones. *Fig. 1*

Gv 4 Below the spinal bone of the 4th lumbar vertabrae. *Fig. 1*

Piriformis Trigger Points:
Half waybetween the sacrum and the hip joint.

Gb 30 This point is directly in the middle of each "cheek" equal distance from all sides. *Fig. 1*

Gb 31 Standing erect with your hands laying the side of the thigh. This point is at the ***tip of the middle finger***. *Fig. 2*

Gb 34 4 fingers width below the outside of the kneecap, and just in front of and below the knobby head of the bone. *Fig. 2*

B 60 This lies in the hollow midway between the tip of the outer ankle bone and the Achilles tendon. *Figs. 2 & 3*

B 36 At the midpoint, just below the gluteal fold. *Fig. 3*

B 37 At the midpoint in the back of the thigh. *Fig. 3*

B 40 On the middle of the crease behind the knee. *Fig. 3*

Jing Well Points
Located on each side of the toenails at the base of the nail. *Fig. 4*

Fig. 1

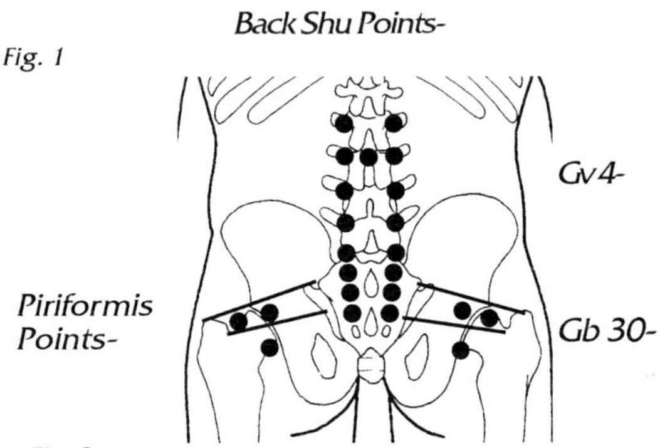

Fig. 2

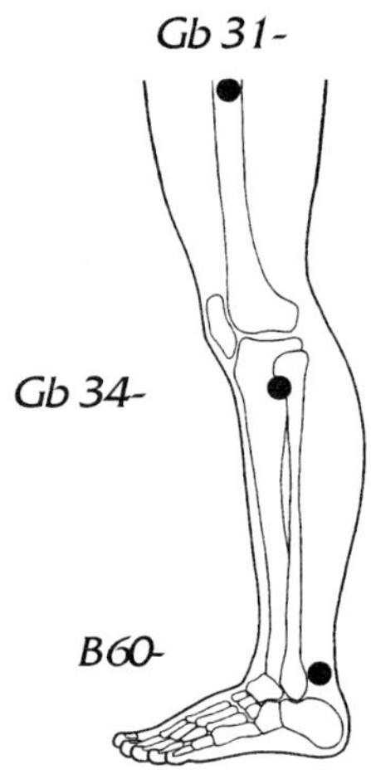

Fig. 3

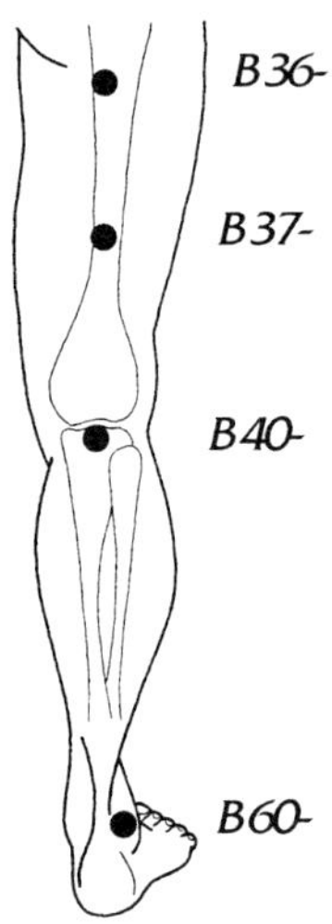

Fig. 4

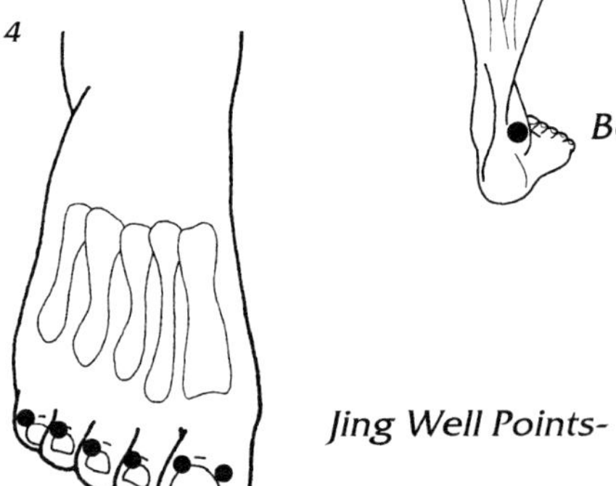

Back Pain - Upper

For upper back pain sedate the following points between the shoulder blades.

Fig. 1

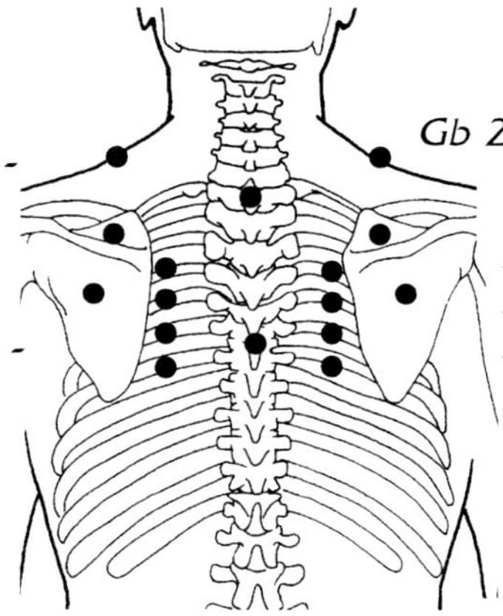

Gb 21 This lies halfway between the knob of bone at the base of the neck and the tip of the shoulder. *Fig. 2*

Gv 14 Just below the most prominent spinal bone at the base of the neck in the midline. *Fig. 2*

Si 13 4 fingers width ***below Gb 21*** just on top of the spine of the shoulder blade. *Fig. 2*

B 42 4 fingers width to each side of the spine at the level of the 3rd thoracic vertebrae. *Fig. 2*

B 43 4 fingers width to each side of the spine at the level of the 4th thoracic vertebrae. *Fig. 2*

Fig. 2

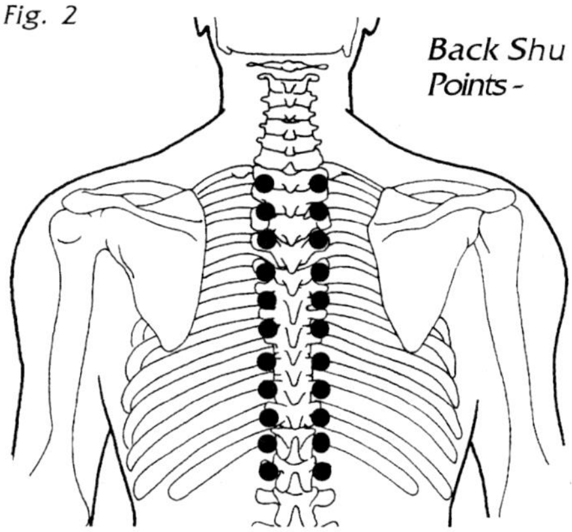

Si 11 Located at the middle of the shoulder blade. ***Tender when pressed***. *Fig. 2*

B 44 4 fingers width to each side of the spinal bone of the 5th thoracic vertebrae. *Fig. 2*

Gv 11 Just below the spinal bone of the 5th thoracic vertebrae. *Fig. 2*

B 45 4 fingers to each side of the spinal bone of the 6th thoracic vertebrae. *Fig. 2*

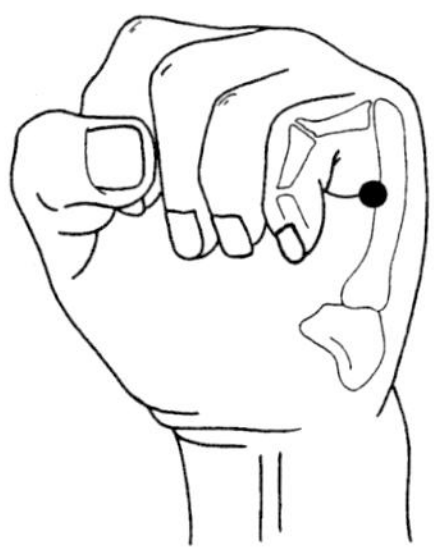

Back Shu
2 fingers width to each side of the spinal bones. *Fig. 2*

Si 3 On the end of the main transverse crease of the hand. ***Best located with the fist clenched***. *Fig. 3*

Fig. 4

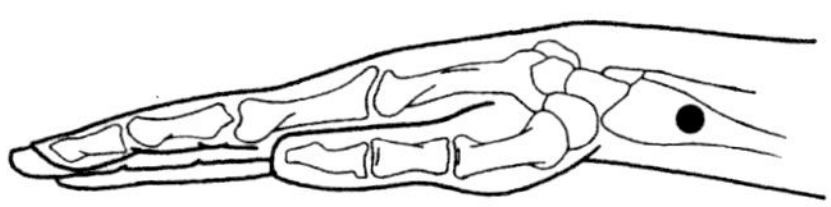

Lu 7 2 fingers width above the base of the thumb, in the small hollow of the bone. *Fig. 4*

Bell's Palsy

***B**ell's Palsy is a swelling of the facial nerves from viral or immune disease. This leads to compression of the nerve where it crosses through the narrow area of the temporal bone, causing pain behind the ear and atrophy of the facial muscles.*

Gb 14 1 fingers width ***above*** the middle of the eyebrows, directly above the pupils. *Fig. 1*

Extra 2 1 fingers width ***back*** from the outside of eye socket, in the hollow. *Figs. 1 & 2*

Gb 8 Located 1 fingers width directly above the upper most tips of the ear. *Fig. 2*

St 7 2 fingers width in front of the ear, in the hollow just ***below*** the upper jaw bone. *Fig. 2*

Si 18 Located below the outer corner of the eye socket, ***directly under the cheek bone.*** *Fig. 2*

St 6 On the highest point of the bulge of the muscle at the angle of the jaw, ***when the jaw is clenched***. *Fig. 2*

Li 4 In the centre of the fleshy mass between the thumb and index finger. *Fig. 3*

Fig. 1

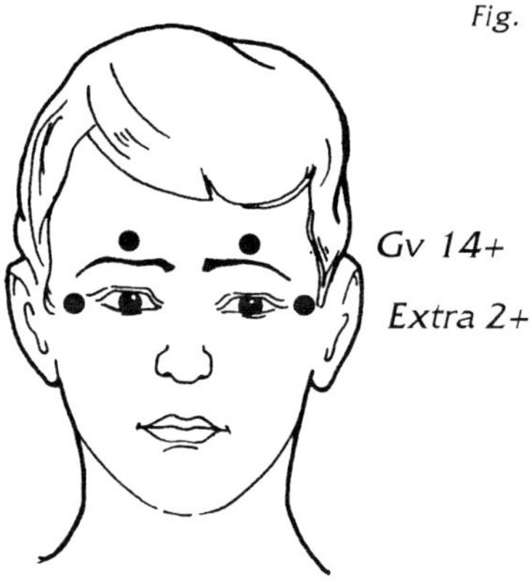

Fig. 2

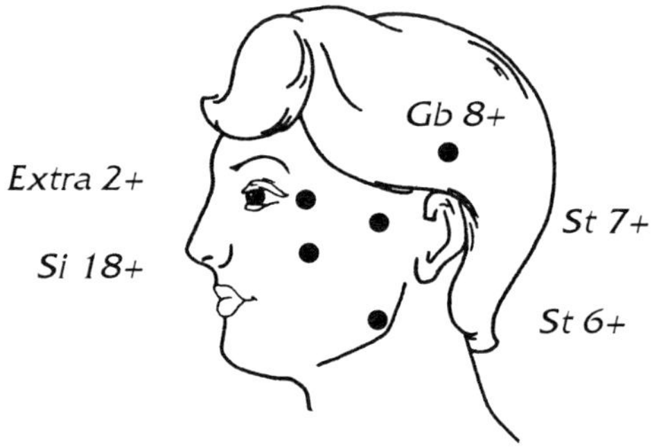

Fig. 3

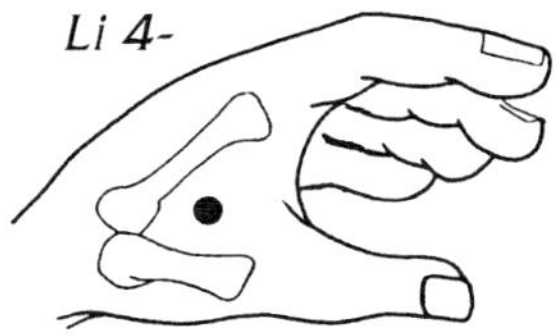

Bell's Palsy

Consult a Doctor before treating any points. For chronic conditions, the lower back region should be treated first. For additional relief, apply ETPS to the points on the following page.

Gb 34 4 fingers width below the outside of the kneecap, just in front of and below the knobby head of the fibula bone. *Fig. 4*

St 44 In the hollow at the base of the 1st and 2nd toes. *Fig. 5*

St 45 Located on the outside base of the second toe nail. *Fig. 5*

Sp 1 Located on the inside base of the big toe nail. *Fig. 5*

Fig. 4

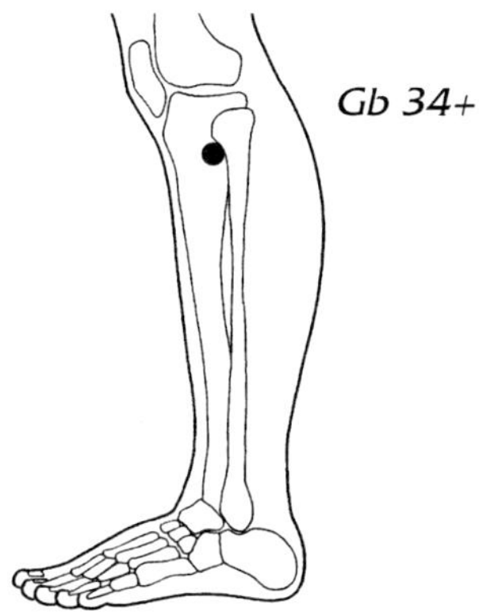

Fig. 5

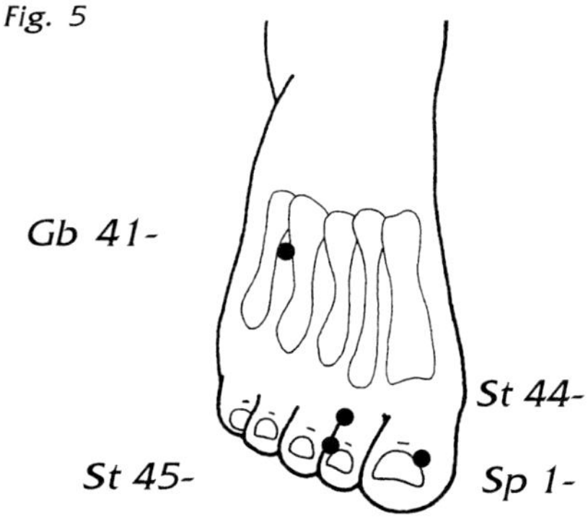

Bursitis of the Shoulder

***B**ursitis is caused by trauma, or repetitive or excessive frictional force. For optimal relief, sedate the following points in order, starting with the points in the legs and feet.*

Gb 34 4 fingers width below the outside of the kneecap, and just in front of and below the knobby head of the fibula bone. *Fig. 1*

St 38 Halfway between the kneecap and ankle, and 1 fingers width to the outside of the shin bone. *Fig. 1*

Gb 41 On top of the foot. In the hollow formed where the 4th and 5th toes bones meet. *Fig.2*

GB 20 Below the base of the skull, in the hollow just outside the spinal muscles of neck. *Fig. 3*

Back Shu Points:
Located 2 fingers width to each side of the spinal bones. *Fig. 3*

Gb 21 This lies halfway between the bone at the base of the neck and the tip of the shoulder, directly on top of the trapezius (shoulder) muscle. *Fig. 3*

Tw 15 1 thumbs width ***below Gb 21.*** *Fig. 3*

Si 3 4 fingers width below GB 21 just above the boney portion of the shoulder blade. *Fig. 3*

Li 18 4 fingers width beside the highest point of the Adam's apple in the prominent muscle at the side of the neck. *Fig. 4*

Tender Points
Stimulate tender points located in the tight muscles at the side of the neck. *Fig. 4*

Fig. 1

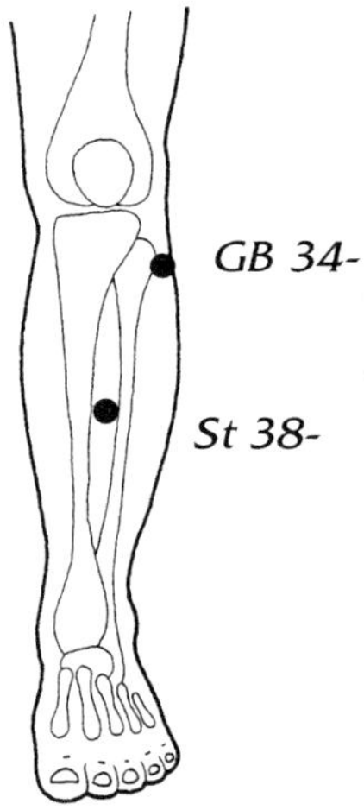

Fig. 2

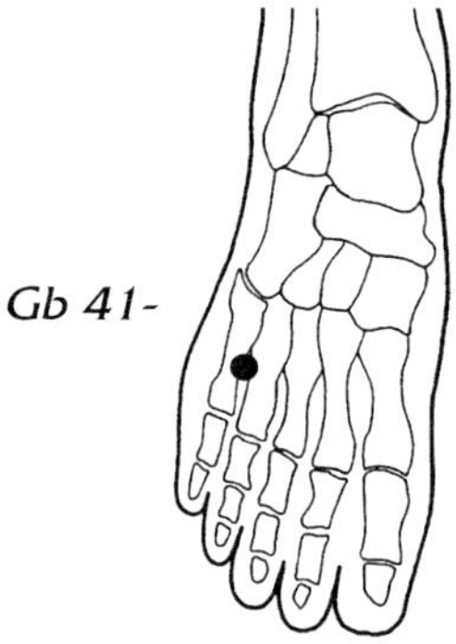

Fig. 3

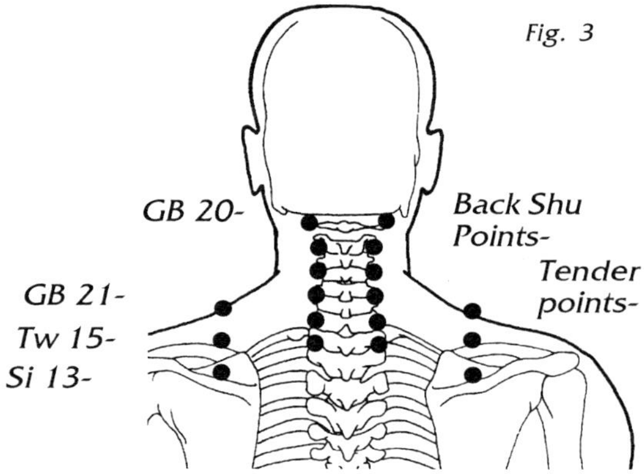

Fig. 4

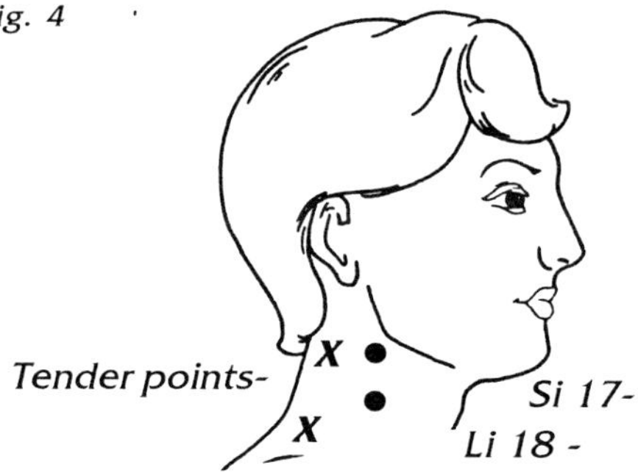

Bursitis of the Shoulder

Bursitis is caused by trauma, or repetitive or excessive frictional force. For optimal relief, sedate the following points in order, starting with the points in the legs and feet.

Tw 15 This point is located in the ***hollow formed in the deltoid muscle crease in the back of the shoulder. Opposite position to Li 15.*** Best located with arm the raised. *Fig. 1*

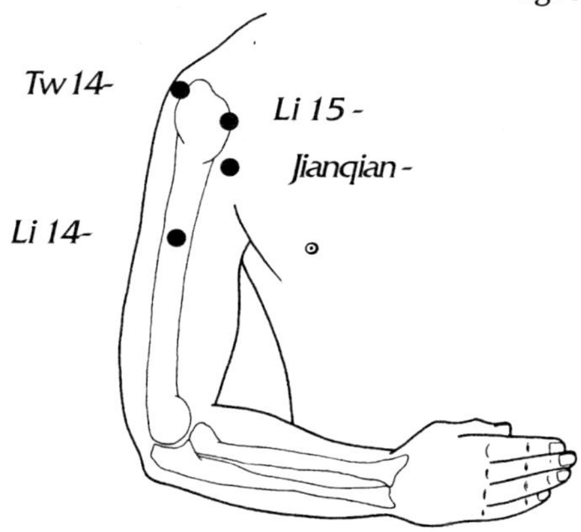

Fig. 1

Li 15 This point is located in the ***hollow formed in the deltoid muscle in front of the shoulder*** *Fig. 1*

Jianqian
Midway between ***Li 15*** and the armpit fold. *Fig. 1*

Li 14 On the ***lower border*** of the deltoid muscle, on the outside of the arm. *Fig. 1*

Fig. 2

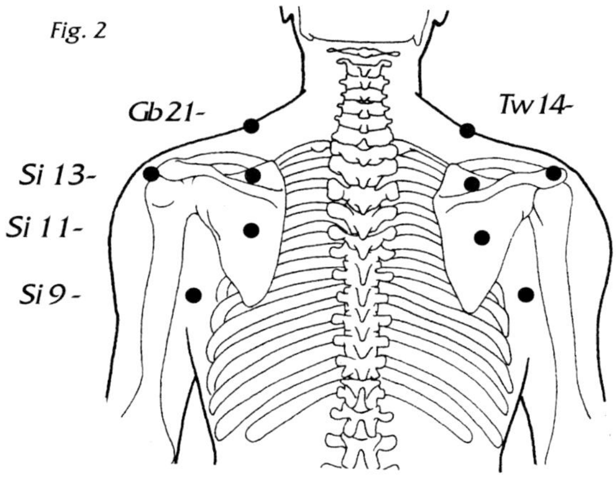

Gb 21 Halfway between the most prominent bone at the bottom of the neck and the outside tip of the shoulder bone. *Fig. 2*

Si 13 Located on the spine of the shoulder blade, ***4 fingers width below Gb 21.*** *Fig. 2*

Si 10 Directly in the middle of the shoulder blade, very tender when pressed. *Fig. 2*

Si 9 With an arm at the side, this point is located 1 thumbs width above the fold. *Fig. 2*

Calf Pain - General

Consult a Doctor before treating any points. For chronic conditions, stimulate at the points on this page first. The distal and local points on the following page may be used after the below points. Sedate points for maximum relief.

Back Shu Points:
Located 2 fingers width to each side of the spinal bones. ***Sedate these points from the middle to the lower back. Above points innervate the affected region and often provide substantial relief.*** *Fig. 1*

Piriformis Trigger Points:
Approximately half way between the sacrum (the triangular bone at the base of the spine) and the outside hip joint. Or, one hands width above GB 30. Press and rub (palpate) the general area until tenderness is detected.

Gb 30 This point is directly in the middle of each "cheek", equal distance from all sides. *Fig. 2*

Gb 31 Stand erect, hands flat along the side of the thigh. This point is at the ***tip of the middle finger***. *Fig. 3*

Gb 34 4 fingers width below the outside of the kneecap, and just in front of and below the knobby head of the fibula bone. *Fig. 3*

Fig. 1

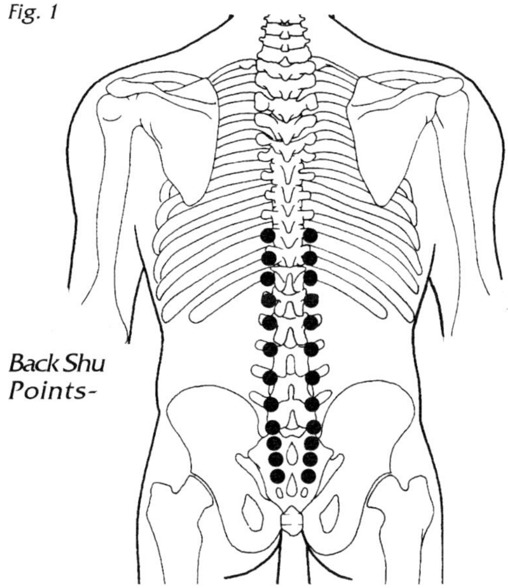

Fig. 2

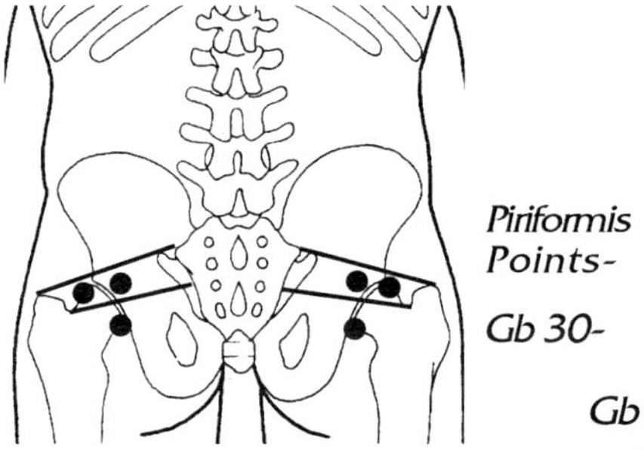

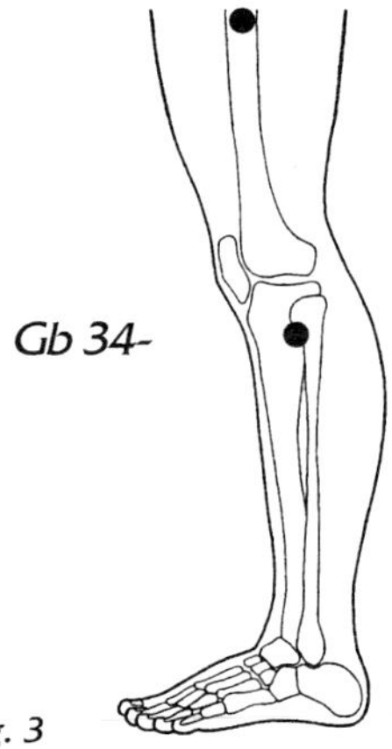

Fig. 3

Calf Pain - General

Calf pain is often successfully treated with stimulation of local points within the calf muscles. For additional relief, stimulate points in the lower back ***(pg. 39-40)*** *and ankle region* ***(pg. 35-36)*** *on negative polarity.*

B 40 On the middle of the crease behind the knee. *Fig. 1*

B 57 At the mid point of the calf where the calf muscle narrows to form the tendon, between the 2 calf muscles. *Fig. 1*

B 58 1 thumbs width below and 1 thumbs width to the outside of ***B 57.*** *Fig. 1*

B 60 This lies in the hollow midway between the tip of the outer ankle bone and the Achilles tendon. *Figs. 1 & 2*

Sp 6 3 fingers above the inner ankle and just behind the prominent shin bone. ***Tender when pressed.*** *Fig. 3*

K 7 2 thumbs width above **K 3.** *Fig. 3*

K 3 In the hollow midway between the tip of the inner ankle bone and the Achilles tendon. *Fig. 3*

Tender Points

Stimulate any tender trigger points found within the tight calf muscles. ***The areas are marked with an "X".*** *Figs. 1, 2, & 3*

Fig. 1

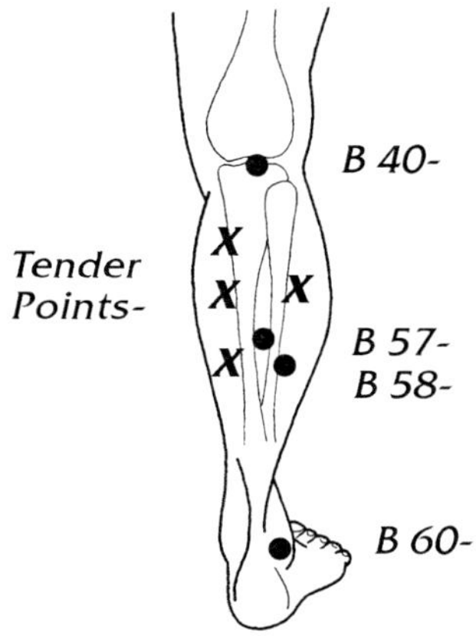

Fig. 2

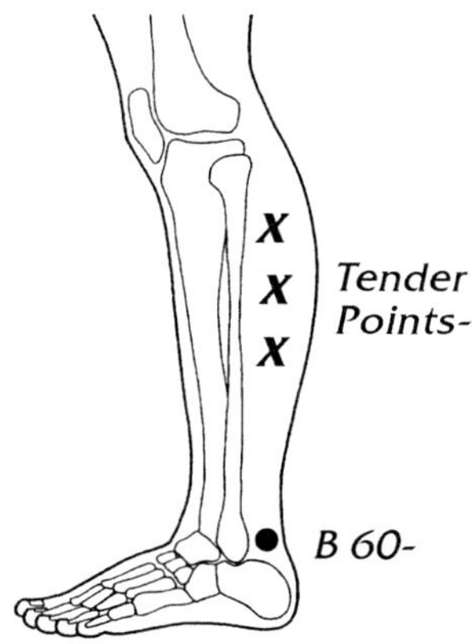

Fig. 3

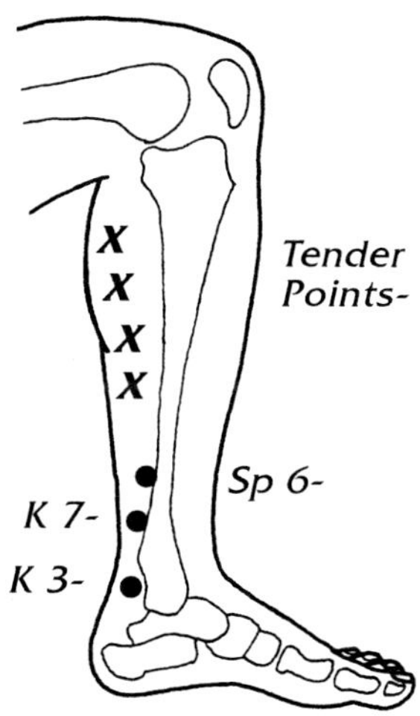

Carpal Tunnel Syndrome

*Treat this condition first in the **lower back and neck regions.** Next, apply to localized tender and acupoints within the wrist area. For painful swelling or circulation problems, also sedate **Sp6.***

Back Shu Points:
Located 2 fingers width to each side of the spinal bones. ***Sedate these points from the middle to the lower back. Above points innervate the affected region and often provide substantial relief.*** *Fig. 1*

Piriformis Trigger Points:
Approximately half way between the sacrum (the triangular bone at the base of the spine) and the outside hip joint. Or, one hands width above GB 30. Press and rub (palpate) the general area until tenderness is detected. *Fig. 2*

Gb 30 This point is directly in the middle of each "cheek", equal distance from all sides. *Fig. 2*

Gb 31 Stand erect, hands flat along the side of the thigh. This point is at the ***tip of the middle finger***. *Fig. 3*

Gb 34 4 fingers width below the outside of the kneecap, and just in front of and below the knobby head of the fibula bone. *Fig. 3*

Sp 6 3 fingers width above the inner ankle and just behind the prominent shin bone. *Fig. 4*

Fig. 1

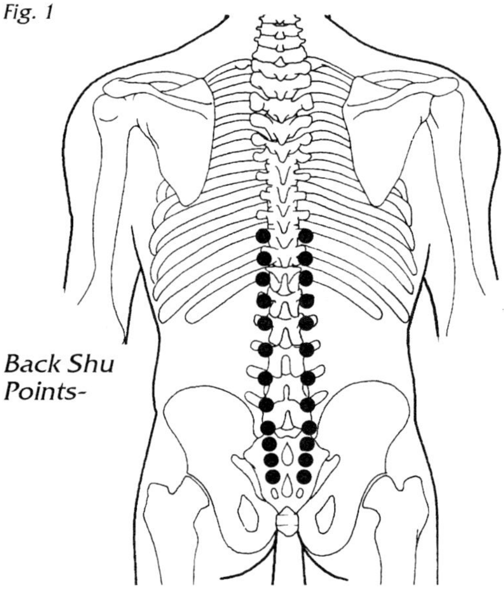

Fig. 2

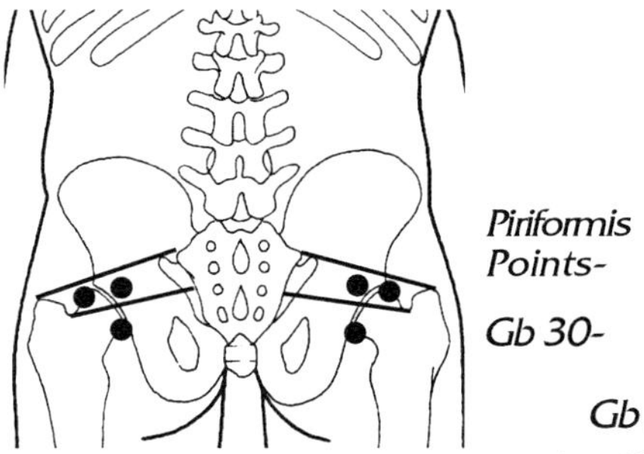

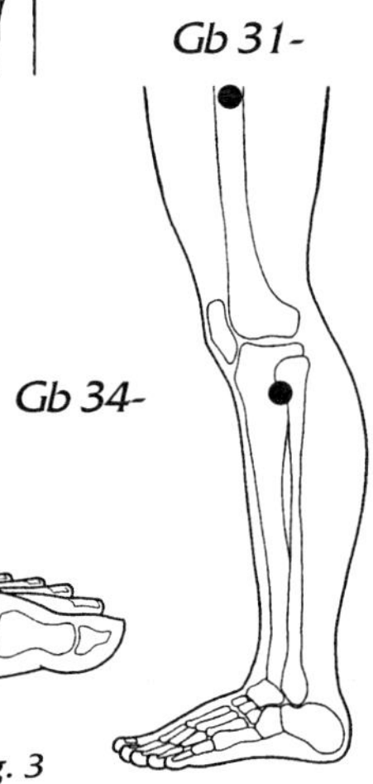

Fig. 3

Fig. 4

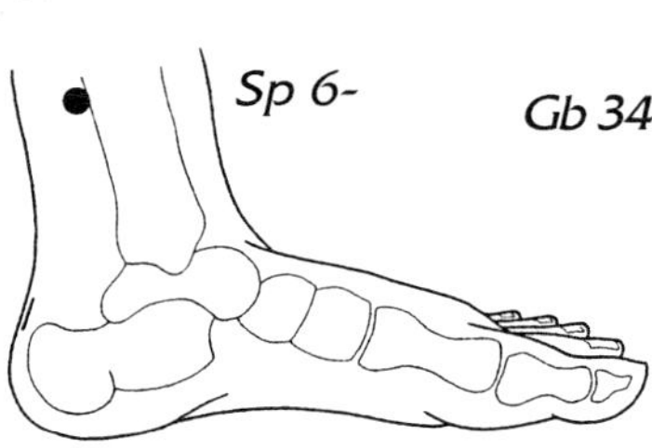

Carpal Tunnel

A**fter first treating the **lower back & neck,** apply ETPS to local acupoints within the wrist area. For painful swelling sedate **Sp 6.

Gb 20 Below the base of the skull, in the hollow just outside the spinal muscles of neck. *Fig. 1*

Back Shu Points
Located 2 fingers width to each side of the spinal bones. *Fig. 1*

Gv 14 This lies just below the most prominent bone at the base of the neck on the midline. *Fig. 1*

Gb 21 This lies halfway between the bone at the base of the neck and the tip of the shoulder, on top of the muscle. *Fig. 1*

Si 13 4 fingers width ***below GB 21*** just on top of the spine of the shoulder blade. *Fig. 1*

Si 17 Above the prominent neck muscle, ***at the level of the corner of the jaw***. *Fig. 2*

Li 18 4 fingers width beside the highest point of the Adam's apple in the prominent muscle at the side of the neck. *Fig. 2*

P 8 With the fist closed, between the tips of the middle & ring fingers. *Fig. 3*

Lu 9 At the base of the thumb in the groove at the end of the wrist crease. *Fig. 3*

P 7 On the wrist crease, in between the tendons. *Fig. 3*

H 7 On the wrist crease, just inside the prominent tendon. *Fig. 3*

P 6 3 fingers width from the most distal wrist crease. *Fig. 3*

Fig. 1

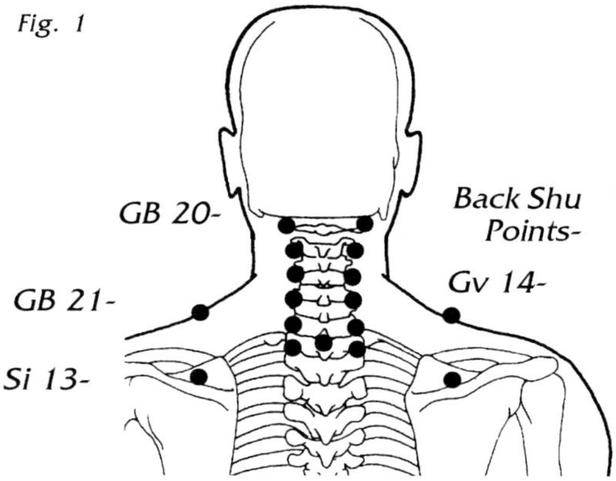

Fig. 2

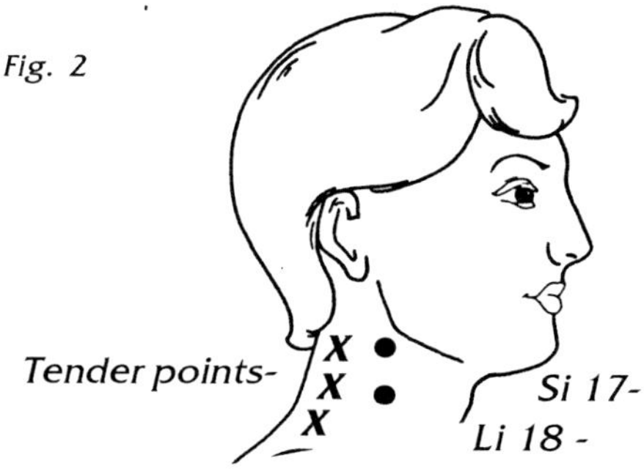

Fig. 3

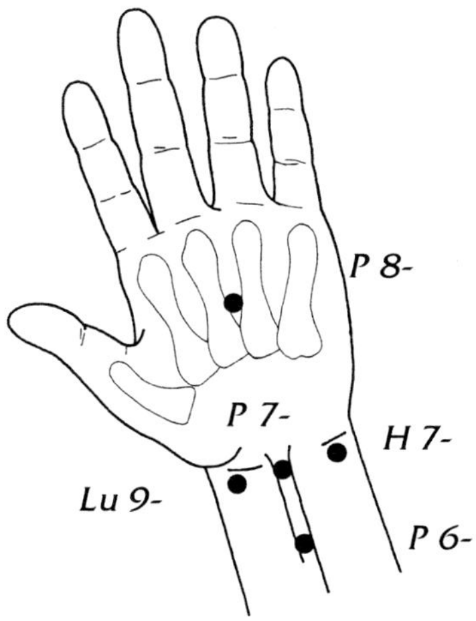

Cervical Spondylosis

Cervical Spondylosis is characterized by restricted neck movements and pain when tilting the head forward or backward. For relief, sedate the following points and test for results. For additional points see next page.

Back Shu Points:
Located 2 fingers width to each side of the spinal bones. ***Sedate these points from the middle to the lower back. Above points innervate the affected region and often provide substantial relief.*** *Fig. 1*

Piriformis Trigger Points:
Approximately half way between the sacrum (the triangular bone at the base of the spine) and the outside hip joint. Or, one hands width above GB 30. Press and rub (palpate) the general area until tenderness is detected. *Fig. 2*

Gb 30 This point is directly in the middle of each "cheek", equal distance from all sides. *Fig. 2*

Gb 31 Stand erect, hands flat along the side of the thigh. This point is at the ***tip of the middle finger***. *Fig. 3*

Gb 34 4 fingers width below the outside of the kneecap, and just in front of and below the knobby head of the fibula bone. *Fig. 3*

Gb 39 4 fingers width above the tip of the outer ankle bone and just ***behind*** the fibula bone. *Fig. 3*

Fig. 1

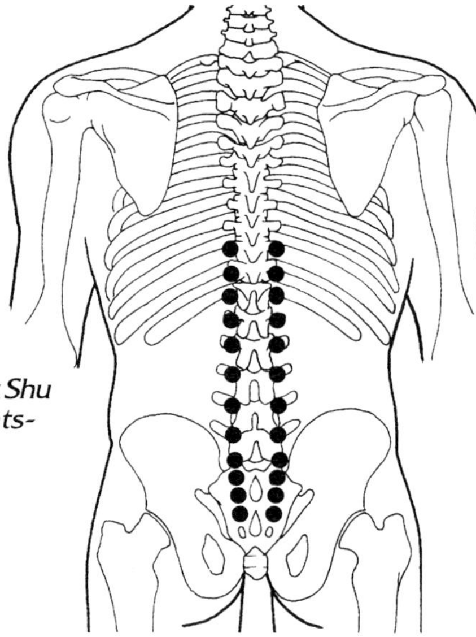

Fig. 2

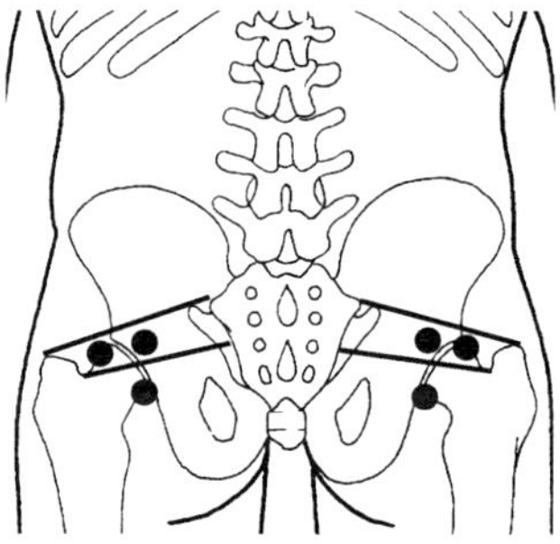

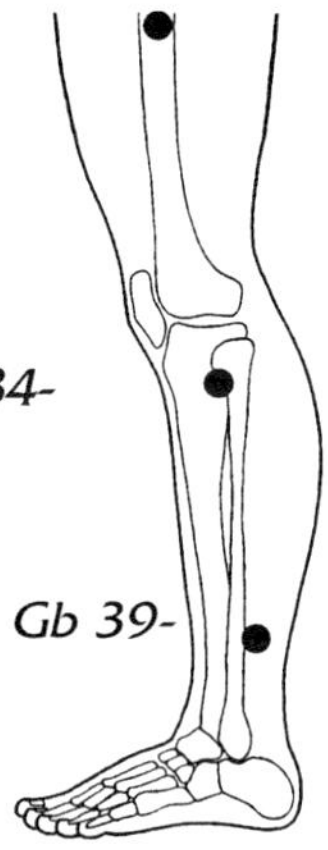

Fig. 3

Cervical Spondylosis

***F**or additional relief to chronic conditions, sedate the following local and distal points on top of the points on the previous page.*

Gb 20 Below the base of the skull, in the hollow just outside the main spinal muscles of neck. *Fig. 1*

Back Shu Points
These lie 2 fingers width to each side of the spinal bones. *Fig. 1*

Gv 14 This lies just below the most prominent bone at the base of the neck on the midline. *Fig. 1*

Gb 21 This lies halfway between the bone at the base of the neck and the tip of the shoulder, directly on top of the trapezius (shoulder) muscle. *Fig. 1*

Si 13 4 fingers width ***below GB 21*** just on top of the spine of the shoulder blade. *Fig. 1*

Si 17 Above the prominent neck muscle, ***at the level of the corner of the jaw***. *Fig. 2*

Li 18 4 fingers width beside the highest point of the Adam's apple in the prominent muscle at the side of the neck ***(below the corner of the jaw)***. *Fig. 2*

Si 3 On the end of the main transverse crease of the hand. ***Best located with the fist clenched***. *Fig. 3*

Tw 5 On the back of the wrist 2 thumbs width above the wrist crease in between the 2 forearm bones. *Fig. 4*

Fig. 1

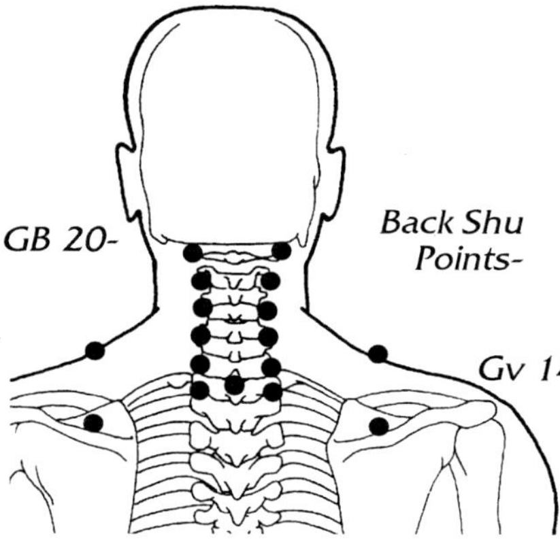

Fig. 2

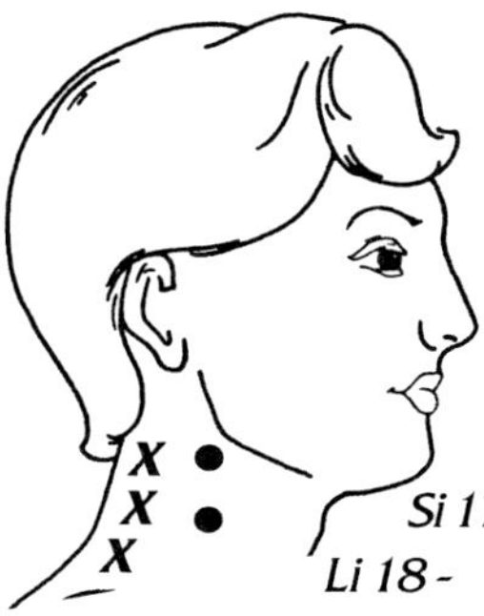

Fig. 3

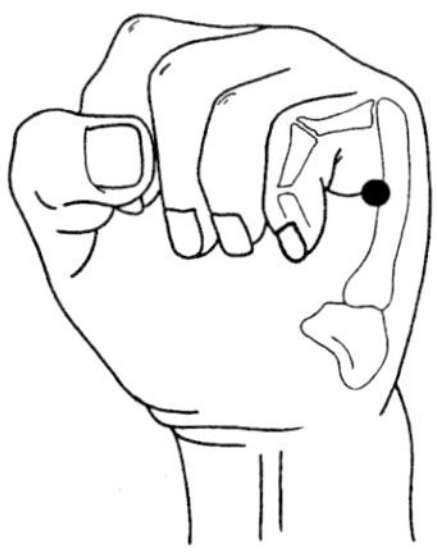

Fig. 4

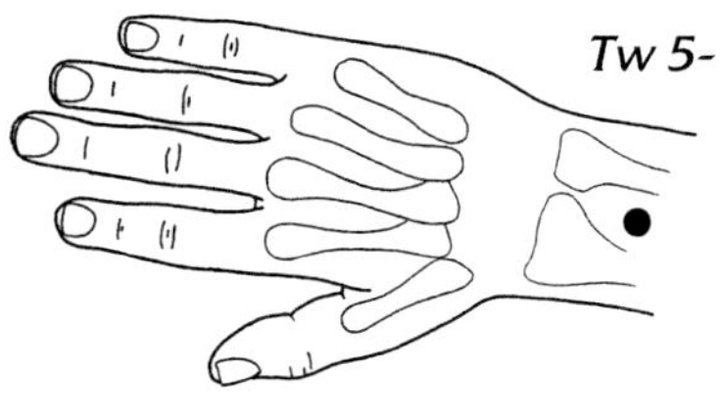

Chronic Fatigue Syndrome

Consult a Doctor before treating any points. For chronic conditions, the sedate the parasympathetic points first, to calm the nerves and relax muscles.

Lu 9 In the groove at the thumb side of the wrist crease, and inside of the tendon. *Fig. 1*

H 7 On the little finger side of the wrist crease, to the inside of the tendon. *Fig. 1*

P 6 3 fingers width from the most distal wrist crease, in between the tendons. *Fig. 1*

Sp 6 3 fingers width above the inner ankle and just behind the prominent shin bone. *Fig. 2*

K 3 Halfway between the Achilles tendon and the inner ankle bone. *Fig. 2*

K 27 2 thumbs width on each side of the sternum, in the hollow just below the collarbone. *Fig. 3*

Cv 17 On the breast bone at the heart level or the 4th rib space. Tender when pressed. *Fig. 3*

B 62 In the depression half a finger below the outer ankle bone. *Fig. 4*

Fig. 1

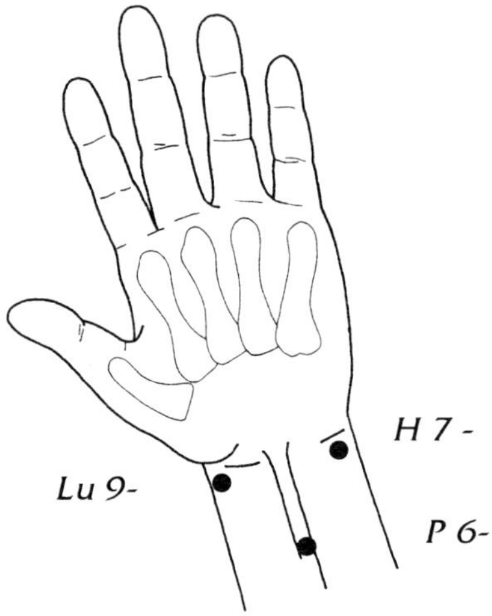

Fig. 2

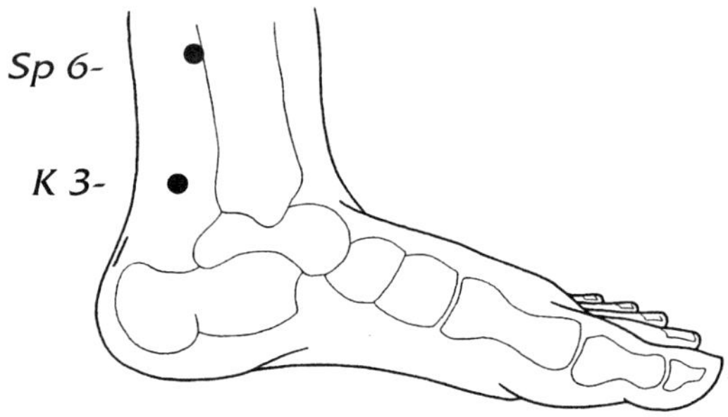

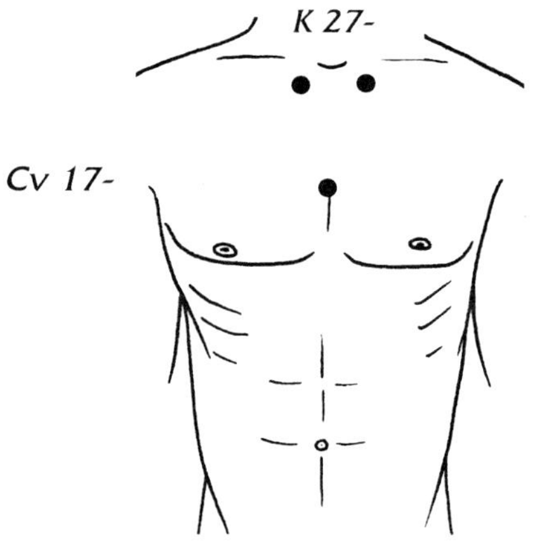

Fig. 3

Fig. 4

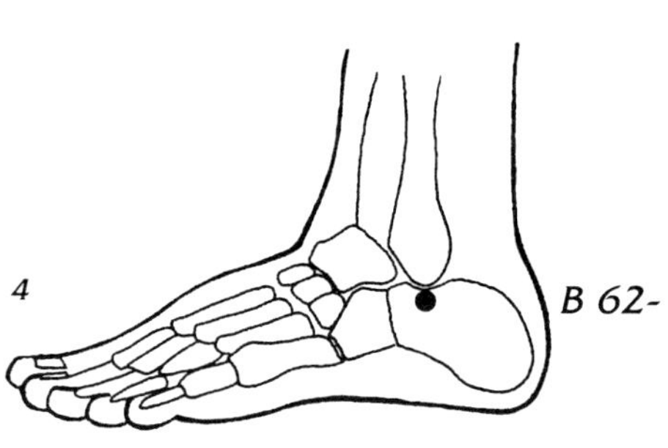

Chronic Fatigue

***O**nce the the patient is calmed, tonify the following points to help increase energy.*

Fig. 1

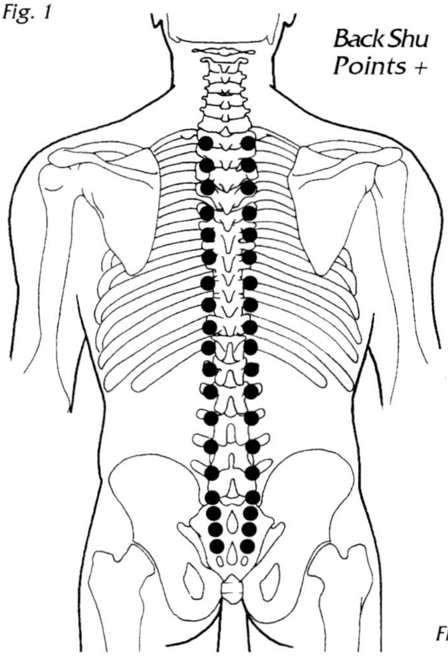

Back Shu Points

Stimulate the following points in the midback range. These are located 2 fingers width to each side of the spine. ***Starting from waist level move upwards to the highest level of the shoulder blade. Tonify the ropy muscles found on each side of the spine.*** *Fig. 1*

St 36 4 fingers width below the kneecap and 1 fingers width to the outside of the shin bone. *Fig. 2*

Li 11 This lies on the end of the outer elbow crease with the arm bent. *Fig. 3*

Cv 6 On the midline 2 fingers width below the belly button. *Fig. 3*

Fig. 2

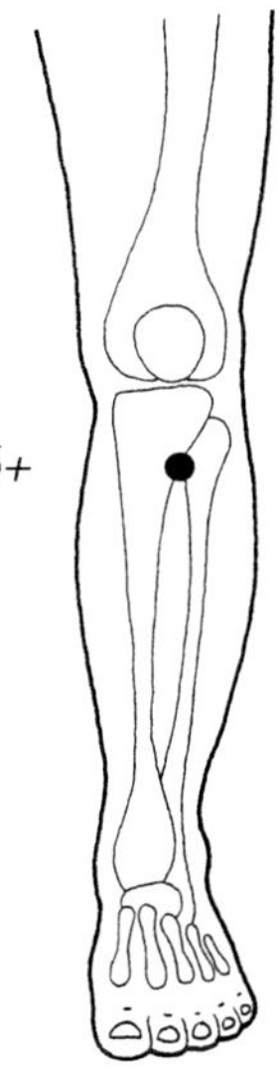

Fig. 4

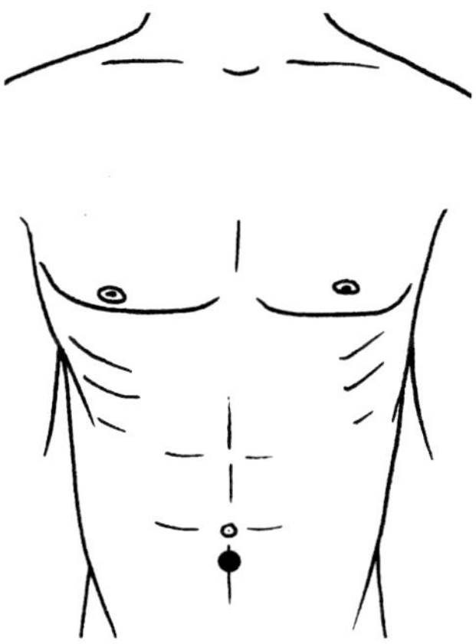

Fig. 3

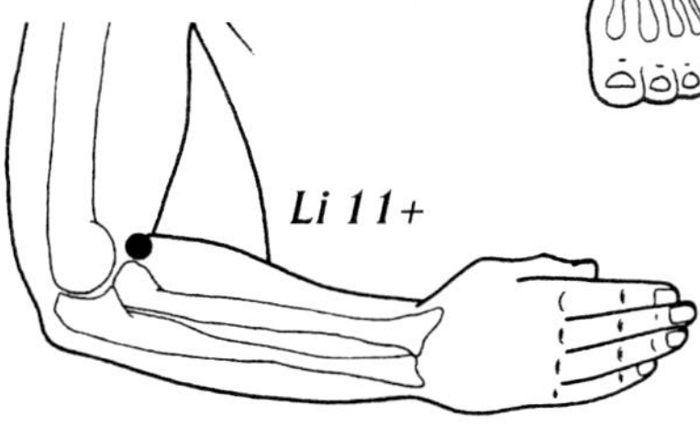

Coccyx Injury

Coccyx injuries may be relieved by first treating acutherapy points in the sacral coccyx area. Finish by sedating points down the leg and in the feet. ***Jing Well Points*** *on the toes have been reported to be very successful in providing relief.*

Back Shu Points:
Located 2 fingers width to each side of the spinal bones. *Fig. 1*

Gb 30 This lies in the upper/outer part of the buttock muscle. *Fig. 1*

Gv 2 **At the junction between the sacrum and the coccyx,** *in the hollow. Fig. 1*

B 31 This lies at the top of the sacral bone and 2 fingers width away from the midline. *Fig. 1*

B 32 This lies 1 thumbs width below ***B 31.*** *Fig. 1*

B 34 At the ***highest level of the upper leg bone***, this point lies 1 thumbs width to each side of the midline. *Fig. 1*

B 40 On the middle of the crease behind the knee. *Fig. 2*

B 60 This lies in the hollow midway between the tip of the outer ankle bone and the Achilles tendon. *Fig. 2*

St 44 At the meeting of the base of 2nd and 3rd toes in between the web. *Fig. 3*

Jing Well Points
At the outer base of the toe nails. *Fig. 3*

Sp 6 3 fingers width above the inner ankle bone and behind the prominent shin bone. *Fig. 4*

Fig. 1

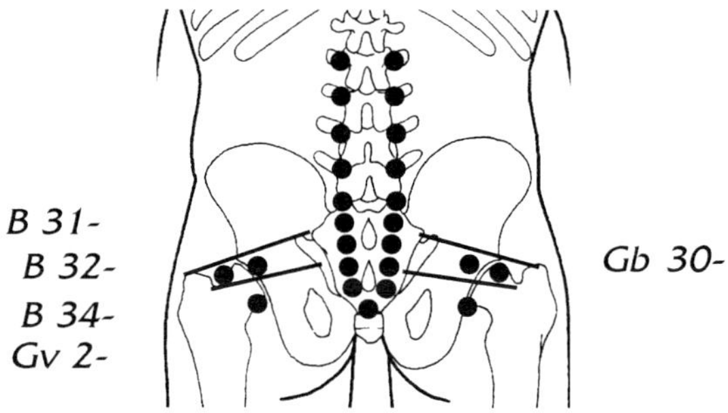

Fig. 2

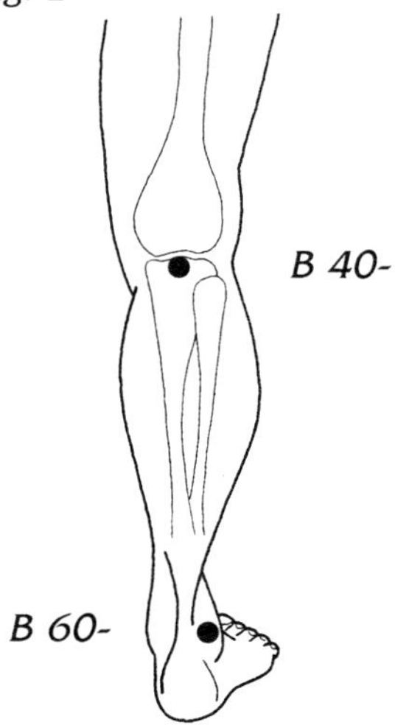

Fig. 3

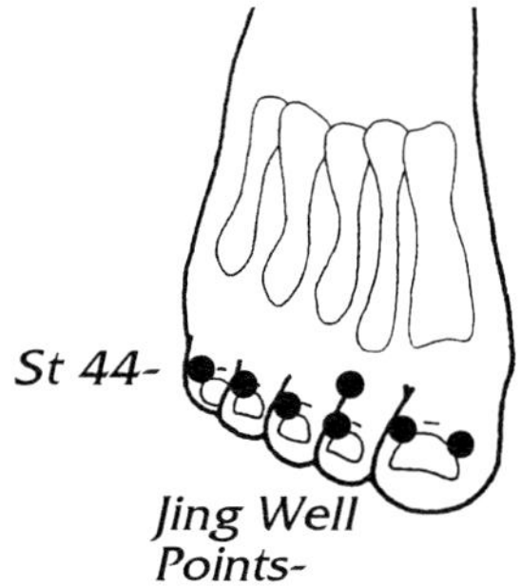

Fig. 4

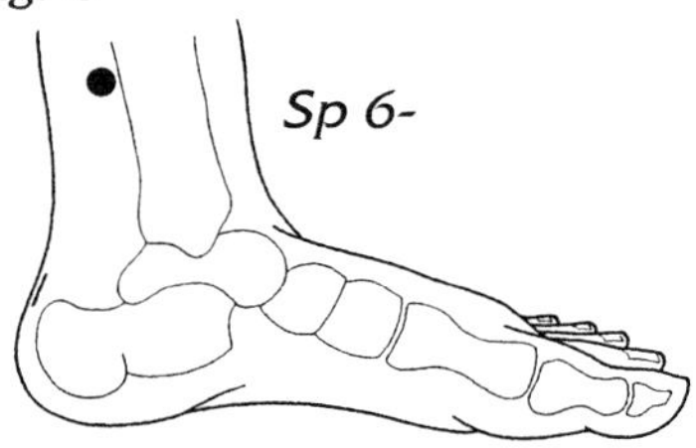

Constipation

***S**tart by sedating **Tw 6 on both arms.** Next, the distal points on the feet, hands and legs should be sedated, followed by the points on the abdomen.*

Li 4 In the fleshy mass between the thumb and index finger. *Fig. 1*

Tw 6 4 fingers width above the transverse wrist crease, in between the 2 forearm bones. *Fig. 1* **

St 36 4 fingers width below the knee cap and 1 fingers width to the outside of the shin bone. *Fig. 2*

Gb 34 4 fingers width below the knee cap on the outside of the leg, and just in front and below the protruding bone. *Fig. 2*

St 37 4 fingers width ***below St 36*** and 1 fingers width to the outside of the shin bone. *Fig. 2*

St 44 On top of the foot, in the hollow where the 1st and 2nd toe bones meet. *Fig. 2*

St 25 2 thumbs width to ***each side*** of the belly button. *Fig. 3*

Sp 15 4 thumbs width to ***each side*** of the belly button. *Fig. 3*

Cv 6 2 fingers width directly below the belly button. *Fig. 3*

Fig. 1

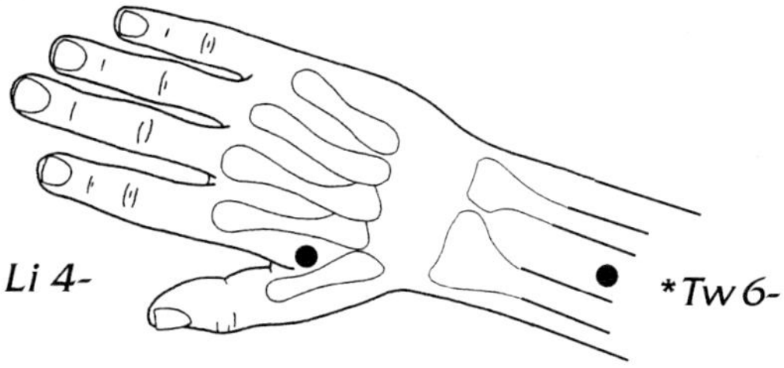

Fig. 2

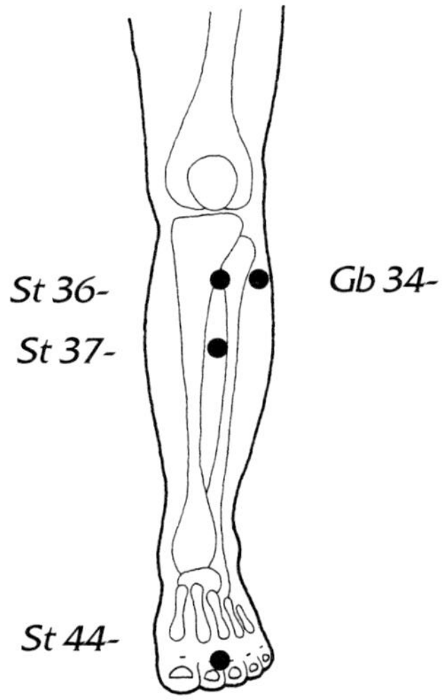

Fig. 3

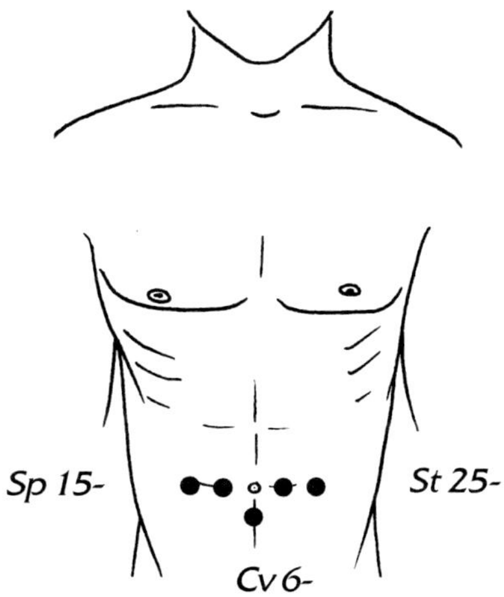

Costochondritis

***C**ostocondritis is characterized by pain n the chest, usually at the front of the rib cage. Start by sedating the points in the wrist and hands, and finish with the local points. If additional relief is required, then sedate the following points in the upper back and spine on next page.*

Lu 9 in the groove at the thumb side of the wrist crease, and inside of the tendon. *Fig. 1*

P 6 3 fingers width from the most distal wrist crease, in between the tendons. *Fig. 1*

H 7 On the little finger side of the wrist crease, in between the 2 wrist tendons. *Fig. 1*

Fig. 1

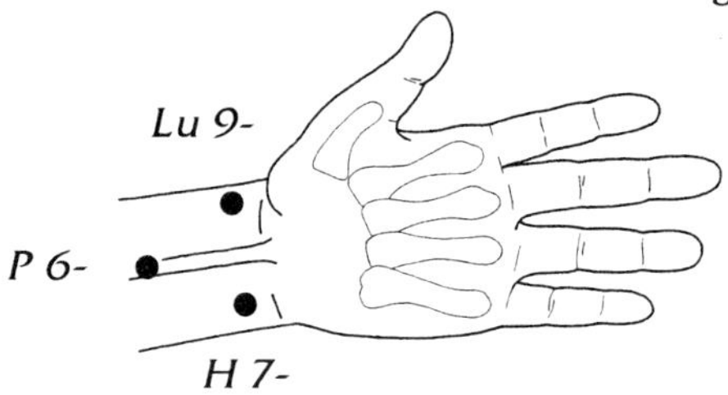

Lu 7 2 fingers width above the base of the thumb, in the small hollow of the bone. *Fig. 2*

Fig. 2

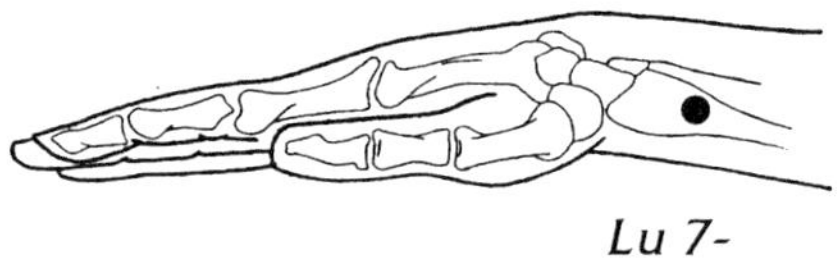

Li 4 In the middle of the fleshy mass between the thumb and index finger and slightly towards the index finger. *Fig. 3*

Fig. 3

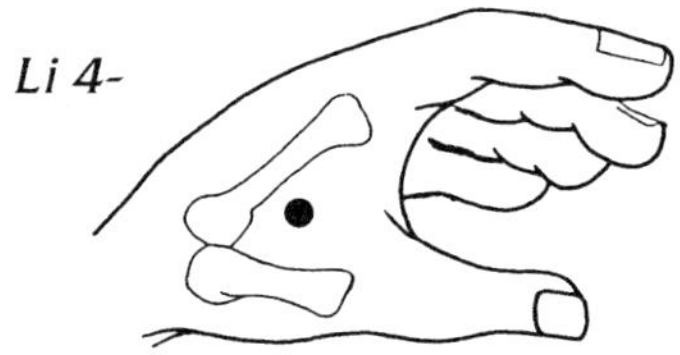

Cv 22 In the hollow just above the upper border of the breastbone. *Fig. 4*

Tender Points

Sedate any tender points that are in the local area or involved with the injured muscles. ***They may feel tender or sore when pressed.*** *Fig. 4*

Cv 17 On the breast bone at the heart level or the 4th rib space. Tender when pressed. *Fig. 4*

Fig. 4

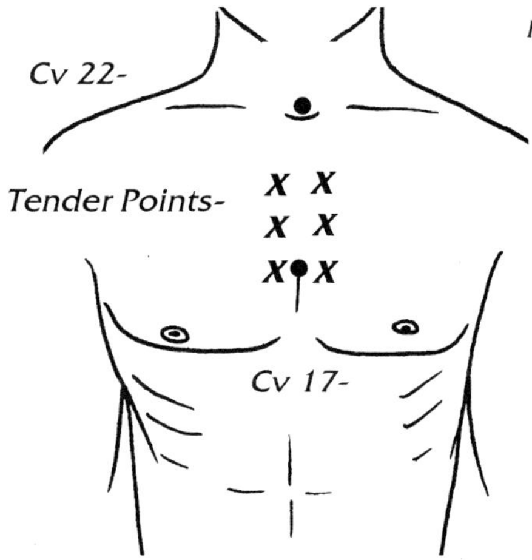

Costochondritis

If additional relief is required, then sedate the following points in the upper back and spine.

Back Shu Points

These points are located 2 fingers width on each side of the bumps in the spine. ***Sedate the back area of tightness or muscular pain. Start from the neck and move downward to the waist level.*** *Fig. 1*

Fig. 1

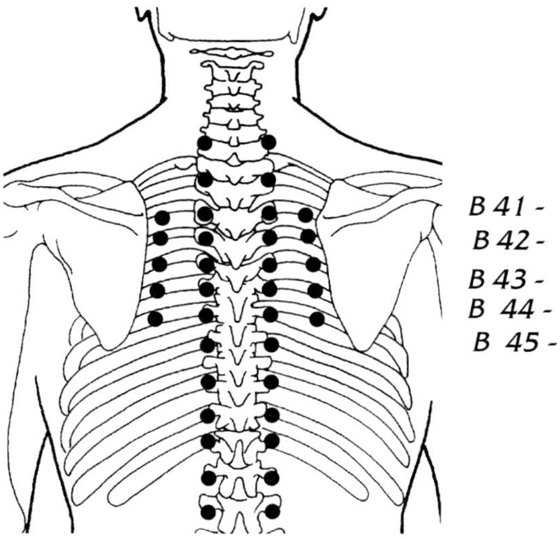

Back Shu Points-

B 41 On the inside of the shoulder blade, at the level of the ***2nd*** thoracic vertabrae. *Fig. 1*

B 42 On the inside of the shoulder blade, at the level of the ***3rd*** thoracic vertabrae. *Fig. 1*

B 43 On the inside of the shoulder blade, at the level of the ***4th*** thoracic vertabrae. *Fig. 1*

B 44 On the inside of the shoulder blade, at the level of the ***5th*** thoracic vertabrae. *Fig. 1*

B 45 On the inside of the shoulder blade, at the level of the ***6th*** thoracic vertabrae. *Fig. 1*

Acu-tips

Always apply the unit to the most tender points involved with an injury. They seem to yield the most effective results with chronic pain management.

Over time, try to reduce the number of points treated. As the body recovers from an injury or illness, the number of tender points and their severity of tenderness should drop dramatically.

Digestive Problems

***A** Doctor should be consulted for a proper diagnosis. Once diagnosed, distal points in the legs and arms should be treated first, followed by the abdomen.*

Back Shu Points:

Located 2 fingers width to each side of the spinal bones. ***Sedate these points from the middle to the lower back. Above points innervate the affected region and often provide substantial relief.*** *Fig. 1*

Fig. 1

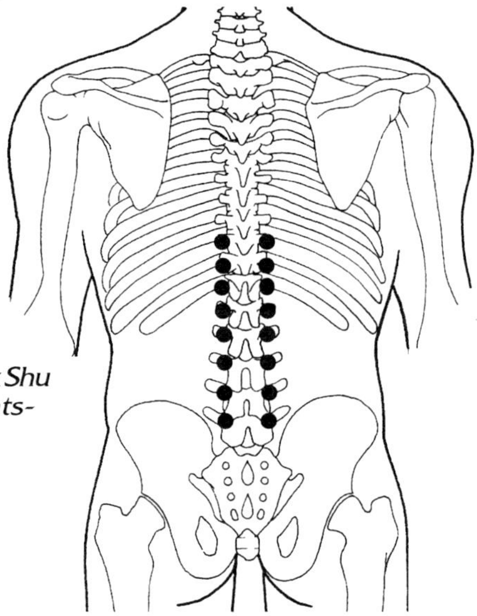

Piriformis Trigger Points:

Approximately half way between the sacrum (the triangular bone at the base of the spine) and the outside hip joint. Or, one hands width above GB 30. Press and rub (palpate) the general area until tenderness is detected. *Fig. 2*

Fig. 2

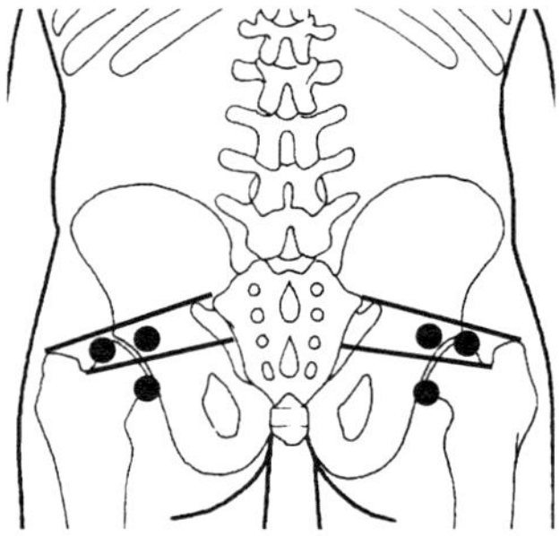

Gb 30 This point is directly in the middle of each "cheek", equal distance from all sides. *Fig. 2*

Gb 31 Stand erect, hands flat along the side of the thigh. This point is at the ***tip of the middle finger***. *Fig. 3*

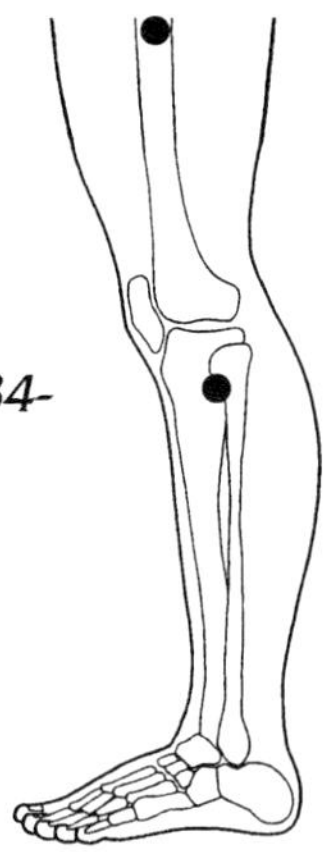

Fig. 3

Gb 34 4 fingers width below the outside of the kneecap, and just in front of and below the knobby head of the fibula bone. *Fig. 3*

Digestive Problems

***A** Doctor should be consulted for a proper diagnosis. Once diagnosed, distal points in the legs and arms should be treated first, followed by the abdomen.*

Cv 12 On the midline, half way between belly button and the lower chest bone. *Fig. 1*

St 25 2 thumbs width ***to each side*** of the belly button. *Fig. 1*

Cv 6 On the midline, 2 fingers width ***below*** the belly button. *Fig. 1*

St 34 2 thumbs width above the upper/outer border of the kneecap. *Fig. 2*

St 36 4 fingers width below the knee cap and 1 fingers width to the outside of the shin bone. *Fig. 2*

St 44 At meeting of the base of 2nd and 3rd toes, in the web. *Fig. 2*

Li 4 In the fleshy mass between the thumb and index finger. *Fig. 3*

Tw 6 4 fingers width above the transverse wrist crease, in between the 2 forearm bones. *Fig. 3* **

P 6 3 fingers width from the most distal wrist crease, in between the tendons. *Fig. 4*

Fig. 1

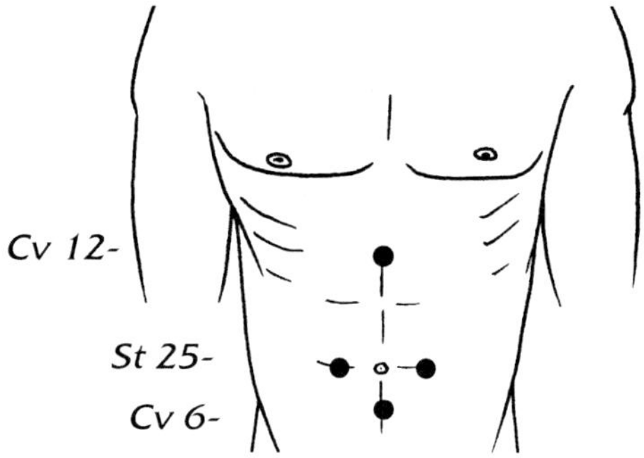

Fig. 2

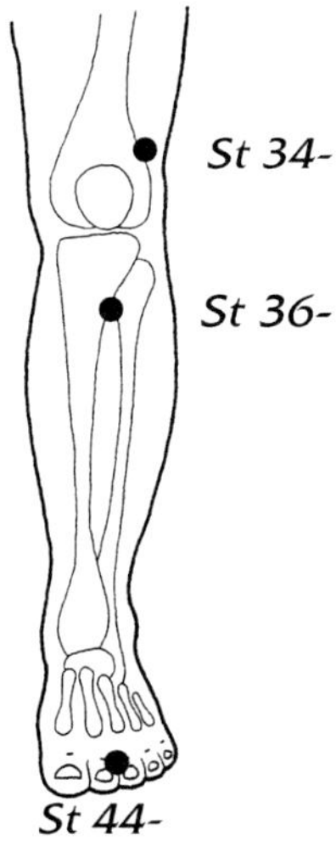

Fig. 3

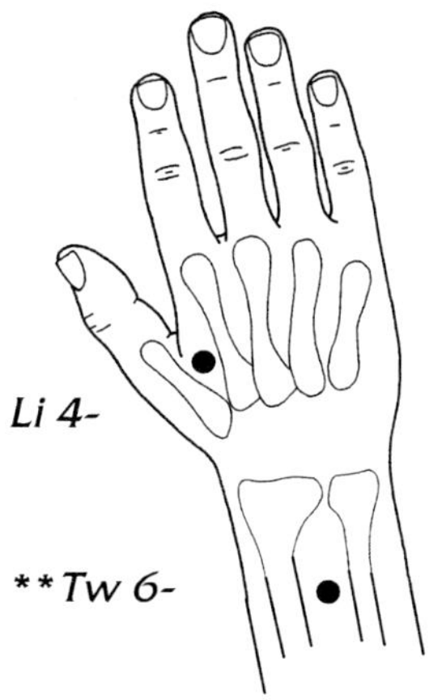

Fig. 4

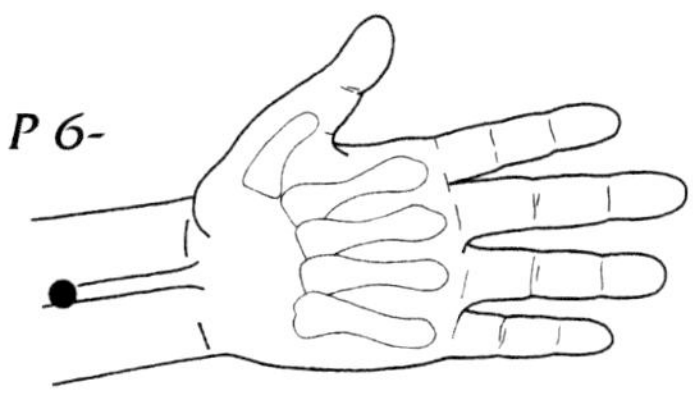

Dupuytren's Contracture

***D**upuytren's Contracture causes problems in bending the fingers and decreases their agility. Sedate the acutherapy and tender points in the neck first, then follow up with the points on the following page.*

Gb 20 Below the base of the skull, in the hollow just outside the main spinal muscles of neck. *Fig. 1*

Back Shu Points
These lie 2 fingers width to each side of the spinal bones. *Fig. 1*

Gv 14 This lies just below the most prominent bone at the base of the neck on the midline. *Fig. 1*

Gb 21 This lies halfway between the bone at the base of the neck and the tip of the shoulder, directly on top of the trapezius (shoulder) muscle. *Fig. 1*

Si 13 4 fingers width ***below GB 21*** just on top of the spine of the shoulder blade. *Fig. 1*

Si 17 Above the prominent neck muscle, ***at the level of the corner of the jaw***. *Fig. 2*

Li 18 4 fingers width beside the highest point of the Adam's apple in the prominent muscle at the side of the neck ***(below the corner of the jaw)***. *Fig. 2*

Si 3 On the end of the main transverse crease of the hand. ***Best located with the fist clenched***. *Fig. 3*

Tw 5 On the back of the wrist 2 thumbs width above the wrist crease in between the 2 forearm bones. *Fig. 4*

Fig. 1

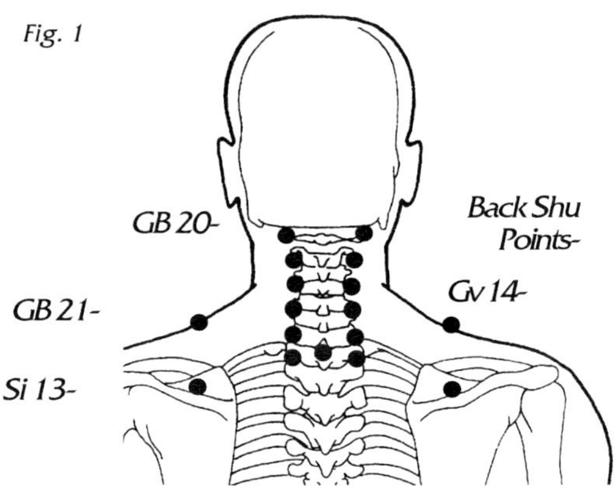

Fig. 2

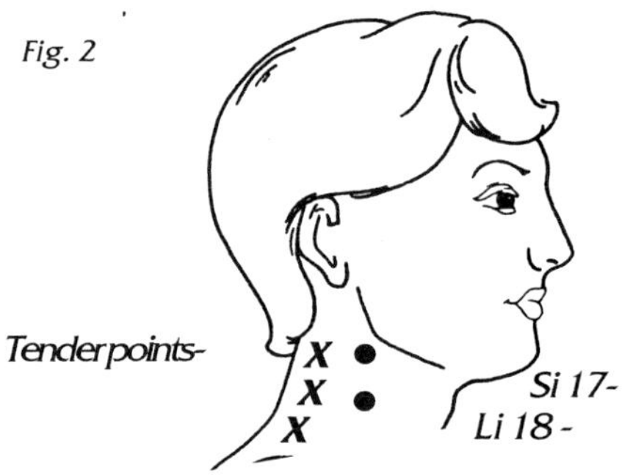

Fig. 3

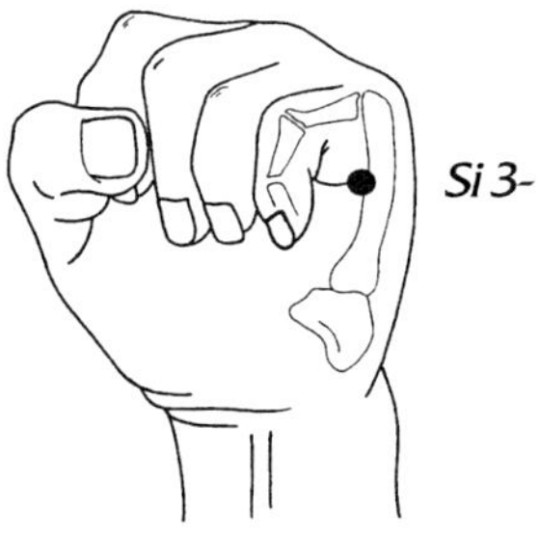

Fig. 4

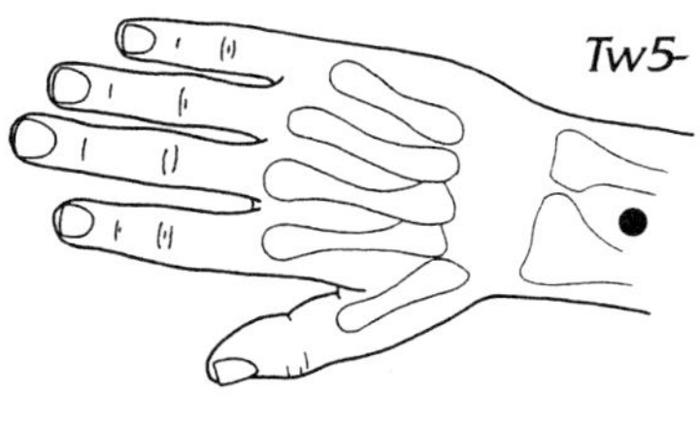

Dupuytren's Contracture

F*or additional relief of Dupuytren's Contracture sedate the following points in the forearm and follow up with points in the wrist and palm.*

Li 11 At the end of the outer elbow crease ***with the* arm slightly bent.** *Fig. 1*

Lu 6 6½ fingers width **away from** the elbow crease on a line drawn from the biceps tendon to the base of the thumb. *Fig. 1*

P 4 6½ fingers width **above** the midpoint of the inner wrist crease, between the 2 wrist tendons. *Fig. 1*

Tender Points

Look for tender points located within tight muscles of the forearm. The suggested areas of these tight muscle bands are marked with an "X" and should be stimulated for a relaxing response. Fig. 1

Fig. 1

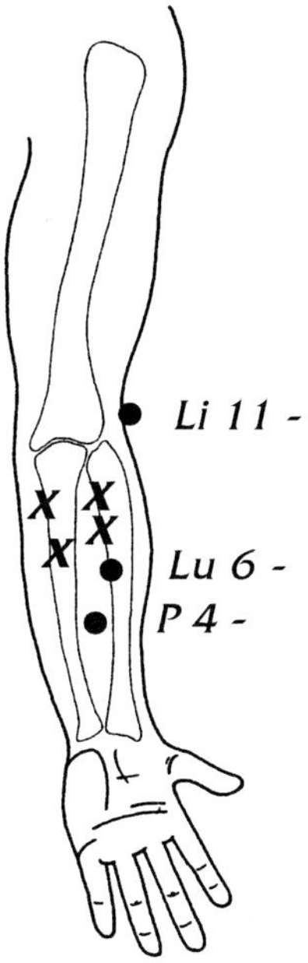

P 8 ***While clenching the fist***, the tip of the middle finger touches this point. *Fig. 2*

H 8 ***Clench the fist***. This point is on the palm between the tips of the 4th and 5th fingers. *Fig. 2*

Lu 10 On the palm side of the hand, in the middle of the large muscle pad near the base of the thumb. *Fig. 2*

P 6 3 fingers width from the most distal wrist crease, inbetween the tendons. *Fig. 2*

Fig. 2

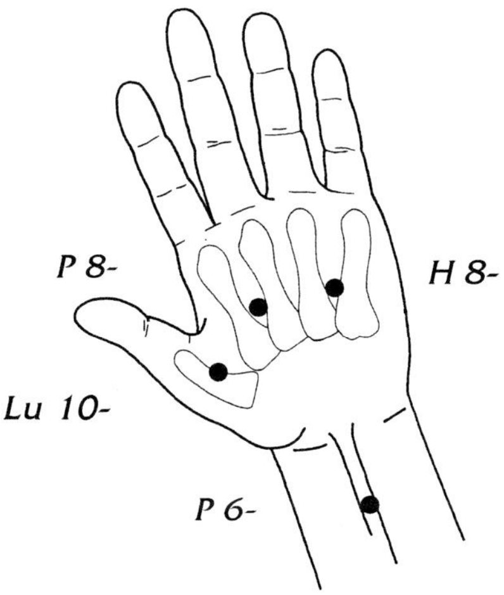

Earache

Consult a Doctor before commencing treatment to ensure a proper diagnosis. Once diagnosed, sedate the neck and the below distal points first.

Gb 20 Below the base of the skull, in the hollow just outside the main spinal muscles of neck. *Fig. 1*

Back Shu Points
These lie 2 fingers width to each side of the spinal bones. *Fig. 1*

Gv 14 This lies just below the most prominent bone at the base of the neck on the midline. *Fig. 1*

Gb 21 This lies halfway between the bone at the base of the neck and the tip of the shoulder, directly on top of the trapezius (shoulder) muscle. *Fig. 1*

Si 13 4 fingers width ***below GB 21*** just on top of the spine of the shoulder blade. *Fig. 1*

Si 17 Above the prominent neck muscle, ***at the level of the corner of the jaw***. *Fig. 2*

Si 3 On the end of the main transverse crease of the hand. ***Best located with the fist clenched***. *Fig. 3*

Li 4 This point is located in the centre of the webbing between the thumb and index finger. *Fig. 4*

Tw 5 On the back of the wrist 2 thumbs width above the wrist crease in between the 2 forearm bones. *Fig. 4*

Fig. 1

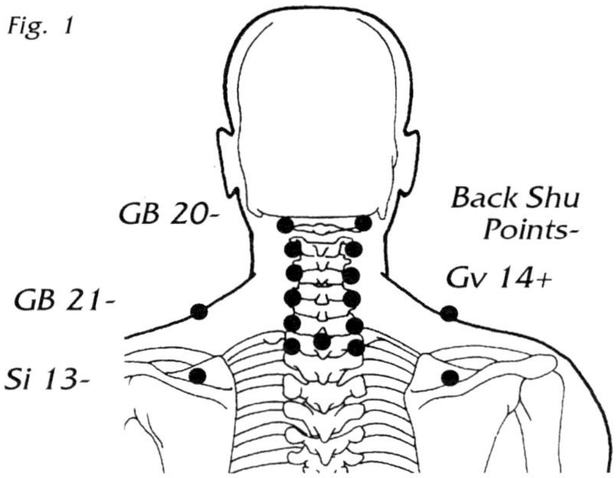

Fig. 2

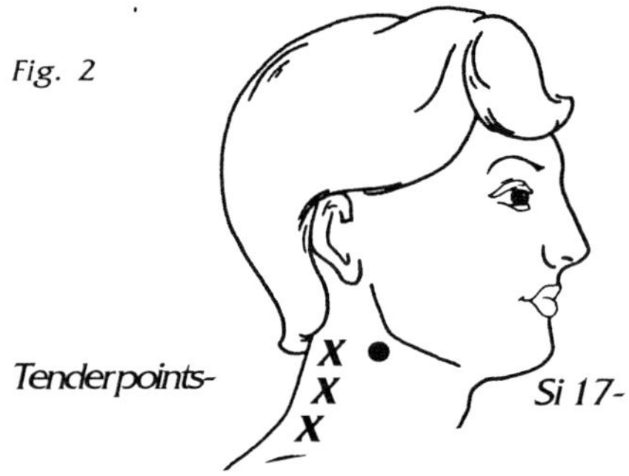

Fig. 3

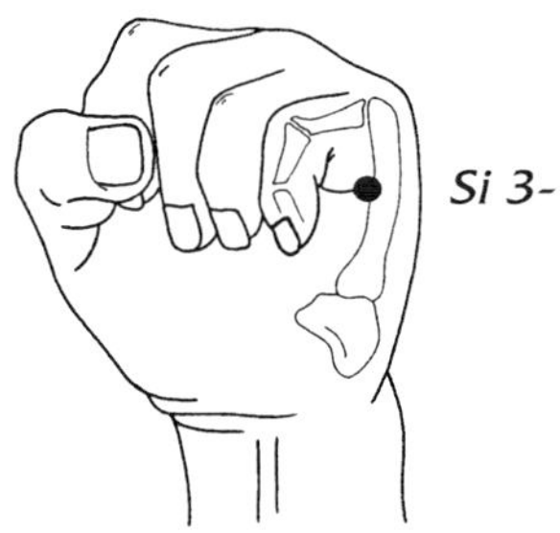

Fig. 4

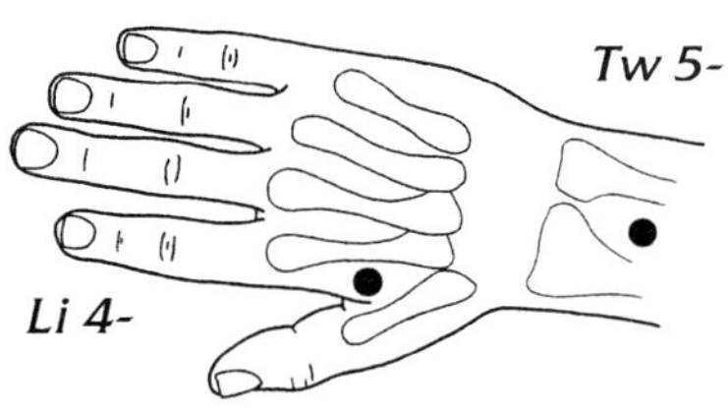

continued on next page

Earache

***F**or additional relief, sedate the following points in order, starting with the distal points and working towards the local points. If there is an infection, **tonify immune points on page 146**.*

Gb 41 In the depression, where the 4th & 5th toe bones meet. *Fig. 1*

B 67 At the outer base of the baby toe nail. *Fig. 1*

Gb 44 At the outer base of the 4th toe nail. *Fig. 1*

Li 11 This lies on the end of the outer elbow crease ***with the arm bent. Tonify.*** *Fig. 2*

Tw 21 In front of the midpoint of the ear in the hollow felt when the ***mouth is opened***. *Fig. 3*

Si 19 Just in front of the upper end of the ear lobe in a hollow formed ***when the mouth is opened***. *Fig. 3*

Gb 2 Just in front of lobe of ear. *Fig. 3*

Tw 17 On the indentation directly ***behind*** the ear lobe. *Fig. 3*

Fig. 1

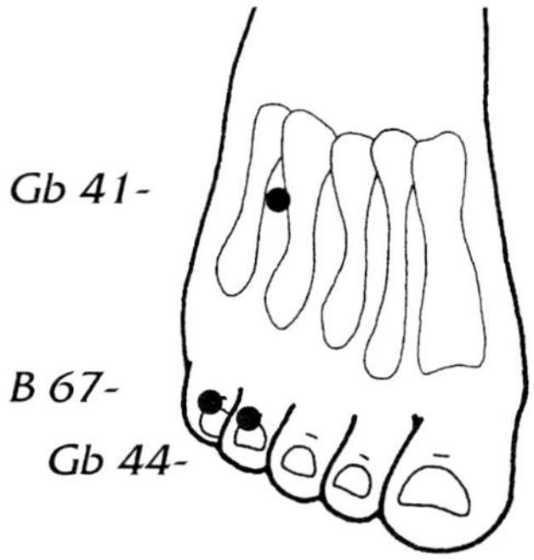

Fig. 2

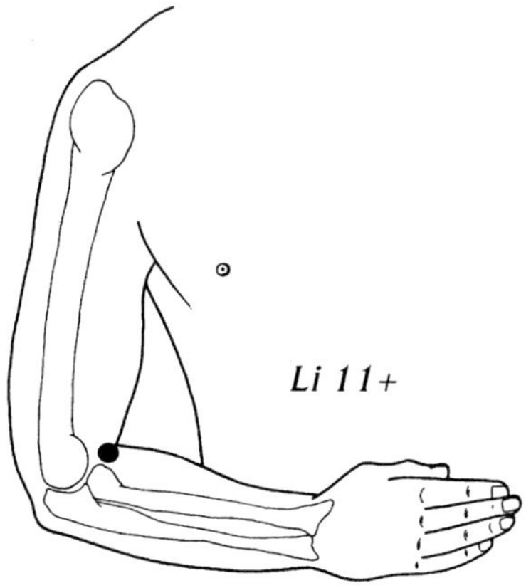

Fig. 3

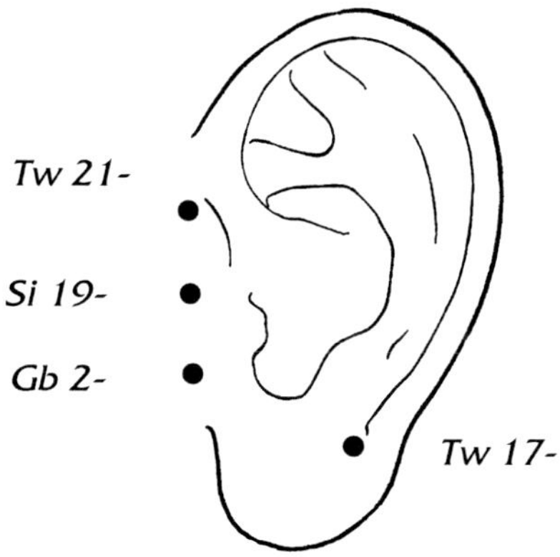

Elbow Pain - Golfer's

Consult a Doctor before treating any points. For chronic conditions, sedate the points in the lower back first. Secondly, the neck should be treated, with local points on final page applied for additional pain relief. Sedate points.

Back Shu Points:
Located 2 fingers width to each side of the spinal bones ***Sedating these points from the lower back to the sacrum often provides substantial relief to the patient.*** *Fig. 1*

Piriformis Trigger Points:
Approximately half way between the sacrum and the hip joint, (1hands width above GB 30). Also located in the upper outer quadrant of the buttocks, approximately one hands width below the iliac crest (hip bone). Press and rub (palpate) the general area until tenderness is detected. *Fig. 1*

Gb 30 This point is directly in the middle of each "cheek", equal distance from all sides. *Fig. 2*

Gb 31 Stand erect, hands flat along the side of the thigh. This point is at the ***tip of the middle finger***. *Fig. 2*

Gb 34 4 fingers width below the outside of the kneecap, and just in front of and below the knobby head of the bone. *Fig. 2*

Gb 41 In the depression, where the 4th & 5th toe bones meet. *Fig. 3*

Jing Well Points
Located on each side of the toenails at the base of the nail. *Fig. 3*

Fig. 1

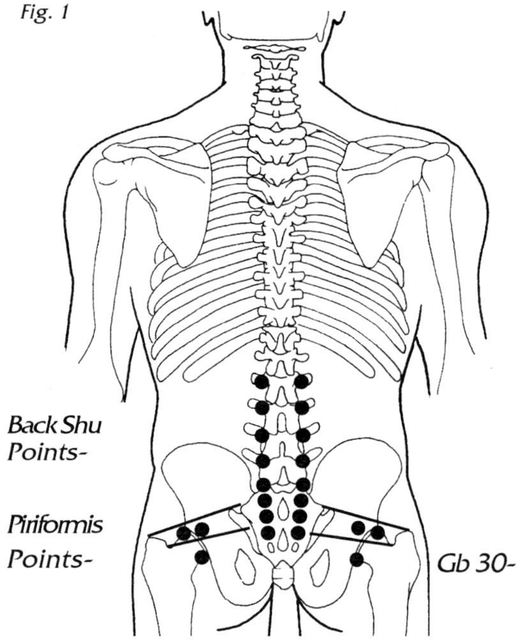

Fig. 2

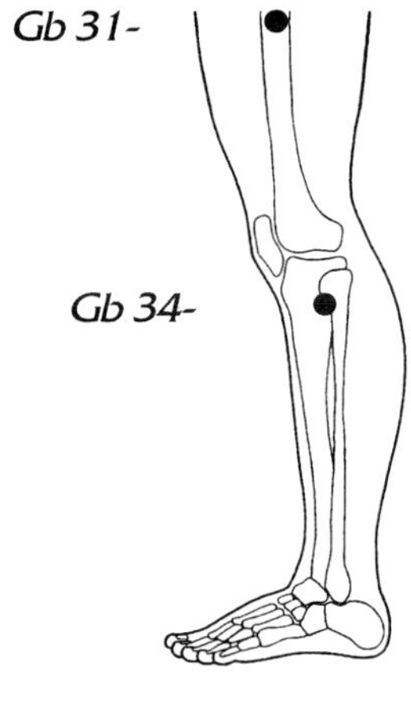

Fig. 3

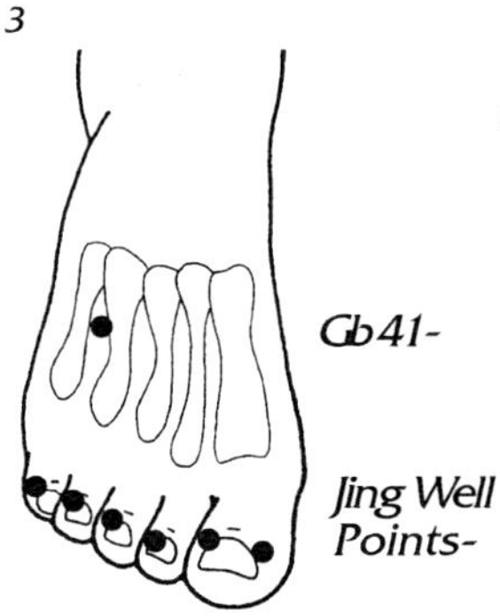

continued on next page

Elbow Pain - continued next page

The following points are for general pain in the neck and upper limbs. Relaxing neck muscles often provides relief to chronic elbow disorders. For additional relief, refer to the local points on the following page.

Gb 20 Below the base of the skull, in the hollow just outside the main spinal muscles of neck. *Fig. 1*

B 10 Located 2 fingers width from the middle of the spine at the level of the natural hairline at the back of the neck. ***In the middle of the ropy muscles on each side of the spine.*** *Fig. 1*

Gb 21 This lies halfway between the bone at the base of the neck and the tip of the shoulder, directly on top of the trapezius (shoulder) muscle. *Fig. 1*

Tw 15 1 thumbs width ***below Gb 21.*** *Fig. 1*

Si 13 4 fingers width ***below GB 21*** just on top of the spine of the shoulder blade. *Fig. 1*

Tender Points Stimulate these tender points located in the tight muscles at the side of the neck. *Fig. 2*

Si 17 Above the prominent neck muscle, ***at the level of the corner of the jaw.*** *Fig. 2*

Li 18 4 fingers width beside the highest point of the Adam's apple in the prominent muscle at the side of the neck ***(below the corner of the jaw).*** *Fig. 2*

Si 3 On the end of the main transverse crease of the hand. ***Best located with the fist clenched.*** *Fig. 3*

Fig. 1

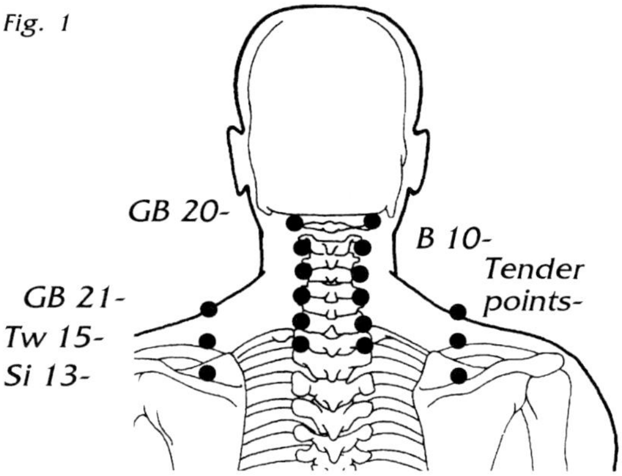

Fig. 2

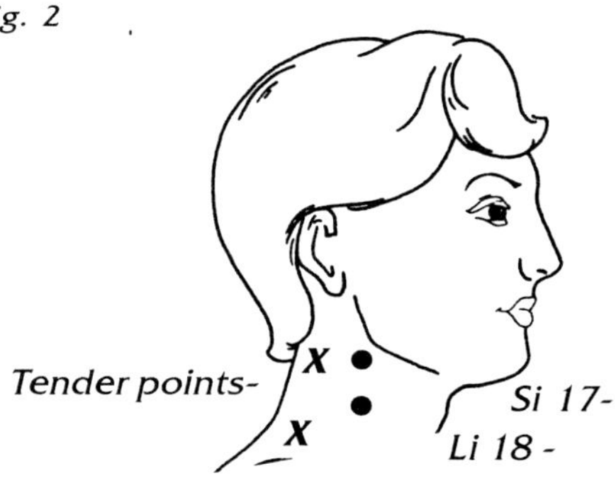

Fig. 3

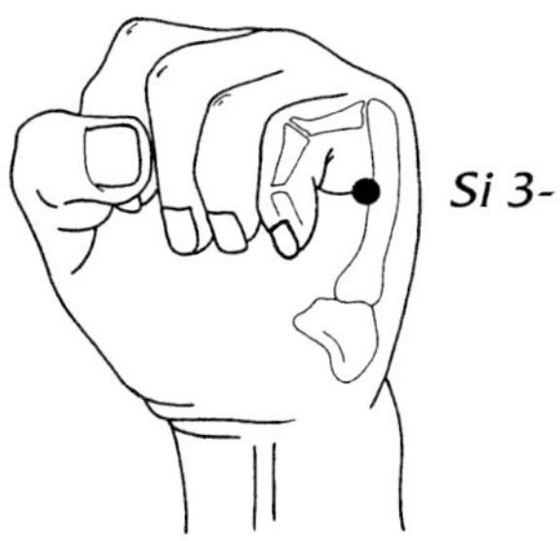

Elbow Pain

***T**his is a condition affecting the inside muscles of the elbow. After sedating the neck points on previous page, for additional relief apply ETPS to local points and tender trigger points throughout muscles (marked with an "X").*

Lu 5 On the elbow crease to the ***outside*** of the biceps tendon. *Fig. 1*

P 3 On the elbow crease just to the *inside* of the biceps tendon. *Fig. 1*

H 3 With the elbow bent, it is ***between*** the inner end of the elbow crease and the inner elbow bone. *Fig. 1*

Si 8 ***Between*** the 2 inner elbow bones, ***best located with the elbow bent***. *Figs. 1 & 2*

Tw 10 In the middle of the arm, 2 fingers width above the back of the protruding elbow bone. *Fig. 2*

Li 11 On the end of the ***outside*** elbow crease with the arm slightly bent. *Fig. 2*

Li 10 2 fingers width ***away from*** Li 11, towards the thumb. *Fig. 2*

Tender Points

Sedate these tender points in the muscles surrounding the elbow, they are marked with an "x". *Figs. 1 & 2*

Li 4 This point is located in the centre of the webbing between the thumb and index finger. *Fig. 3*

Fig. 1

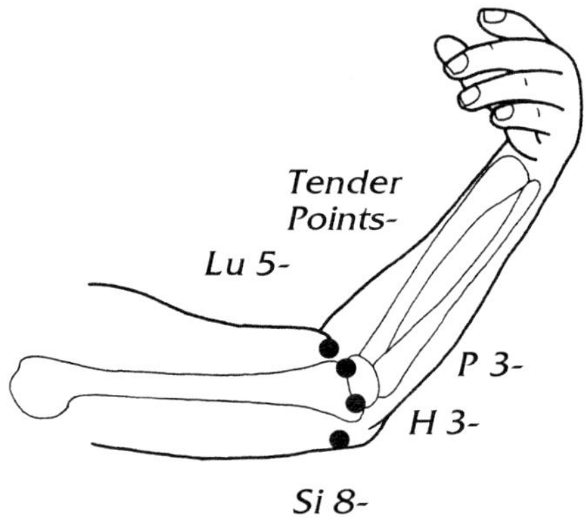

Fig. 2

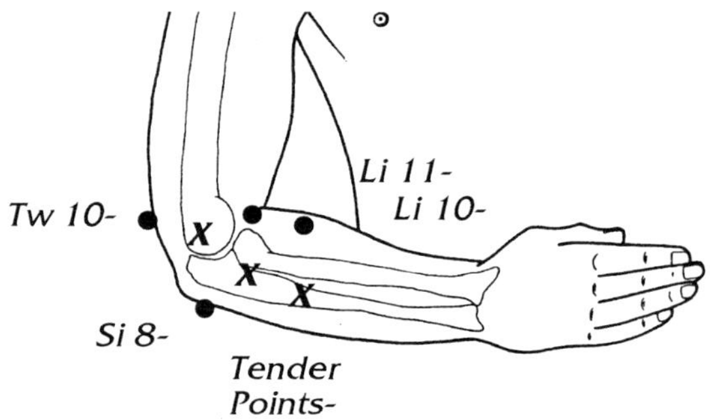

Fig. 3

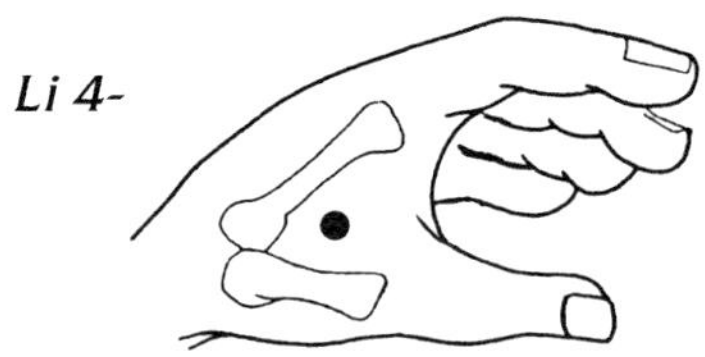

Facial Neuralgia - continued next page

***F**acial Neuralgia or **Facial Tic** is a pain that can be very severe and intense. For chronic conditions, sedate these parasympathetic points first. For additional relief, sedate the sequence of points on the following page.*

Lu 9 In the groove at the thumb side of the wrist crease, and inside of the tendon. *Fig. 1*

H 7 On the little finger side of the wrist crease, to the inside of the tendon. *Fig. 1*

P 6 3 fingers width from the most distal wrist crease, in between the tendons. *Fig. 1*

Sp 6 3 fingers width above the inner ankle and just behind the prominent shin bone. *Fig. 2*

K 3 Halfway between the Achilles tendon and the inner ankle bone. *Fig. 2*

B 62 In the depression half a finger below the outer ankle bone. *Fig. 3*

Cv 17 On the breast bone at the heart level or the 4th rib space. Tender when pressed. *Fig. 4*

Fig. 1

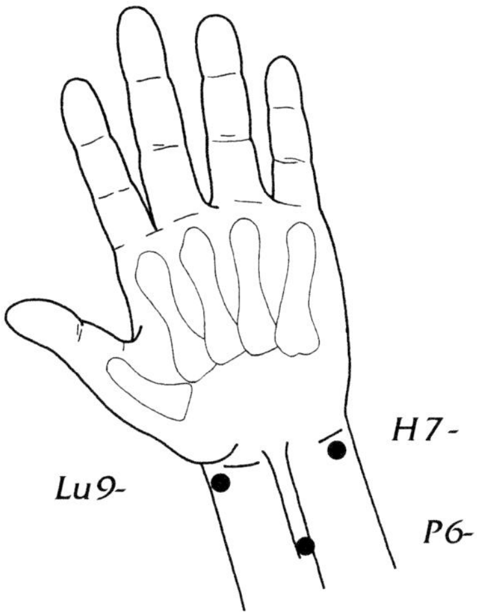

Fig. 2

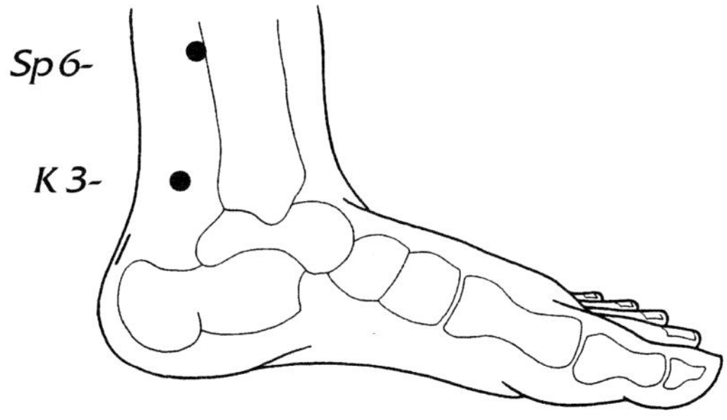

Fig. 4

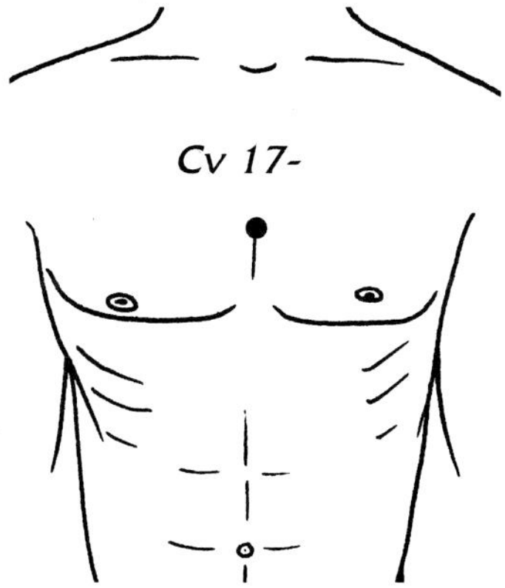

Fig. 3

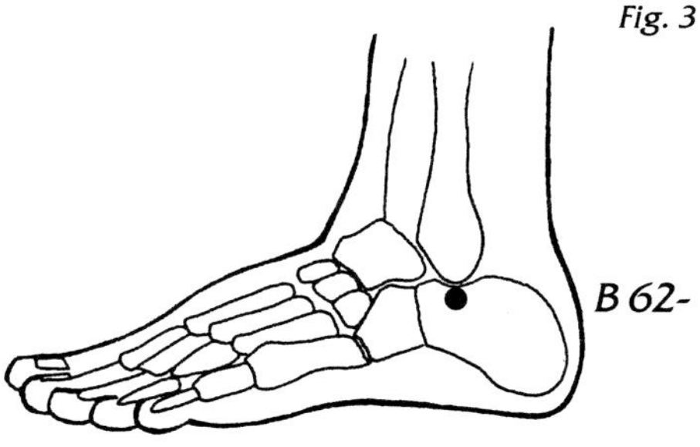

Facial Neuralgia & Tic

F*or additional relief sedate the distal points on the wrists & hands before attempting local points on the face.*

Fig. 1

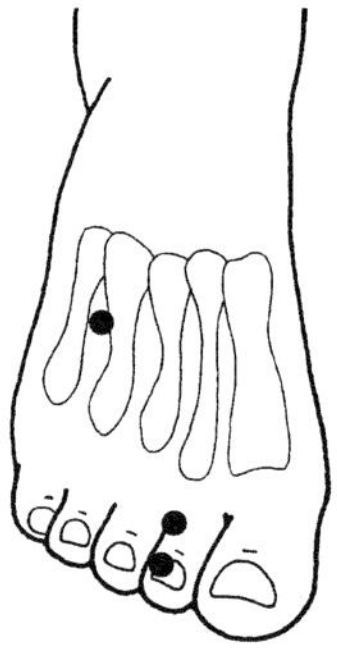

Gb 41 In the depression, where the 4th & 5th toe bones meet. *Fig. 1*

St 44 In the hollow between the base of the 2nd and 3rd toes. *Fig. 1*

St 45 On the outside base of the 2nd toe nail. *Fig. 1*

Fig. 2

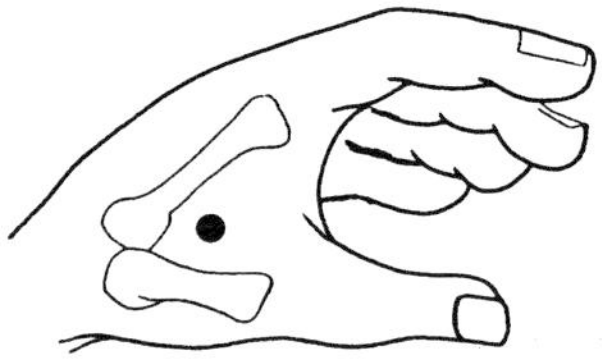

Li 4 In the middle of the fleshy mass between the thumb and index finger. *Fig. 2*

Fig. 3

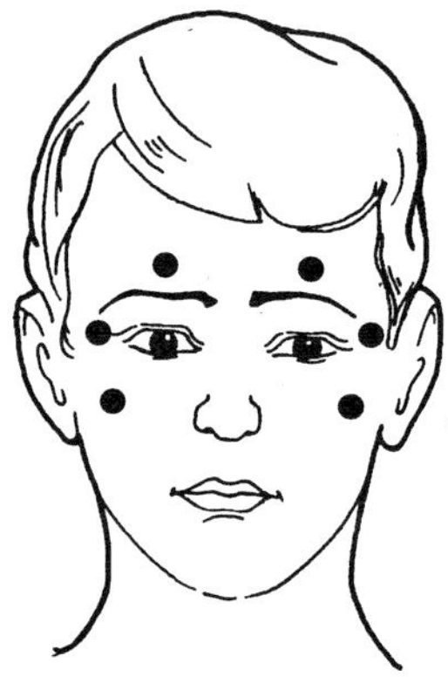

Gv 14 1 fingers width above the eyebrow, directly above the pupil. *Fig. 3*

Extra 2
1 fingers width back from the outside of eye socket, in the hollow. *Figs. 3 & 4*

Si 18 Directly below the outer corner of the eye socket, ***under the cheek bone***. *Figs. 3 & 4*

Fig. 4

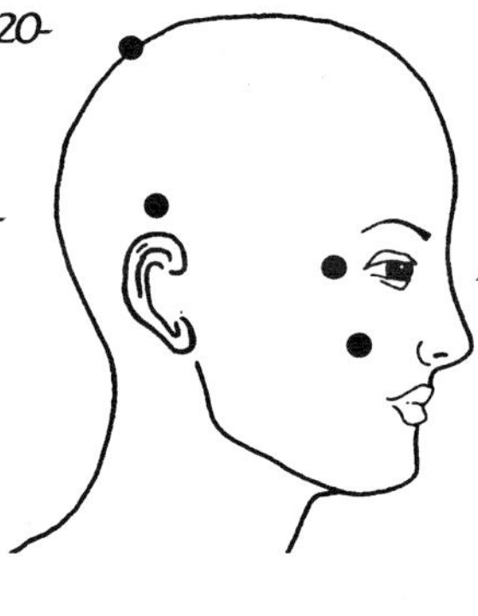

Gv 20 In the middle of the top of the head, halfway between the ears. *Fig. 4*

Gb 8 Located 1 fingers width directly above the uppermost tips of the ear. *Fig. 4*

Facial Pain - Toothache

The following points are for general pain and stiffness in the neck region. Relaxing these neck muscles often provides relief to facial pain disorders. If additional relief is required, refer to the local points on the following page.

Gb 20 Below the base of the skull, in the hollow just outside the main spinal muscles of neck. *Fig. 1*

B 10 Located 2 fingers width from the middle of the spine at the level of the natural hairline at the back of the neck. ***In the middle of the ropy muscles on each side of the spine.*** *Fig. 1*

Gb 21 This lies halfway between the knob of bone at the base of the neck and the tip of the shoulder, in the fleshy mass of muscle. *Fig. 1*

Tw 15 1 thumbs width ***below Gb 21.*** *Fig. 1*

Si 13 4 fingers width ***below GB 21*** just on top of the spine of the shoulder blade. *Fig. 1*

Extra Points
Stimulate these tender points located in the tight muscles at the side of the neck. *Fig. 2*

Si 17 Above the prominent neck muscle, ***at the level of the corner of the jaw.*** *Fig. 2*

Li 18 4 fingers width beside the highest point of the Adam's apple in the prominent muscle at the side of the neck ***(below the corner of the jaw).*** *Fig. 2*

Si 3 On the end of the main transverse crease of the hand. ***Best located with the fist clenched.*** *Fig. 3*

Fig. 1

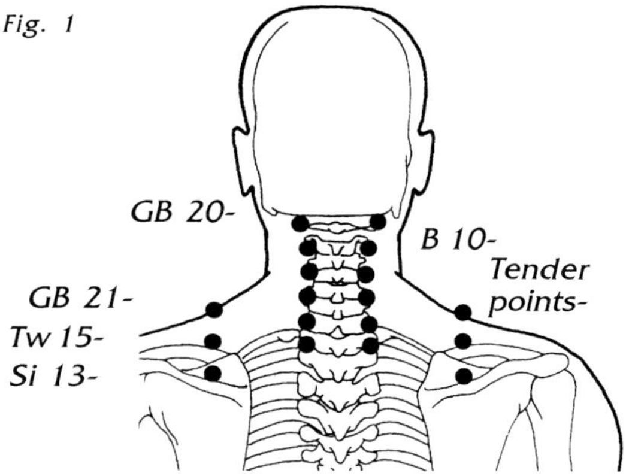

Fig. 2

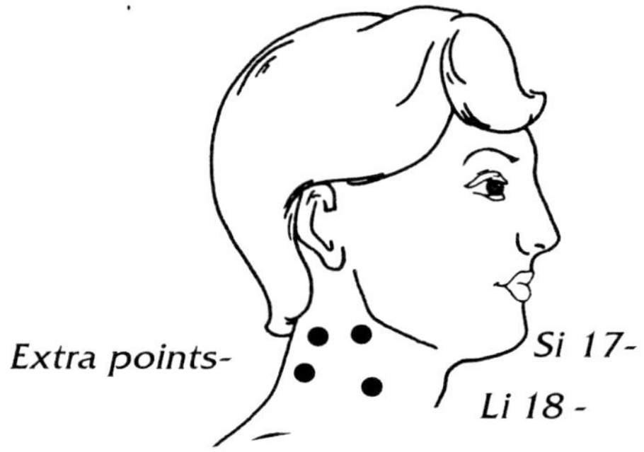

Fig. 3

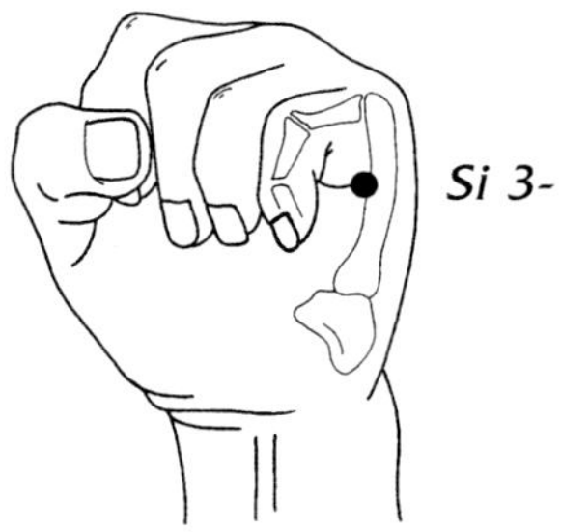

Facial Pain - Toothache

If additional pain relief is required in the face after treating the neck, sedate the following points. It is recommended to sedate the distal points before local points for optimal relief.

Li 4 In the middle of the fleshy mass of muscle between the thumb and index finger, and slightly towards the index finger bone. *Fig. 1*

Gb 8 Located 1 fingers width directly above the uppermost tip of the ear. *Fig. 2*

St 7 2 fingers width in front of the ear, in the hollow ***just below*** the upper jaw bone. *Fig. 2*

Si 18 Below the outer corner of the eye socket, ***directly under cheek bone.*** *Figs. 2 & 3*

St 6 Over the highest point of the bulge of the muscle at the angle of the jaw ***when the jaw is clenched.*** *Fig. 2*

Gb 14 Located 1 fingers width ***above the midpoint*** of the eyebrows. *Fig. 3*

Extra 1 (Yintang) At the midpoint between the ***inner ends*** of the eyebrows. *Fig. 3*

Cv 24 Midway between the lip and the tip of the chin, on the midline. *Fig. 3*

Fig. 1

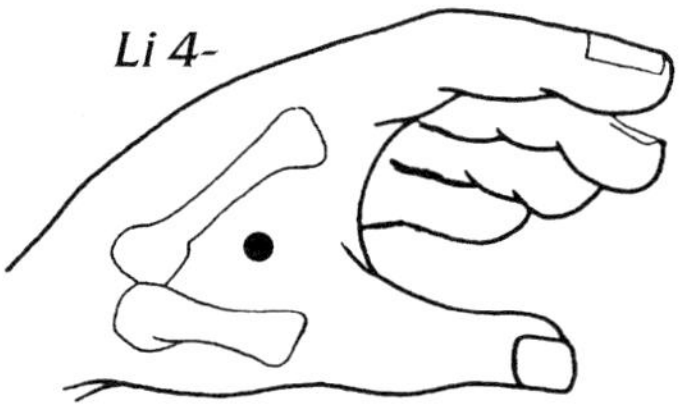

Fig. 2

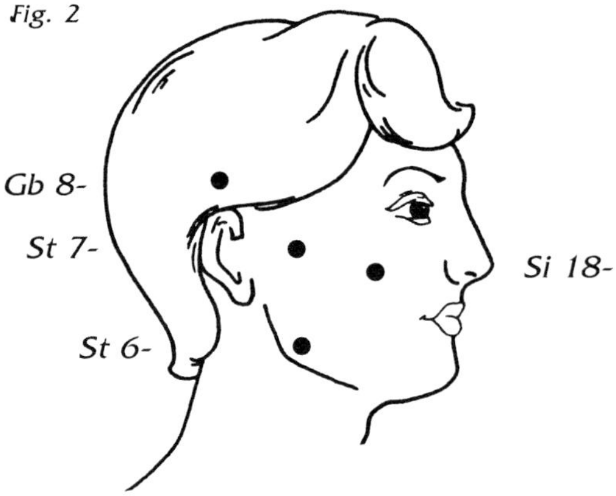

Fig. 3

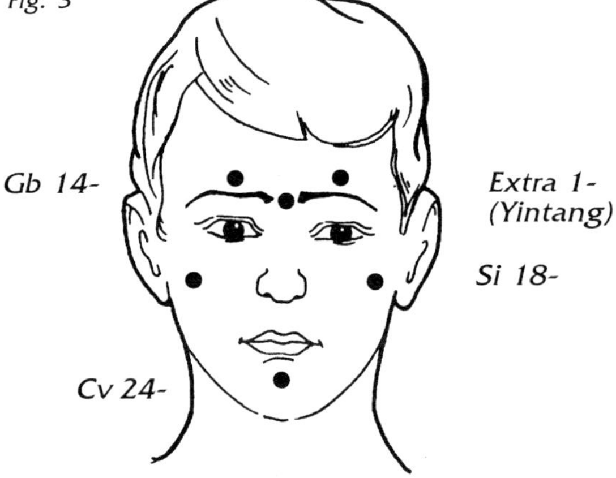

Fibromyalgia - continued next page

***C**onsult a Doctor before treating any points. For chronic conditions, sedate these parasympathetic points to calm the nerves and relax muscles. It has been reported that FM patients respond positively to sedation of these points.*

Lu 9 In the groove at the thumb side of the wrist crease, and inside of the tendon. *Fig. 1*

H 7 On the little finger side of the wrist crease, to the inside of the tendon. *Fig. 1*

P 6 3 fingers width from the most distal wrist crease, in between the tendons. *Fig. 1*

Sp 6 3 fingers width above the inner ankle and just behind the prominent shin bone. *Fig. 2*

K 3 Halfway between the Achilles tendon and the inner ankle bone. *Fig. 2*

K 27 2 thumbs width on each side of the sternum, in the hollow just below the collarbone. *Fig. 5*

Cv 17 On the breast bone at the heart level or the 4th rib space. Tender when pressed. *Fig. 3*

B 62 In the depression half a finger below the outer ankle bone. *Fig. 4*

Fig. 1

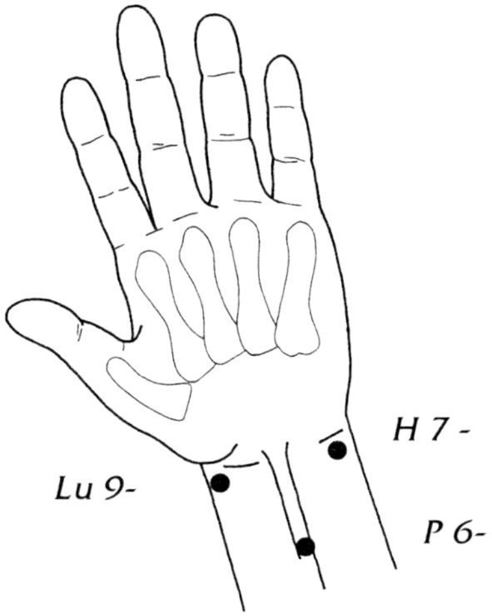

Fig. 2

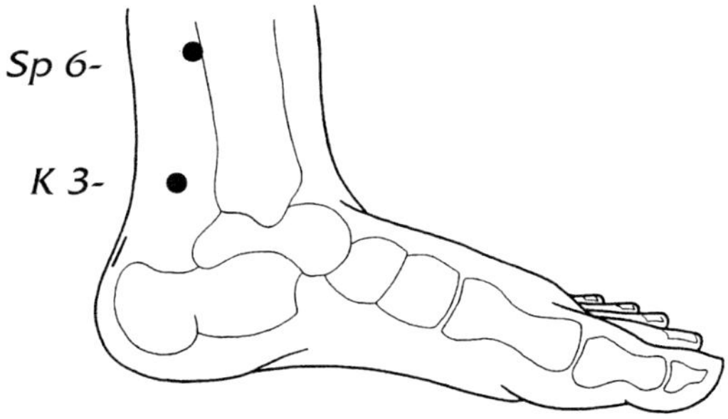

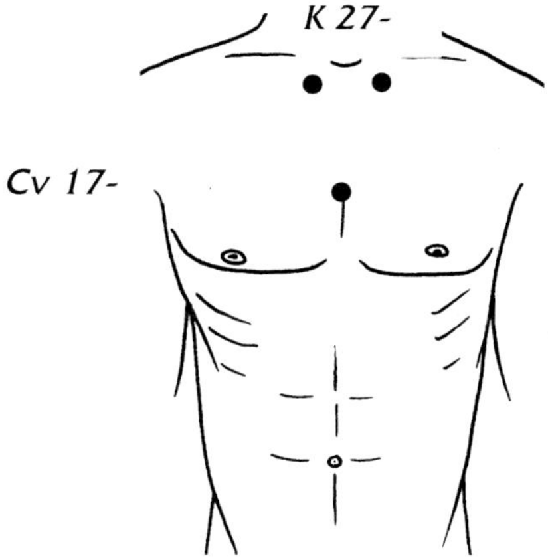

Fig. 3

Fig. 4

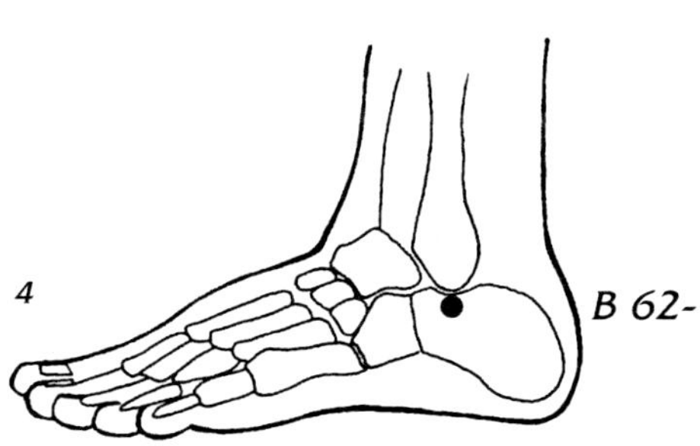

Fibromyalgia

***O**nce the the patient is calmed, tonify the paraspinal points to help relax paraspinal muscles, for decreased muscular pain and increased organ energy. The remaining points are for tonifying and general homeostatics.*

Back Shu Points

Stimulate the following points in the midback range. These are located 2 fingers width to each side of the spine. ***Starting from waist level move upwards to the highest level of the shoulder blade. Tonify the ropy muscles found on each side of the spine.*** *Fig. 1*

St 36 4 fingers width below the kneecap and 1 fingers width to the outside of the shin bone. *Fig. 2*

Li 11 This lies on the end of the outer elbow crease with the arm bent. *Fig. 3*

Cv 6 On the midline 2 fingers width below the belly button. *Fig. 4*

Fig. 1

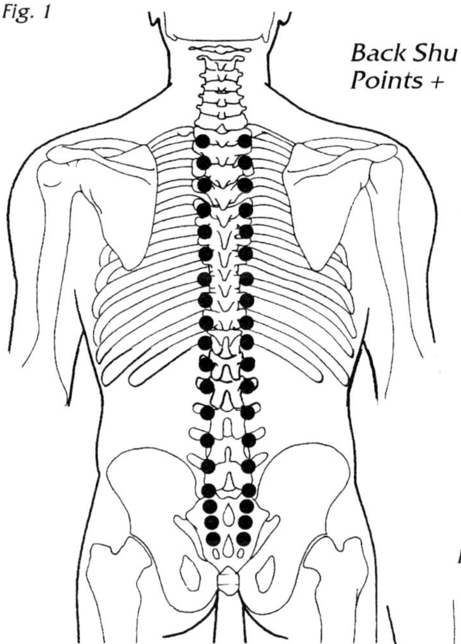

Fig. 2

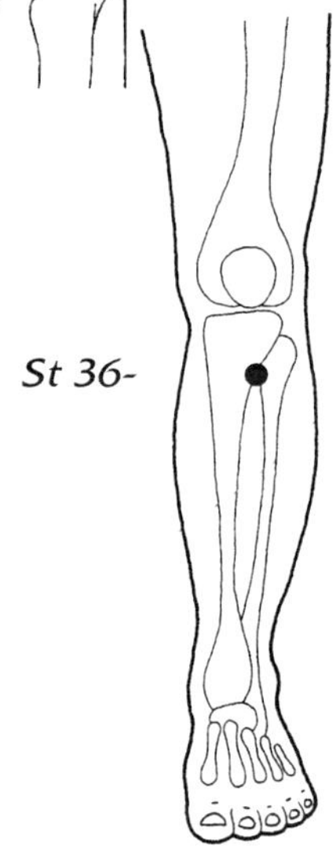

Fig. 4

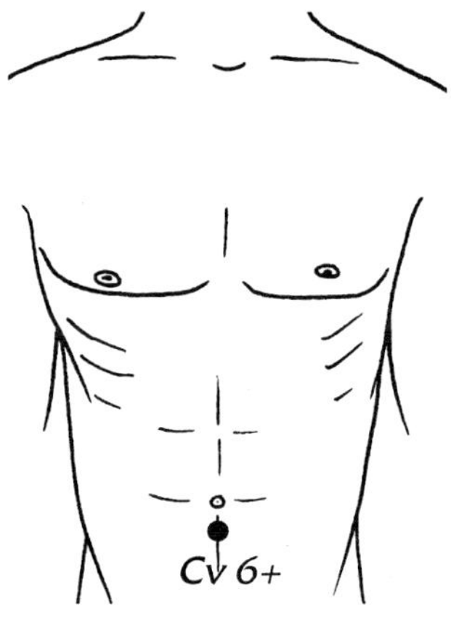

Fig. 3

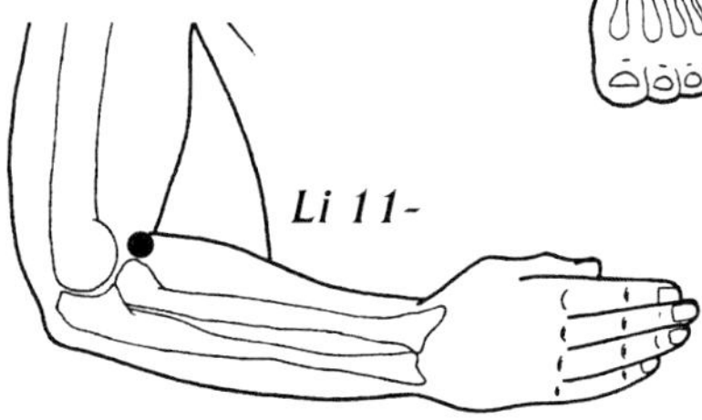

Finger Pain

F**inger pain may be from degenerative source (arthritis) or from an acute injury. For both, sedate the following points.* ***For additional relief, see wrist pain (pg. 99) and elbow pain (also see "X"s in elbow pain, page 68).

Jing Well Points- *Fig. 1*

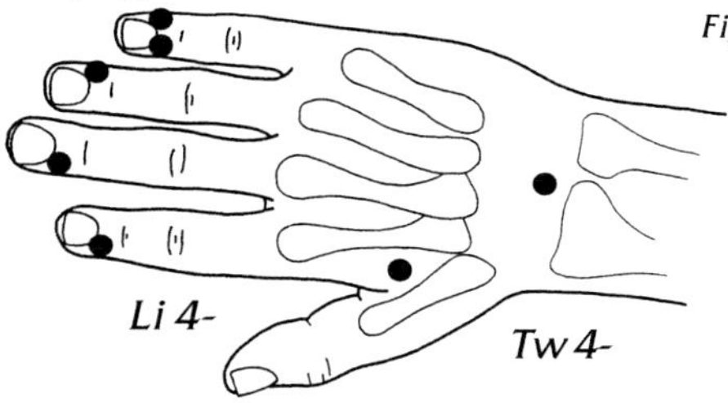

Jing Well Points
At the outer base of the finger nails. *Fig. 1*

Li 4 In the middle of the fleshy mass between the thumb and the index finger, closer to the index finger bone. *Fig. 1*

Tw 4 At the midpoint of the crease on the back of the wrist. *Fig. 1*

Finger Points- *Fig. 2*

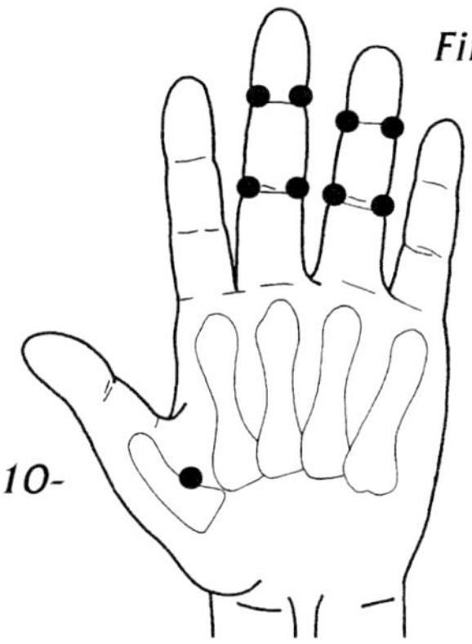

Lu 10-

Finger Points
Located at each end of the outer fingers knuckle crease. ***Stimulate these points for individual painful knuckles.*** *Fig. 2*

Lu 10 On the palm side of the hand, in the middle of the muscle at the base of the thumb. *Fig. 2*

Knuckle Points - *Fig. 3*

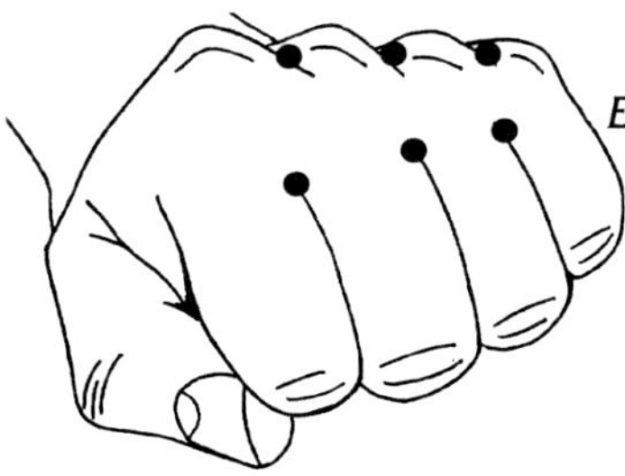

Extra 28-

Knuckle Points
In the hollow between each set of knuckles. ***These are best located with the fist closed.*** *Fig. 3*

Extra 28 Points
With the fist closed, just above the crease where the fingers meet. *Fig. 3*

Fig. 4

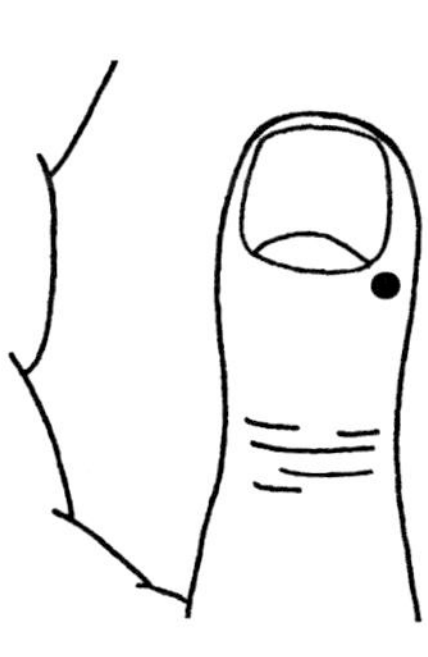

Lu 11-

Lu 11 At the outer/lower corner of the thumb nail. *Fig. 4*

Foot Pain

*For pain of the foot, sedate the following areas. For **Plantar fasciitis** also treat the **back pain points (pg. 28) & calf muscle points (pg. 64),** along with tender points throughout the bottom of the foot.*

St 41 On the front of the ankle, in the crease in between the 2 ankle tendons. *Fig. 1*

Gb 41 In the depression, where the 4th and 5th toe bones meet. *Fig. 1*

Liv 3 On the top of the foot in the hollow between the 1st and 2nd toes, ***where the bones meet.*** *Fig. 1*

Web points In the web at the base of the toes. *Fig. 1*

B 60 This lies in the hollow midway between the tip of the outer ankle bone & the Achilles tendon. *Fig. 2*

B 62 In the depression, ½ fingers width below the outer ankle bone. *Fig. 2*

B 67 Outer/inner corner of the baby toe nail. *Fig. 2*

Sp 6 4 fingers width above the inner ankle and just behind the prominent shin bone. *Fig. 3*

Sp 3 Just proximal to the "Bunion" bone at the base of the big toe, ***at the junction of the red and white skin.*** *Fig. 3*

K 1 In the middle of the sole of the foot, between the ***inner and outer balls of the foot.*** *Fig. 4*

Fig. 1

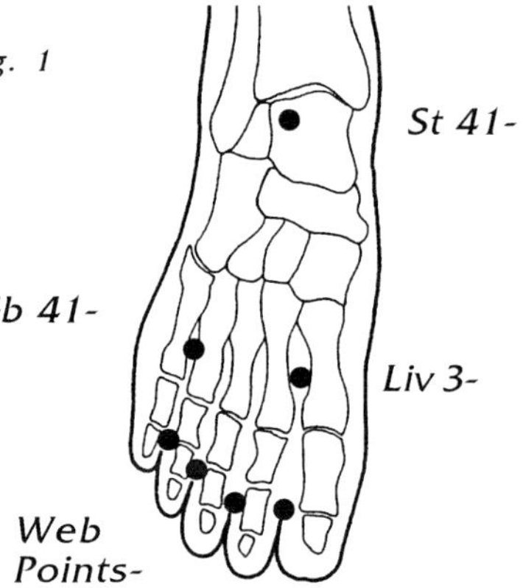

Fig. 2

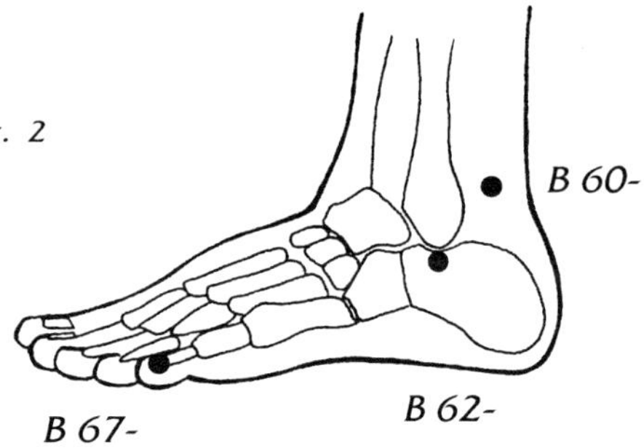

Fig. 3

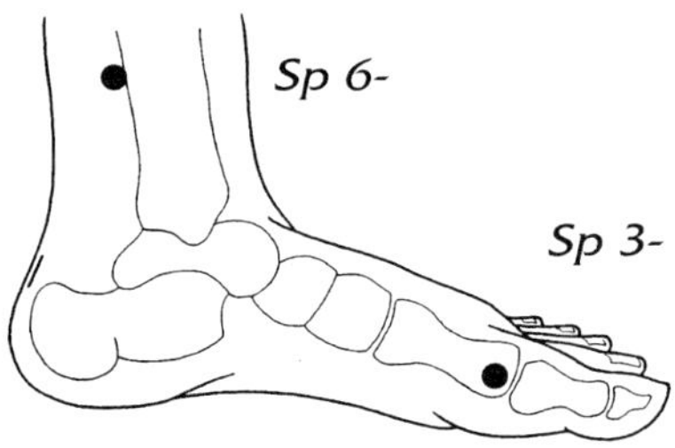

Fig. 4

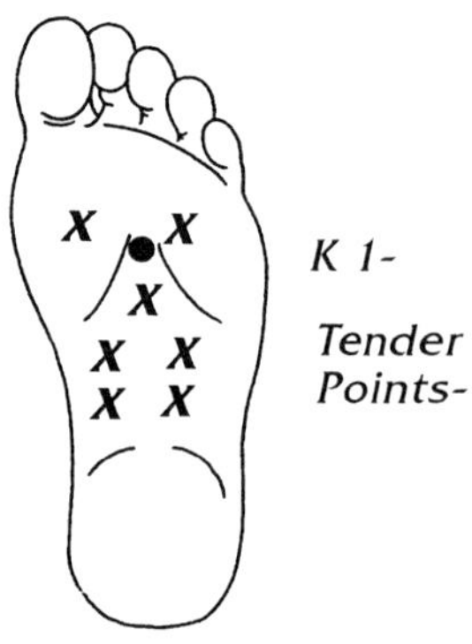

Ganglion

A** ganglion is a fluid-filled sack, on a tendon or on the end of a muscle, often on the back of the wrist. Ganglions are caused by repetitive trauma to the area and/or overuse. Symptoms include a soft, often tender, palpable mass and pain upon applying pressure to the area. For best results, first sedate the points surrounding the Ganglion for relief of pain and swelling. For additional relief, add points **(Li 4, Li 5, Tw 5, Sp 6 and K 3).

Li 4 This lies on the middle of the fleshy mass between the thumb and index finger. *Figs. 1 & 2*

Li 5 At the base of the thumb, in between the 2 thumb tendons. *Figs. 1 & 2*

Tw 4 In the middle of the ***outer*** wrist crease. *Fig. 2*

Tw 5 2 thumbs width above the middle of the ***outer*** wrist crease. *Fig. 2*

Surrounding the "Dragon"
Stimulate tender points surrounding the ganglion. ***This is called surrounding the "dragon".*** *Fig. 2*

Sp 6 3 fingers width above the inner ankle and just behind the prominent shin bone. *Fig. 3*

K 3 Halfway between the Achilles tendon and the inner ankle bone. *Fig. 3*

Fig. 1

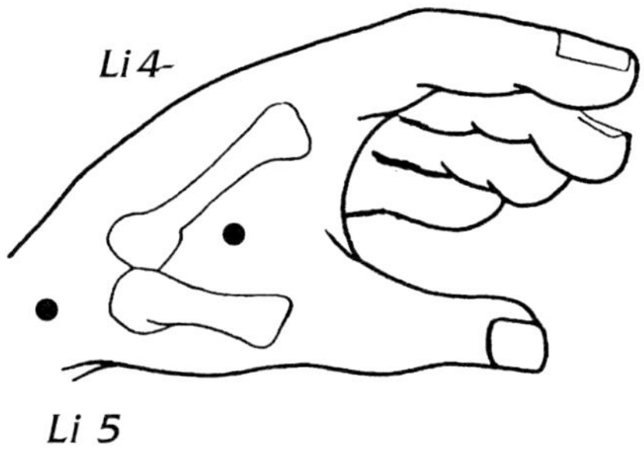

Fig. 2

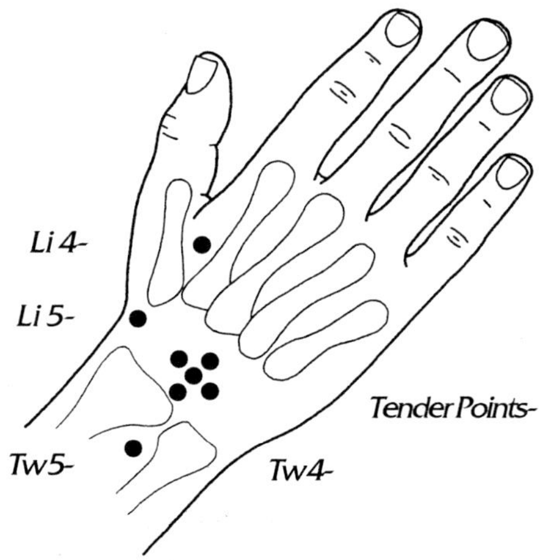

Fig. 3

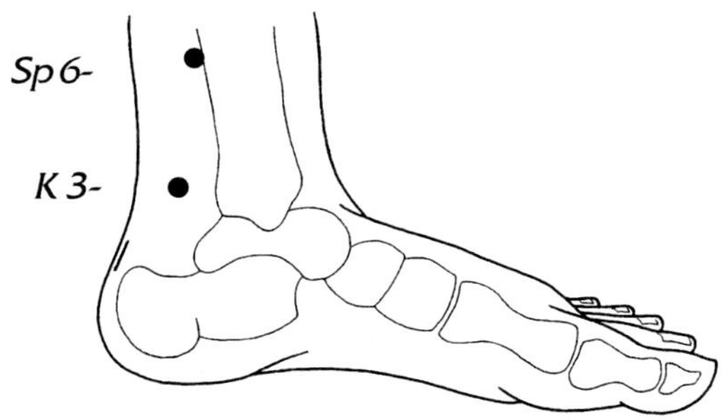

Gout

***G**out is a disorder of metabolism causing recurrent acute arthritis of the peripheral joints, often the big toe. Sedating the following points should provide relief. For additional relief, include local points on the next page.*

Back Shu Points:
Located 2 fingers width to each side of the spinal bones. ***Sedate these points from the lower back to the sacrum. Above points innervate the affected region(s) and often provide substantial relief to the patient.*** *Fig. 1*

Fig. 1

Back Shu Points-

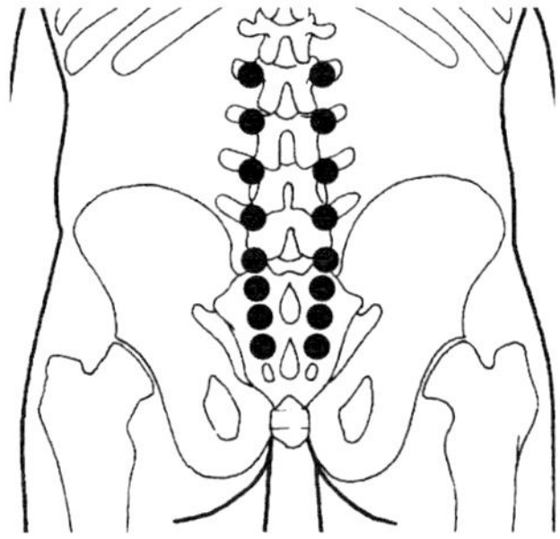

Piriformis Trigger Points:
Approximately half way between the sacrum (the triangular bone at the base of the spine) and the hip joint, or one hands width above GB 30. *Fig. 2*

Fig. 2

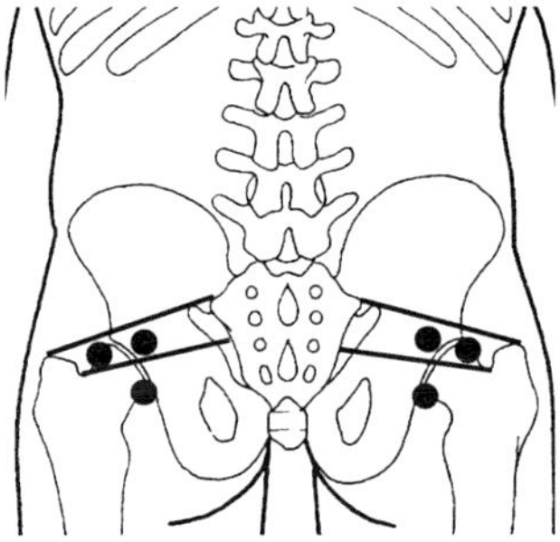

Gb 30-

Gb 30 This point is directly in the middle of the each "cheek" equal distance from all sides. *Fig. 2*

Gb 31 Standing erect with your hands laying the side of the thigh. This point is at the ***tip of the middle finger***. *Fig. 3*

Fig. 3

Gb 31-

Gb 34-

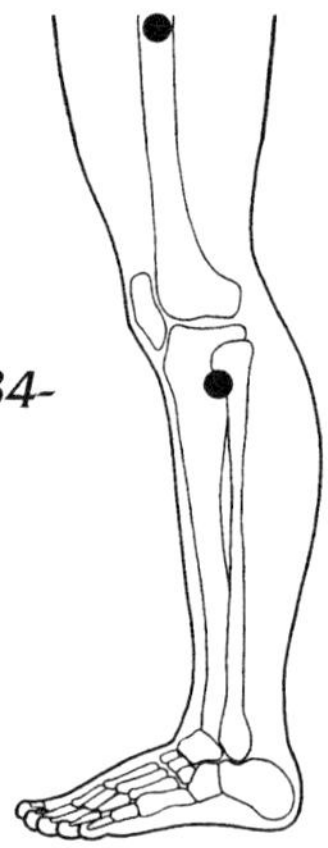

Gb 34 4 fingers width below the outside of the kneecap, and just in front of and below the knobby head of the fibula bone. *Fig. 3*

Gb 41 In the depression, where the 4th & 5th toe bones meet. *Fig. 4*

Fig. 4

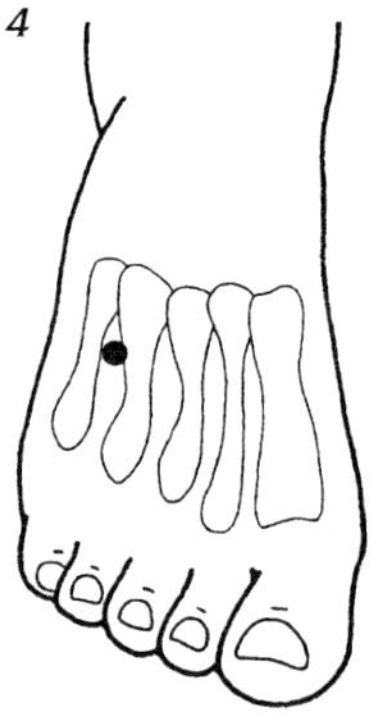

Gb 41-

Gout - continued next page

In this acute condition the following local points are likely to be sensitive. Sedating them should provide welcome relief. For additional response, include low back pain point on previous page.

Sp 6 Three fingers above the highest point of the ankle bone, just behind the shin bone. *Fig. 1*

Sp 5 Below and in front of the tip of the inner ankle bone in the depression. *Fig. 1*

Sp 3 Just proximal to the "Bunion" bone at the base of the big toe, ***at the junction of the red and white skin***. *Fig. 1*

Sp 2 Just distal to the "Bunion" bone at the base of the big toe, ***at the junction of the red and white skin***. *Fig. 1*

St 41 On the front of the ankle, on the crease in between the 2 ankle bones. *Fig. 2*

Liv 3 On top of the foot. In the hollow where the 1st and 2nd toe bones meet. *Fig. 2*

Liv 1 At the ***outer bottom corner*** of the big toe nail. *Fig. 2*

Sp 1 Located on the ***inner bottom corner*** of the big toe nail. *Fig. 2*

Jing Well Points
At the outer base of the toe nails. *Fig. 2*

Fig. 1

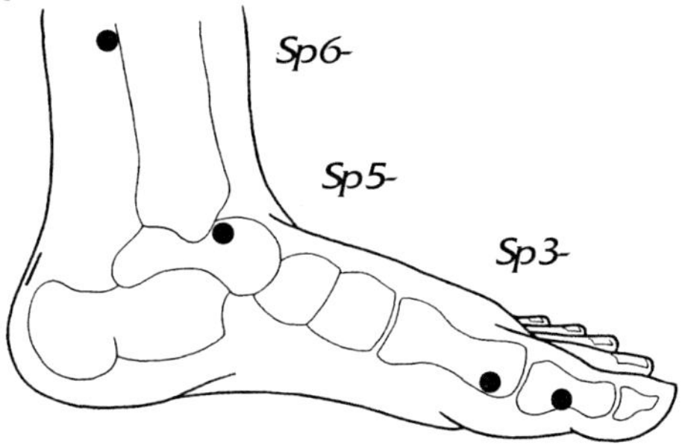

Fig. 2

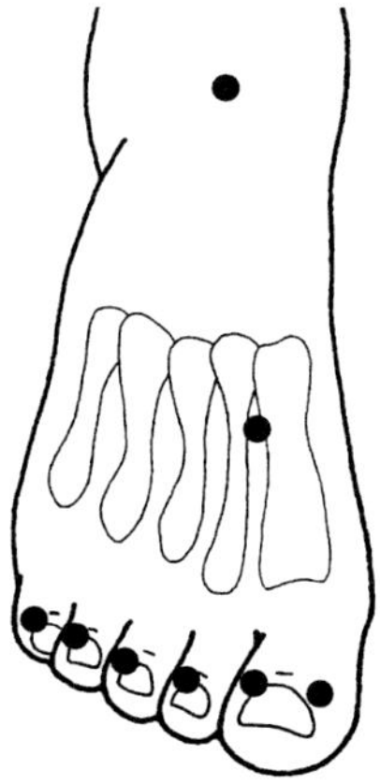

Groin Injury

***G**roin injuries are often caused by overuse or a traumatic sports injury. Sedating the following points should help relax the tightened muscles and balance out the hips.*

Back Shu Points

Located 2 fingers width to each side of the spinal bones. ***Sedate these points from the lower back to the sacrum. Above points innervate the affected region(s) and often provide substantial relief to the patient.*** *Fig. 1*

Piriformis Trigger Points

Approximately half way between the sacrum (the triangular bone at the base of the spine) and the hip joint, or one hands width above GB 30. *Fig. 1*

Gb 30 This point is directly in the middle of the each "cheek" equal distance from all sides. *Fig. 1*

Gb 31 Standing erect with your hands laying the side of the thigh. This point is at the ***tip of the middle finger***. *Fig. 2*

Gb 34 4 fingers width below the outside of the kneecap, and just in front of and below the knobby head of the fibula bone. *Fig. 2*

Liv 3 In the depression, where the 1st & 2nd toe bones meet. *Fig. 1*

Sp 1 At the inner base of the big toe nail. *Figs. 3**

Fig. 1

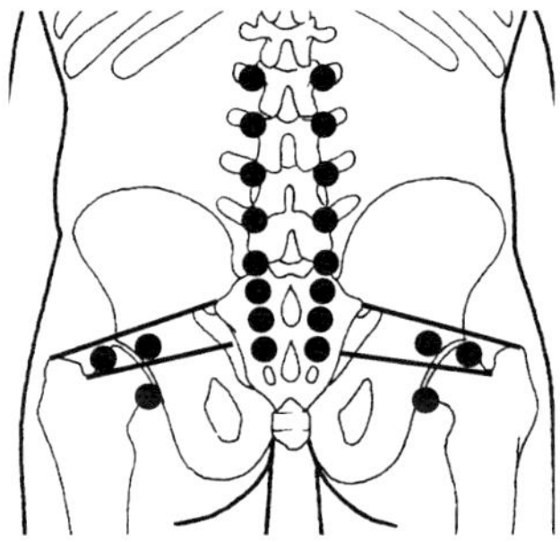

Fig. 2

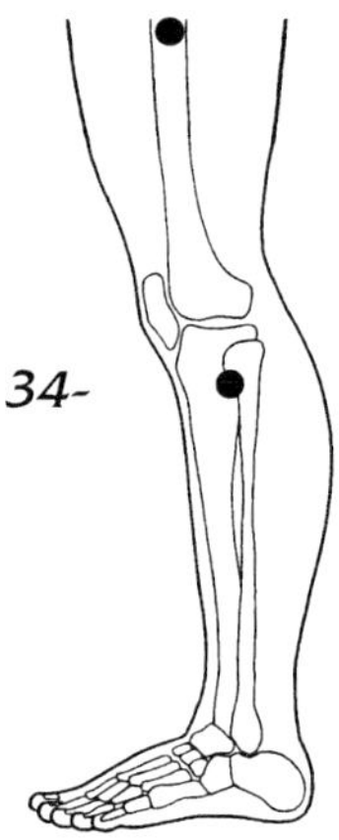

Fig. 3

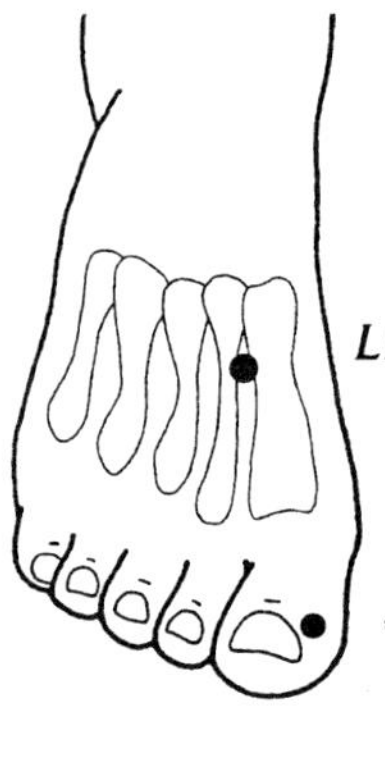

Groin Injury

Groin injury symptoms include pain, local tenderness and, in some cases, swelling. Sedating the following points should help expedite recovery and release provide additional pain relief.

Tender Points

Stimulate any tender points in the local area that are sore to the touch or tight. ***The probable areas for their location are marked with an "X".*** *Fig. 1*

St 31 At the junction of a line drawn down from the hip bone and across the pubic bone. *Fig. 1*

St 32 8 fingers width above the upper/outer border of the kneecap. *Fig. 1*

St 44 In the web at meeting of the 2nd and 3rd toes. *Fig. 1*

Gb 34 4 fingers width below the outside of the knee and just in front of and below the knobby head of the fibula bone. *Fig. 2*

B 60 This lies in the hollow midway between the tip of the outer ankle bone and the Achilles tendon. *Fig. 2*

Jing Well Points

Located on each side of the toenails at the base of the nail. *Fig. 3*

Sp 6 3 fingers width above the inner ankle bone and behind the prominent shin bone. *Figs. 4*

Sp 5 In the depression below and in front of the inner ankle bone. *Fig. 4*

Fig. 4

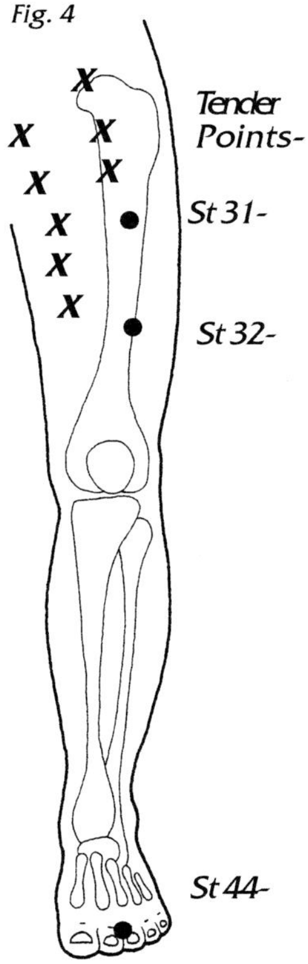

Fig. 4

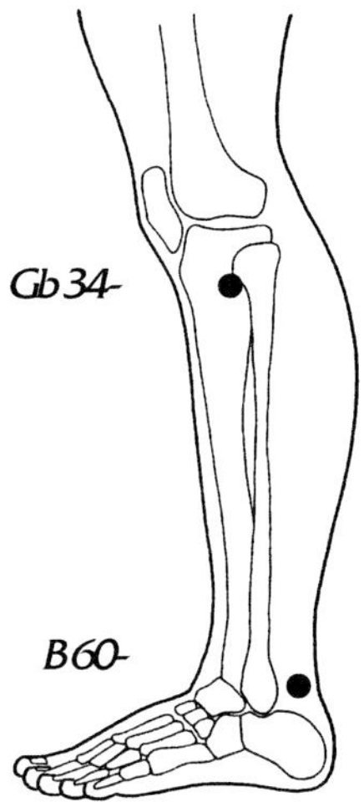

Fig. 3

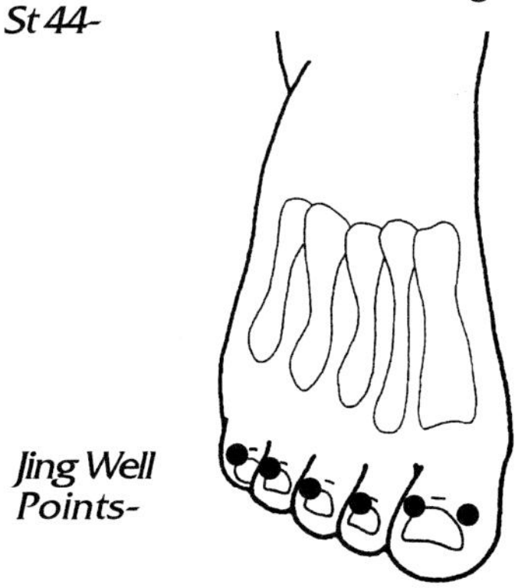

Fig. 4

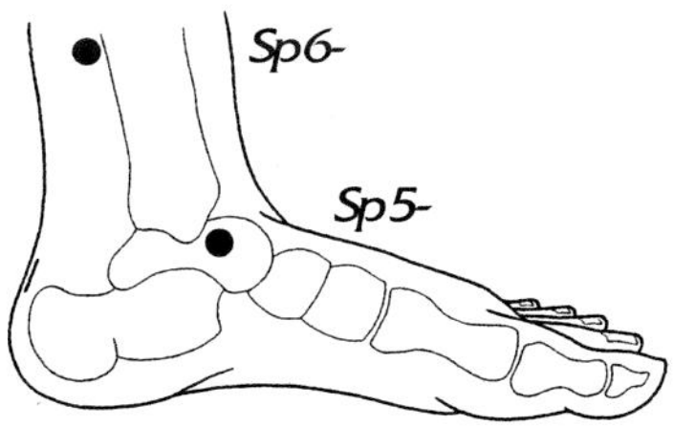

Hand Pain - continued next page

The** following points are recommended for painful conditions of the hand, including arthritic stiffness. For additional relief, stimulate the elbow pain points* ***on page 66.

Li 4 In the middle of the fleshy web between the thumb and index finger, closer to the index finger bone. *Figs. 1 & 2*

Jing Well Points
At the outer base of the finger nails. *Fig. 2*

Tw 4 In the middle of the transverse wrist crease. *Fig. 2*

Tw 5 2 thumbs width from the middle of the transverse wrist crease. *Fig. 2*

Knuckle Points
In the hollow between each set of knuckles. ***These are best located with fist closed.*** *Fig. 3*

Extra 28 Points
With the fist closed, just above the crease where the fingers meet. *Fig. 3*

Lu 11 Very close to the outer/lower corner of the thumb nail. *Fig. 4*

Fig. 1

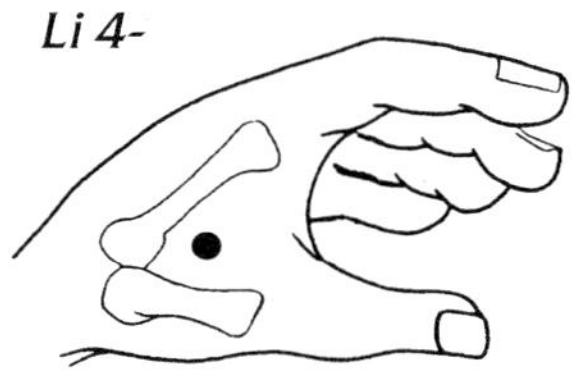

Fig. 2

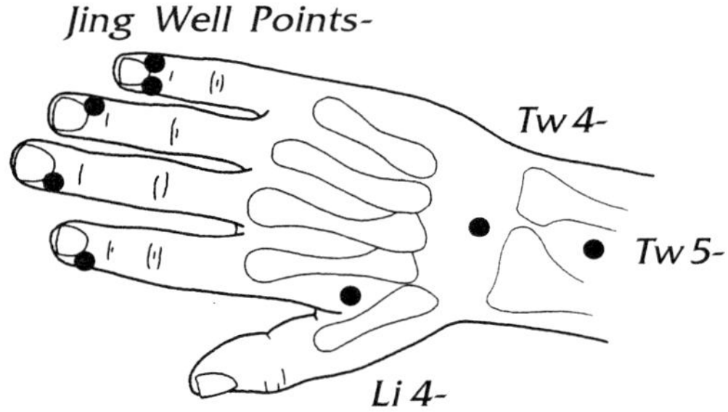

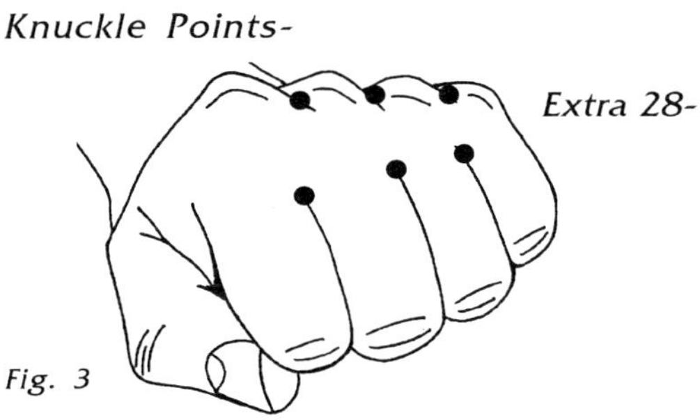

Fig. 3

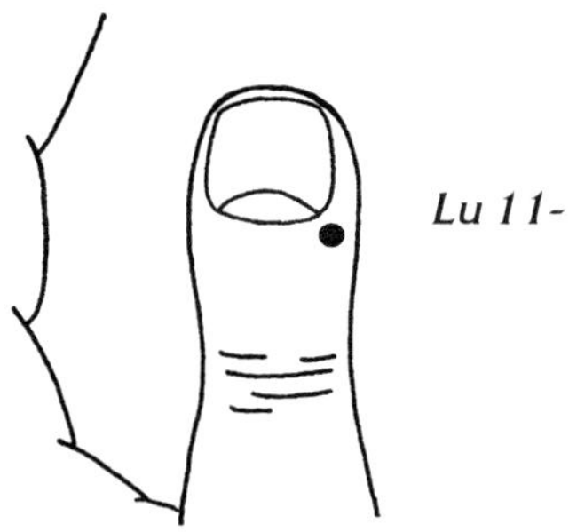

Fig. 4

Hamstring Injuries

***H**amstring injuries are often caused by over-exertion during work or sport. It is advised to start sedating the following back pain points before attempting local points on the next page.*

Back Shu Points:
Located 2 fingers width to each side of the spinal bones. ***Sedate these points from the lower back to the sacrum.*** . *Fig. 1*

Piriformis Trigger Points:
Approximately half way between the sacrum (the triangular bone at the base of the spine) and the hip joint, or one hands width above GB 30.

Gb 30 This point is directly in the middle of the each buttocks half, equal distance from all sides. *Fig. 2*

Gb 31 Standing erect with your hands laying the side of the thigh. This point is at the ***tip of the middle finger***. *Fig. 3*

Gb 34 4 fingers width below the outside of the kneecap, and just in front of and below the knobby head of the fibula bone. *Fig. 3*

B 57 At the mid point of the calf where the calf muscle narrows to form the tendon, between the 2 calf muscles. *Fig. 4*

B 60 In the hollow between the outer ankle bone andthe achilles tendon. *Fig. 4*

Fig. 1

Back Shu Points-

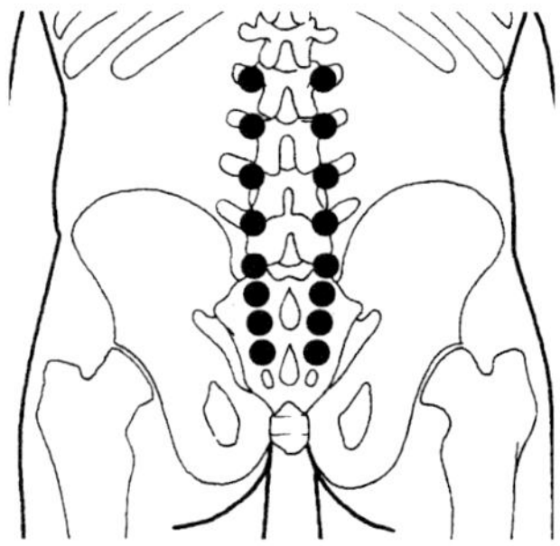

Fig. 2

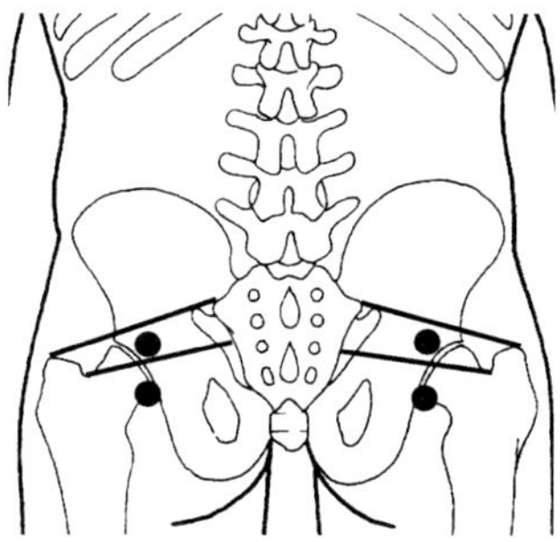

Gb 30-

Fig. 3

Gb 31-

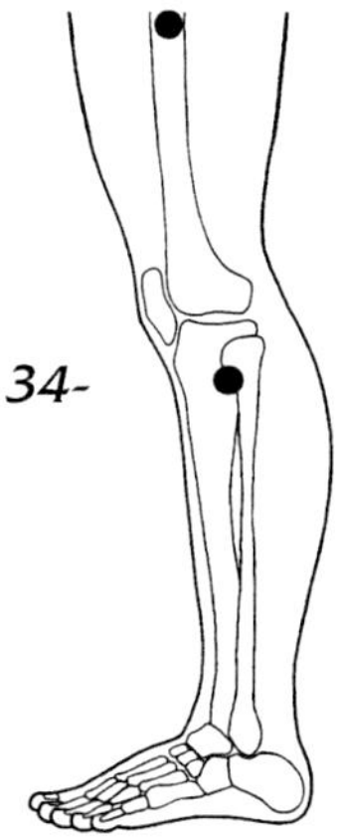

Gb 34-

Fig. 4

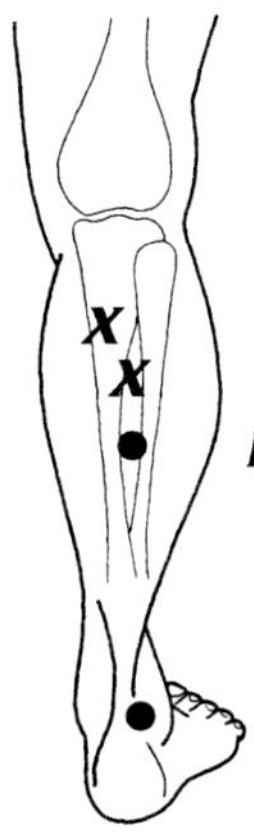

B 57-

B 60-

Heel Pain

F**or painful heel sedate the following points. For additional pain relief, sedate Calf pain points* ***(pg. 64) *and lower back pain points* ***(pg. 28).***

B 60 This lies in the hollow midway between the tip of the outer ankle bone and the Achilles tendon. *Fig. 1*

B 62 In the depression, ½ a finger below the outer ankle bone. *ig. 1*

Gb 40 Just in front and below the outside ankle bone. *Fig. 1*

Sp 6 3 fingers width above the inner ankle and just ***behind*** the prominent shin bone. *Fig. 2*

K 3 In the hollow midway between the tip of the inner ankle bone and the Achilles tendon. *Fig. 2*

K 4 ½ fingers width below and ½ fingers width ***behind K 3.*** *Fig. 2*

K 5 1 thumb width ***below K 3.*** *Fig. 2*

Sp 5 Below and in front of the tip of the inner ankle bone in the depression. *Fig. 2*

Sp 4 3 fingers width towards the ankle from ***Sp 3***. *Fig. 2*

Sp 3 Just proximal to the "Bunion" bone at the base of the big toe, at the junction of the red and white skin. *Fig. 2*

Liv 3 On the top of the foot, in the hollow between the 1st and 2nd toes, where the bones meet. *Fig. 3*

St 41 On the front of the ankle, on the midline between the 2 ankle tendons. *Fig. 3*

Web points
These are located in the fleshy web ***between the toes***. *Fig. 3*

Fig. 1

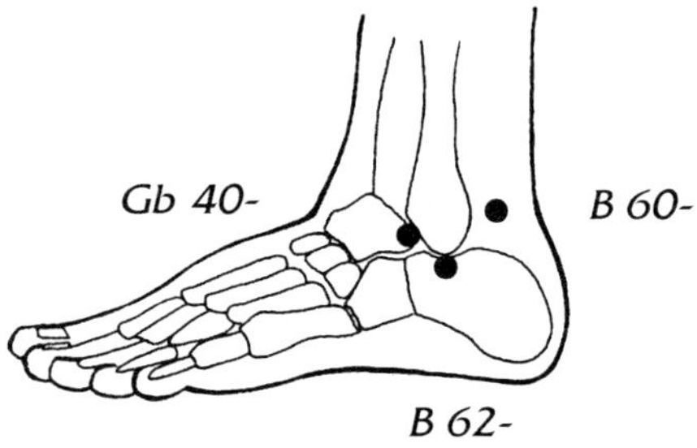

Fig. 2

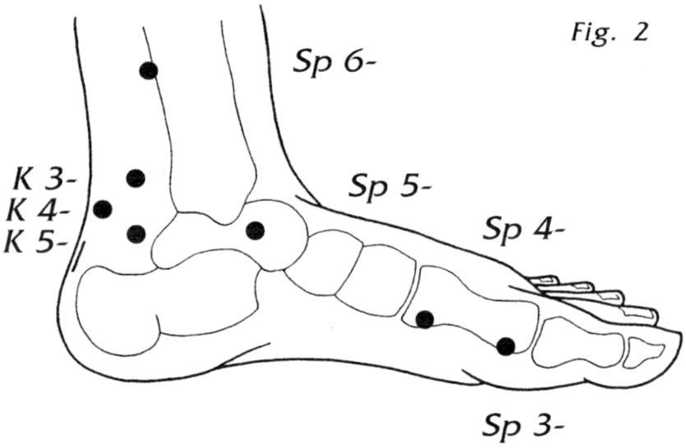

Fig. 3

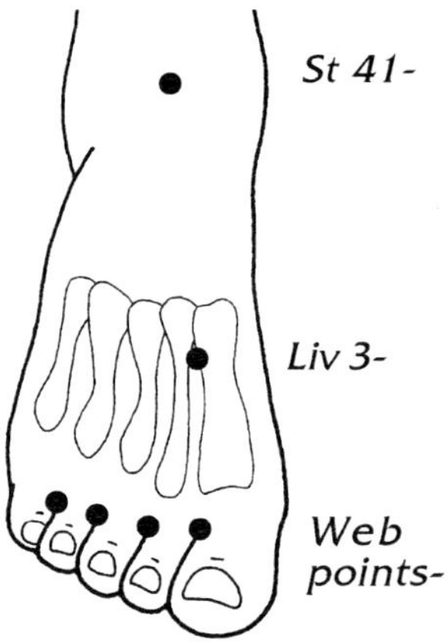

Hernia

***H**ernia injuries are often sports related. Sedate the low back pain points before sedating locally for enhanced benefits.*

Back Shu Points:
Located 2 fingers width to each side of the spinal bones. ***Sedate these points from the lower back to the sacrum. Above points innervate the affected region(s) and often provide substantial relief to the patient.*** *Fig. 1*

Piriformis Trigger Points:
Approximately half way between the sacrum (the triangular bone at the base of the spine) and the hip joint, or one hands width above GB 30. *Fig. 1*

Gb 30 This point is directly in the middle of the each buttocks half, equal distance from all sides. *Fig. 1*

Gb 31 Standing erect with your hands laying the side of the thigh. This point is at the ***tip of the middle finger***. *Fig. 2*

Gb 34 4 fingers width below the outside of the kneecap, and just in front of and below the knobby head of the fibula bone. *Fig. 2*

Liv 3 In the depression, where the 1st & 2nd toe bones meet. *Fig. 3*

Sp 6 Located 3 fingers width above the highest part of the inner ankle bone, and behind the shin bone. *Fig. 4*

Fig. 1

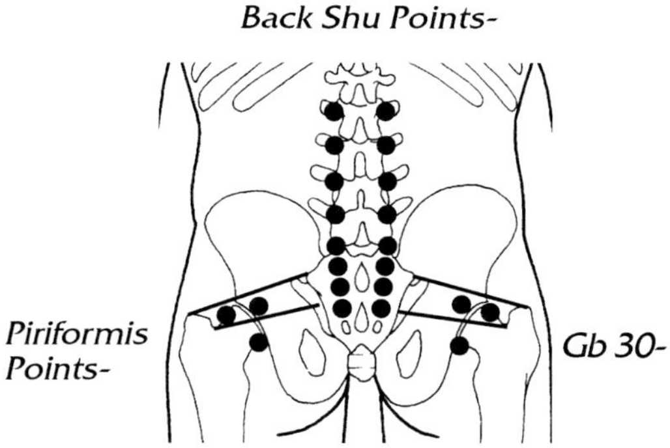

Fig. 2

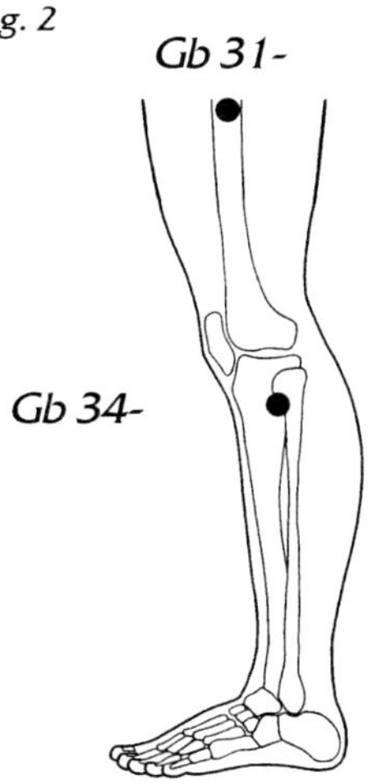

Fig. 3

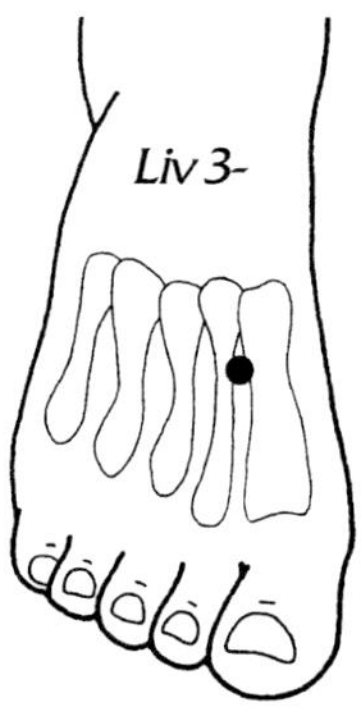

Fig. 4

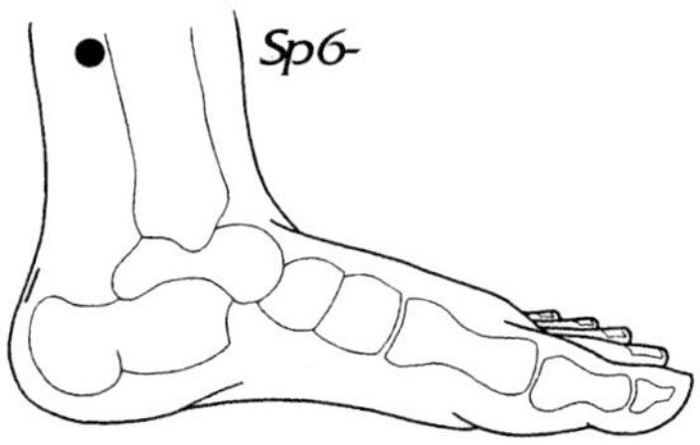

Hernia

***C**hronic groin injuries may include the following distal points points. Sedate for optimal relief.*

Fig. 1

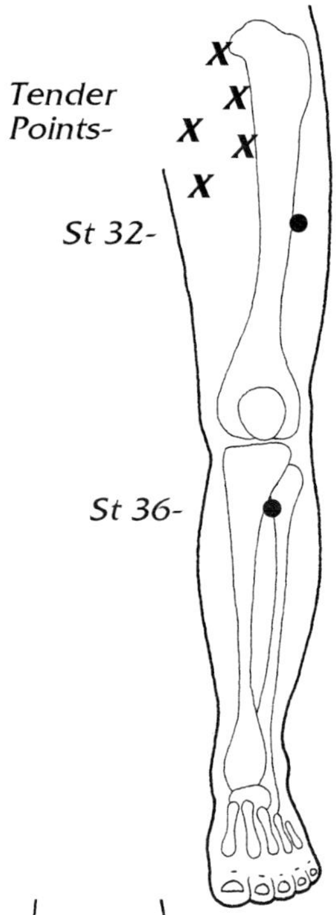

Tender Points
Sedate any tender points in the local area that are involved with the injured muscles. *Fig. 1*

St 32 8 fingers width above the upper/outer kneecap. *Fig. 1*

St 36 4 fingers width below the kneecap, and 1 fingers width to the outside of the shinbone. *Fig. 1*

St 44 At meeting of the base of 2nd and 3rd toes in the web. *Fig. 2*

Fig. 2

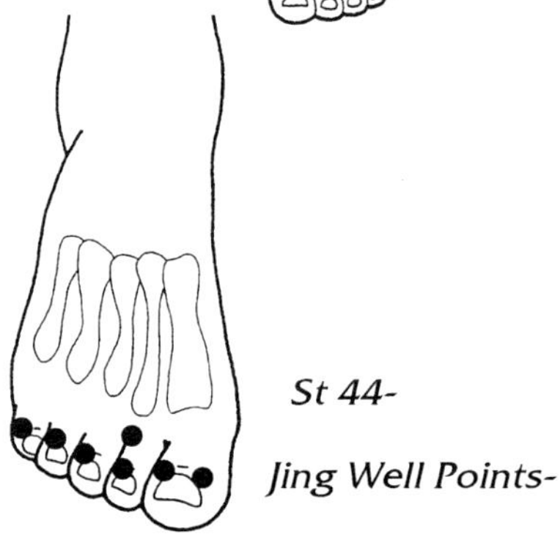

Jing Well Points
At the outer base of the toe nails. *Fig. 2*

Li 4 In the centre of the fleshy mass between the thumb and index finger. *Fig. 3*

Tw 5 This lies on the back of the wrist, 2 thumbs width above the wrist crease. *Fig. 3*

Fig. 3

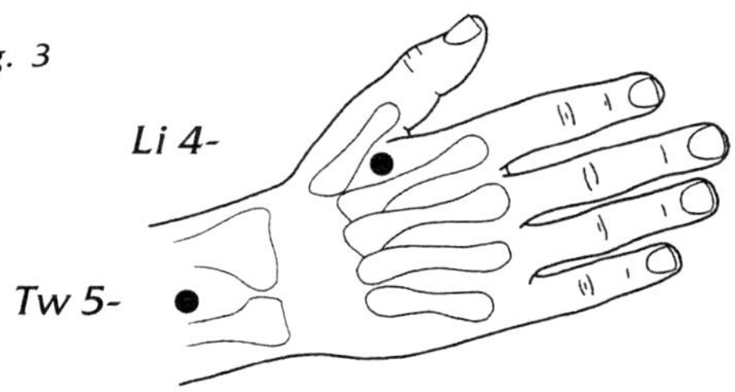

Hips

***H**ip pain is often caused by long term degeneration of the tissues surrounding the hip joint. The low back pain point are often effective in managing chronic hip pain. For additional relief refer to the points on the next page.*

Back Shu Points:
Located 2 fingers width to each side of the spinal bones. ***Sedate these points from the lower back to the sacrum. Above points innervate the affected region(s) and often provide substantial relief to the patient.*** *Fig. 1*

Fig. 1

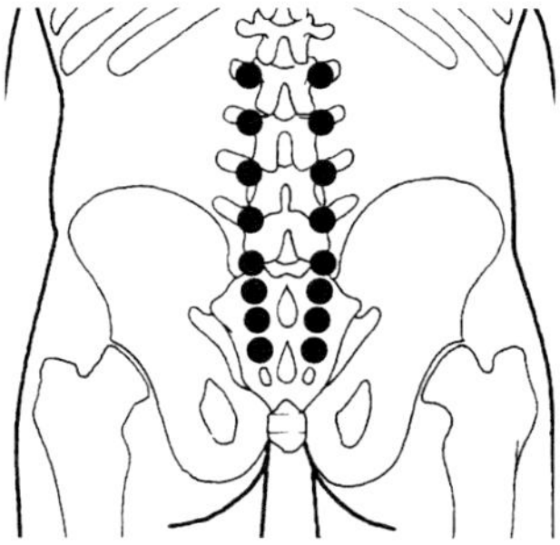

Back Shu Points-

Piriformis Trigger Points:
Approximately half way between the sacrum (the triangular bone at the base of the spine) and the hip joint, or one hands width above GB 30. *Fig. 2*

Gb 30 This point is directly in the middle of the each "cheek" equal distance from all sides. *Fig. 2*

Fig. 2

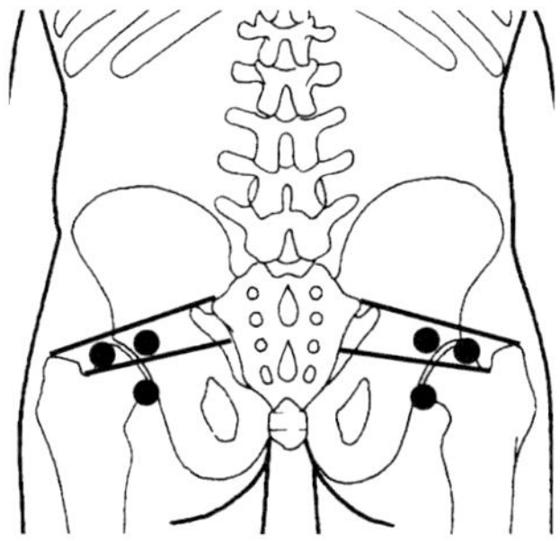

Gb 30-

Gb 31 Standing erect with your hands laying the side of the thigh. This point is at the ***tip of the middle finger***. *Fig. 3*

Gb 34 4 fingers width below the outside of the kneecap, and just in front of and below the knobby head of the fibula bone. *Fig. 3*

Fig. 3

Gb 31-

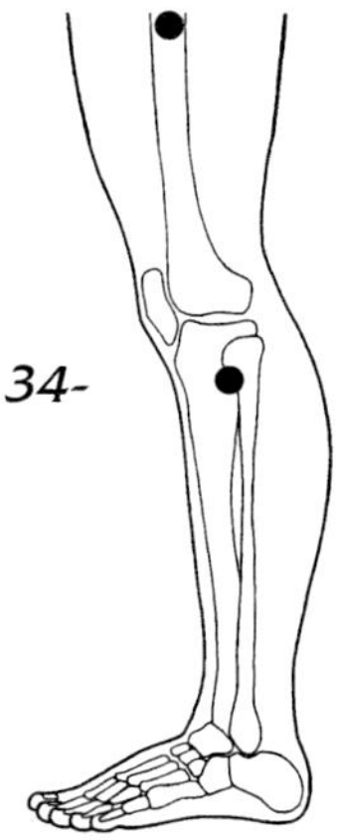

Gb 34-

Jing Well Points
Located on each side of the toenails at the base of the nail. *Fig. 4*

Fig. 4

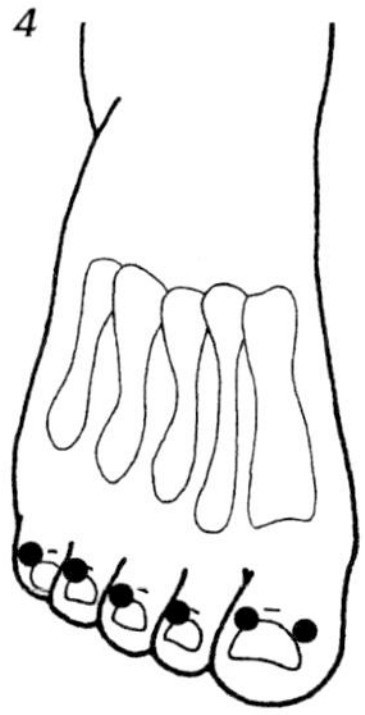

Jing Well Points-

Hips

***F**or additonal hip pain relief beyond the treatment of the lower back pain points, include the following local and distal points.*

Fig. 1

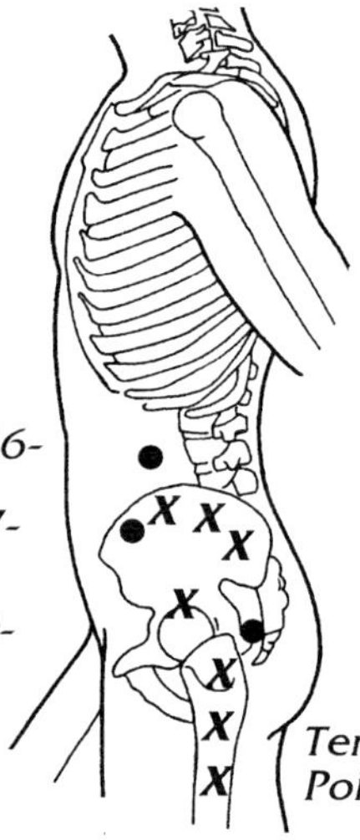

Gb 26 Directly below the "free" ***11th*** rib at the ***same level of the belly button***. *Fig. 1*

Gb 27 Just below the ***highest point*** of the outside hip bone. *Fig. 1*

Gb 30 This lies in the upper/outer part of the buttock muscle. ***It is usually tender on deep finger tip pressure.*** *Fig. 1*

Tender Points

Sedate any tender points located within tight muscles of the hip. Areas of these tight muscle bands are marked with an "X". Fig. 1

Fig. 2

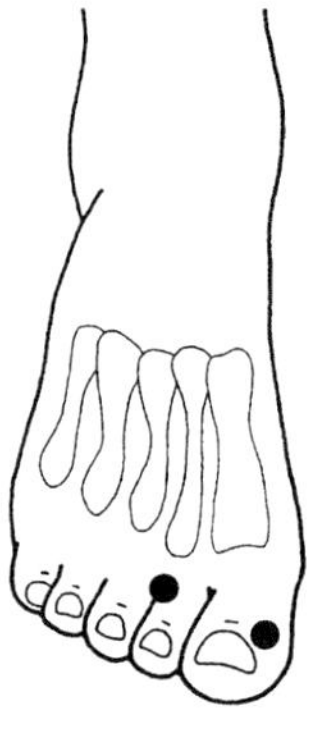

St 44 At the base of the 2nd and 3rd toes in the web. *Fig. 2*

Sp 1 At the base of the big toe nail on the iside corner. *Fig. 2*

Fig. 3

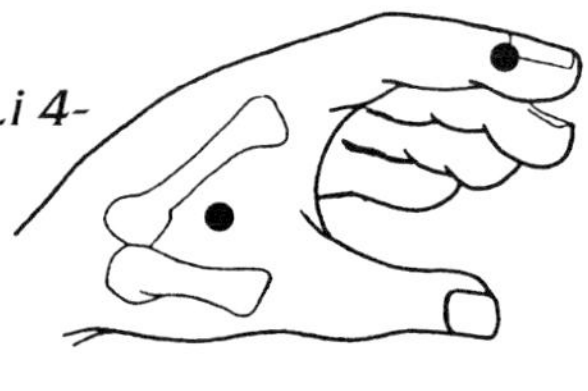

Li 4 Located in the centre of the webbing between the thumb and index finger. *Fig. 3*

Li 1 At the outer base of the index finger nail. *Fig. 3*

Immunity - To Enhance

The following points are suggested to provide enhancement to the immune system if stimulated on a regular basis. Patients with immune deficient disorders should stimulate these points regularly for enhanced benefits. Additional strengthening points include, ***(Cv 2, Cv 4, Cv 6 - page 88),*** *located on the abdomen, illustrated on the next page.*

GV 14 Just below the most prominent bone at the base of the neck, easily located with the ***chin pressed towards chest.*** *Fig. 1*

Fig. 1

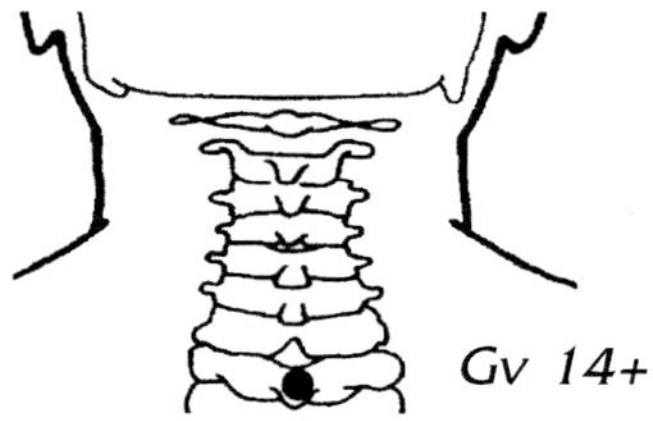

Li 11 This lies at the outer end of the elbow crease, with the ***arm slightly bent.*** *Fig. 2*

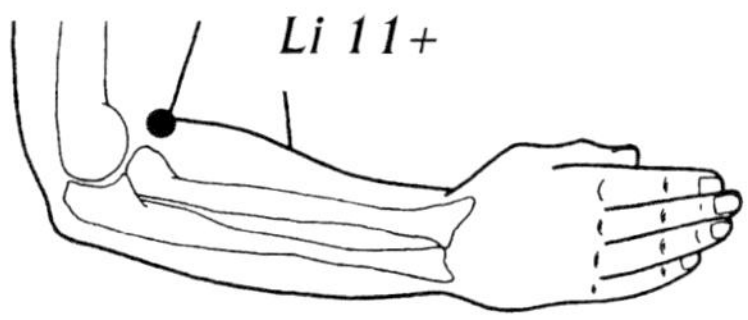

Fig. 2

St 36 4 fingers width below the kneecap and 1 fingers width to the outside of the shin bone. *Fig. 3*

Fig. 3

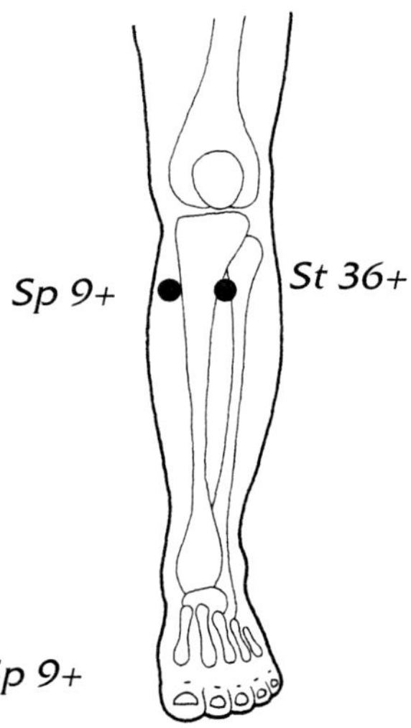

Sp 9 On the inside of the leg, 3 fingers width below the kneecap, in the depression between the bone and the calf muscle. *Fig. 3*

Sp 10 2 thumbs width above the upper/inner border of the kneecap. ***This tender spot is at the highest spot of the inner thigh muscle.*** *Fig. 3*

Sp 6 This point lies 3 fingers width above the inner ankle bone and is located behind the prominent shin bone. ***Usually very tender when pressed.*** *Fig. 4*

Fig. 4

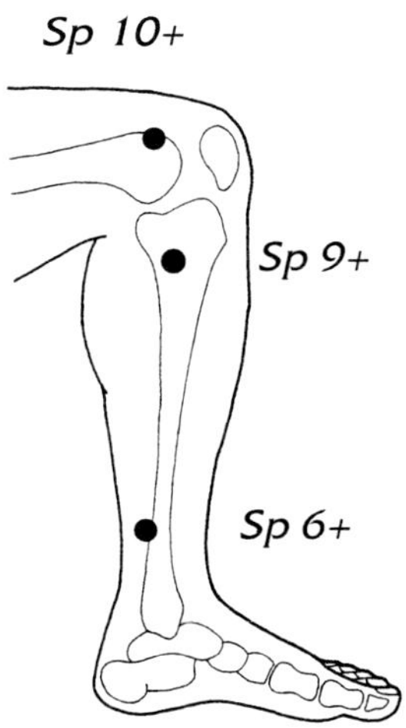

Impotence - Male

S**timulate the following points on positive with a frequency of at least 3 times per week. For additional benefits, sedate the* ***stress points on page 89.

Gv 4 In between the spinal bones of the 2nd and 3rd vetebrae. ***At the waist level.*** *Fig. 1*

Back Shu Points
2 fingers width to each side of the spine ***sedate from the waist level to lower sacrum***. *Fig. 1*

St 36 4 fingers width below the lower kneecap and 1 fingerswidth to the outside of the shin bone. *Fig. 2*

Cv 6 2 fingers width ***below*** the belly button, on the midline. *Fig. 3*

Cv4 4 fingers width ***below*** the belly button, on the midline. *Fig. 3*

Cv 2 Immediately ***above*** the upper border of the pubic bone, on the midline. *Fig. 3*

Liv 8 On the transverse knee, just to the innerside of the large tendon ***with the knee flexed***. *Fig. 4*

Sp 6 This point lies 3 fingers width ***above the inner ankle*** bone and is located behind the prominent shin bone. *Fig. 4*

K 3 Located in the hollow ***between*** the inner ankle bone and the Achilles tendon.* *Fig. 4*

Fig. 1

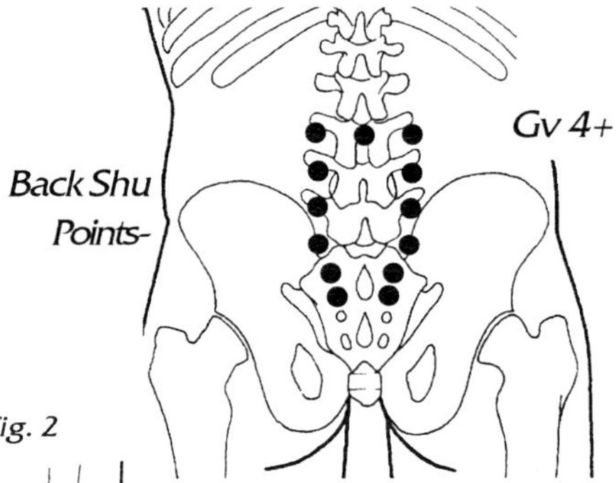

Fig. 2

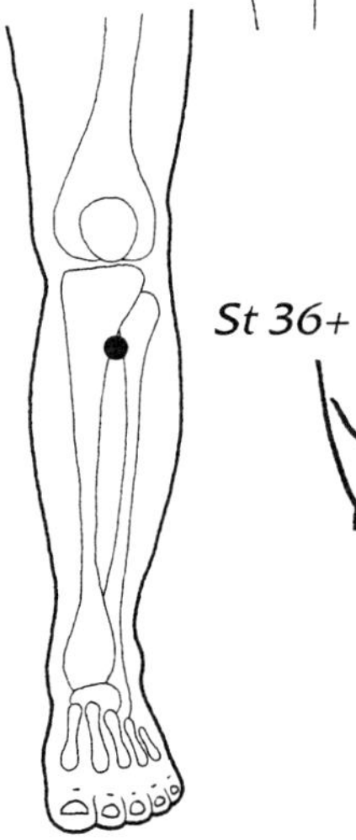

Fig. 3

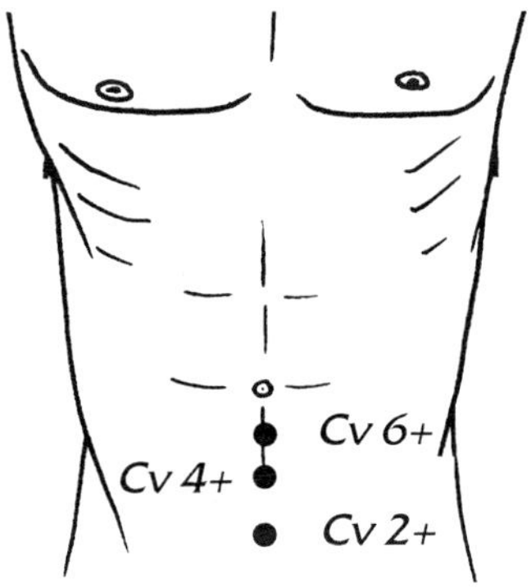

Fig. 4

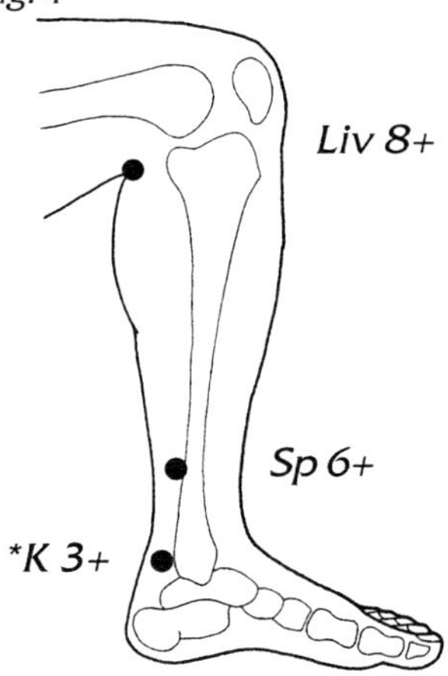

Insomnia - Stress & Apnea

F**or chronic insomnia sedate the following points. For additional relief and relaxation, or to treat slep apnea, sedate the **parasympathetic points on page 116.

For Insomina add:

Gv 20 On the middle of the top of the head, halfway between the ears. *Fig. 1*

Extra 1 (Yintang)
At the midpoint of the inner end of the eyebrows. *Fig. 1*

Extra 8 Located on the forward side of the bony protrusion immediately behind the ear. *Figs. 1 & 2*

Shenman
Located in the lower triangular fossa (Little triangle) of the upper ear. *Figs. 2*

Extra 9 Located opposite to ***Extra 8,*** on the bony protrusion immediately behind the ear. *Figs. 1 & 2*

For Stress add:

H 9 On the thumb side of the base of the baby finger nail. *Fig. 3*

Si 1 Opposite to ***H 9*** on the outside base of the baby finger nail. *Fig. 3*

K 6 1 thumbs width below the inner ankle bone. *Fig. 4*

Fig. 1

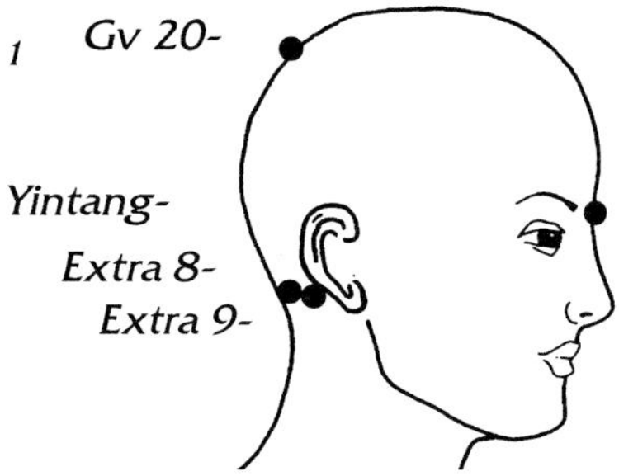

Fig. 2

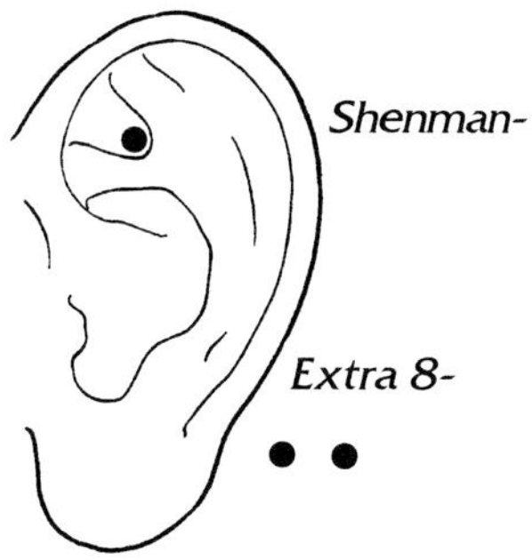

Fig.3

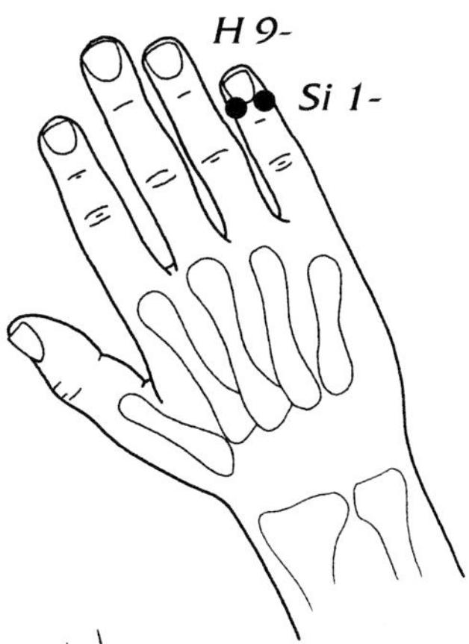

Fig. 4

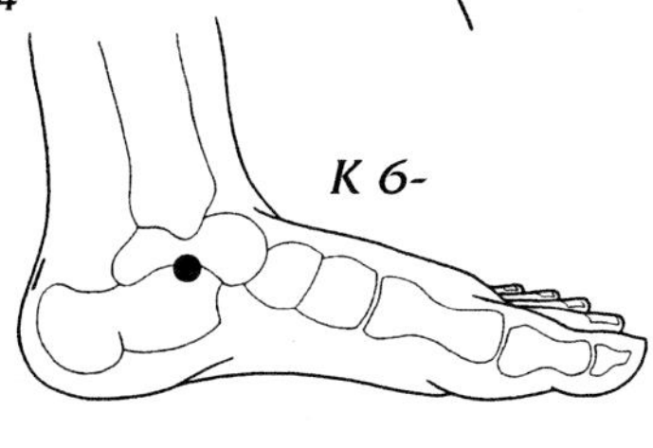

Intercostal Neuralgia -continued

Intercostal neuralgia is pain that runs between the ribs. It is usually initiated by trauma, such as a car accident. Sedate the following spinal points for symptomatic relief of pain.

Back Shu Points:
Located 2 fingers width to each side of the spinal bones. ***Sedate these points from the upper back to the lower back. Above points innervate the affected region(s) and often provide substantial relief to the patient.*** *Fig. 1*

Scapular Points:
These points are located on the inside border of the shoulder blade, inbetween the ribs. *Fig. 1*

Piriformis Trigger Points:
Approximately half way between the sacrum (the triangular bone at the base of the spine) and the hip joint, or one hands width above GB 30. Palpate the area until tenderness is detected. *Fig. 2*

Gb 30 This point is directly in the middle of the each "cheek" equal distance from all sides. *Fig. 2*

Gb 31 Stand erect, hands flat along the side of the thigh. This point is at the ***tip of the middle finger***. *Fig. 3*

Gb 34 4 fingers width below the outside of the kneecap, and just in front of and below the knobby head of the fibula bone. *Fig. 3*

Fig. 1

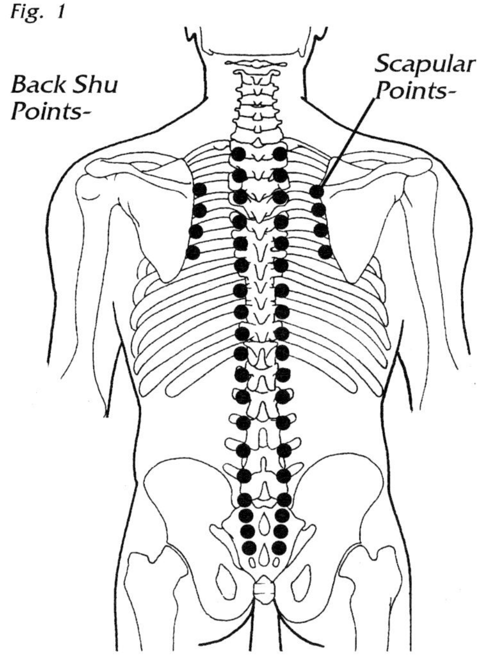

Fig. 2

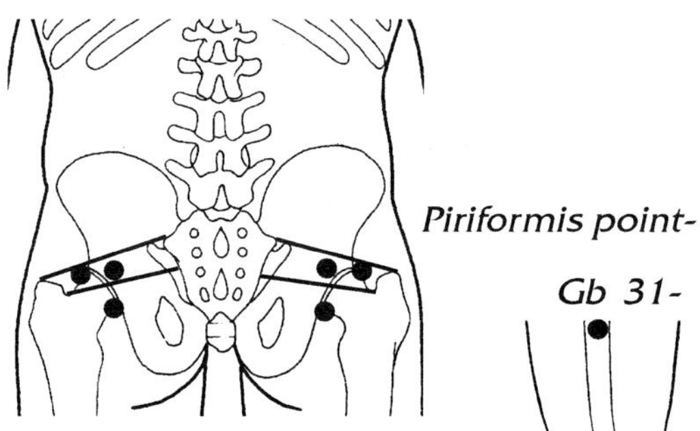

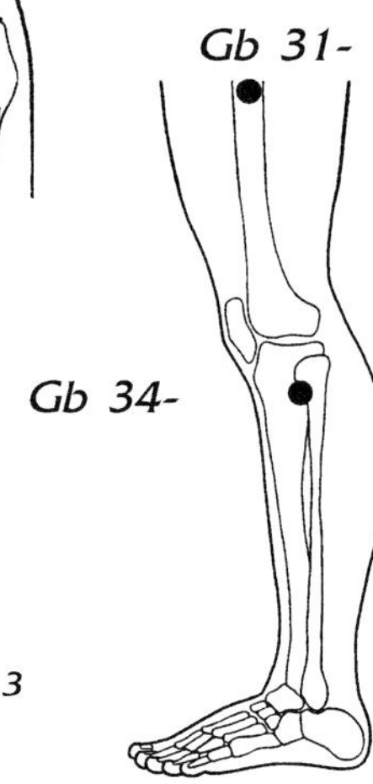

Fig. 3

Intercostal Neuralgia

For additional relief of intercostal neuralgia sedate the following local and distal points. Consult a Doctor before treating this condition. Sedate points for best results. The following points are also effective for upper back pain.

P 6 3 fingers width from the most distal wrist crease, in between the tendons. *Fig. 1*

H 9 On the upper/inner corner of the little finger nail *Fig. 2*

Li 4 In the middle of the fleshy mass between the thumb and forefinger. *Fig. 2*

Lu 7 2 fingers width above the base of the thumb, in the small hollow of the wrist bone. *Fig. 2*

Tw 5 2 fingers width above the wrist crease in between the 2 forearm bones. *Fig. 2*

Lu 1 In the hollow below the shoulder, 3 fingers width below the collarbone. *Fig. 3*

Tender Points

Stimulate any tender points found between the ribs in the muscles. ***The likely areas are marked with an "X".***
Fig. 3

Cv 17 On the breast bone at the heart level or the 4th rib space. Tender when pressed. *Fig. 3*

Cv 12 On the midline, midway between the belly button and the lower end of the breast bone. *Fig. 3*

Fig. 1

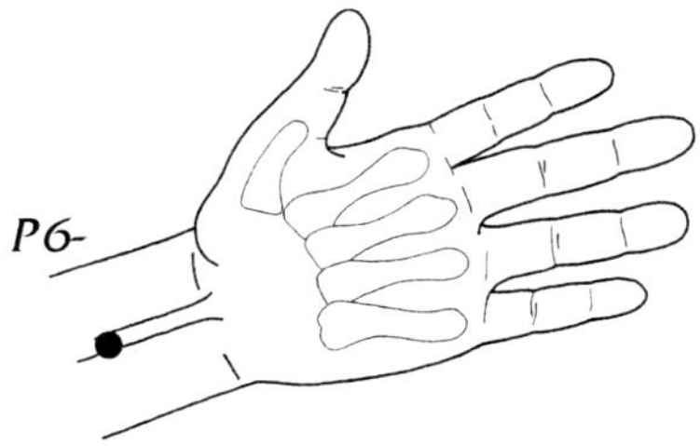

Fig. 2

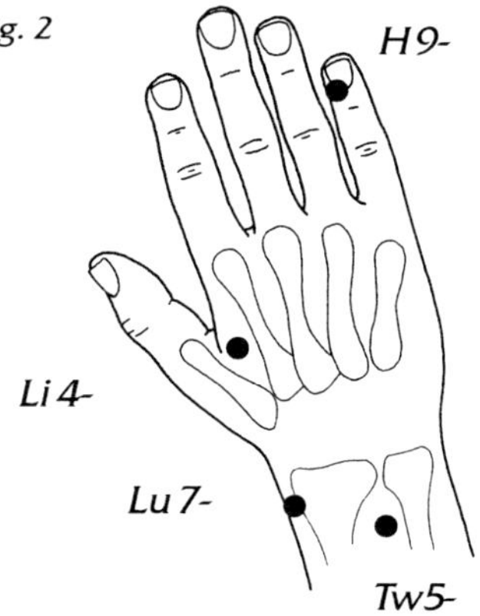

Fig. 3

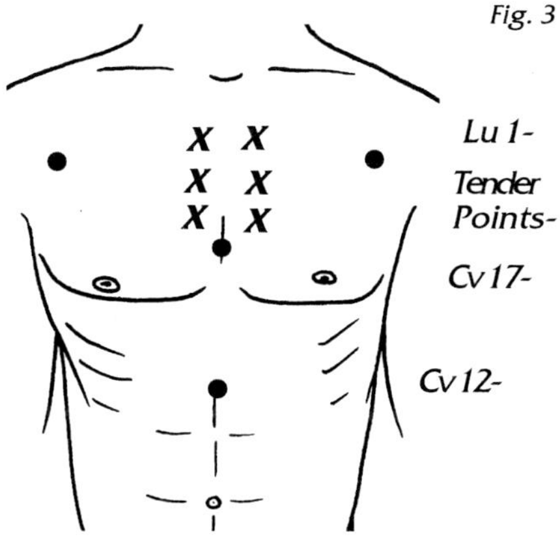

Irritable Bowel - continued next page

C*onsult a Doctor before treating* ***Irritable Bowel Syndrome.*** *For chronic IBS, the lower back region should be treated first, followed by the jing points in the toes. For additional relief, sedate the local on the following page.*

Back Shu Points:
Located 2 fingers width to each side of the spinal bones. ***Sedate these points from the lower back to the sacrum. Above points innervate the affected region(s) and often provide substantial relief to the patient.*** *Fig. 1*

Piriformis Trigger Points:
Approximately half way between the sacrum (the triangular bone at the base of the spine) and the hip joint, or one hands width above GB 30. *Fig. 2*

Gb 30 This point is directly in the middle of the each "cheek" equal distance from all sides. *Fig. 2*

Gb 31 Standing erect with your hands laying the side of the thigh. This point is at the ***tip of the middle finger***. *Fig. 3*

Gb 34 4 fingers width below the outside of the kneecap, and just in front of and below the knobby head of the fibula bone. *Fig. 3*

Jing Well Points
Located on each side of the toenails at the base of the nail. *Fig. 4*

Fig. 1

Back Shu Points-

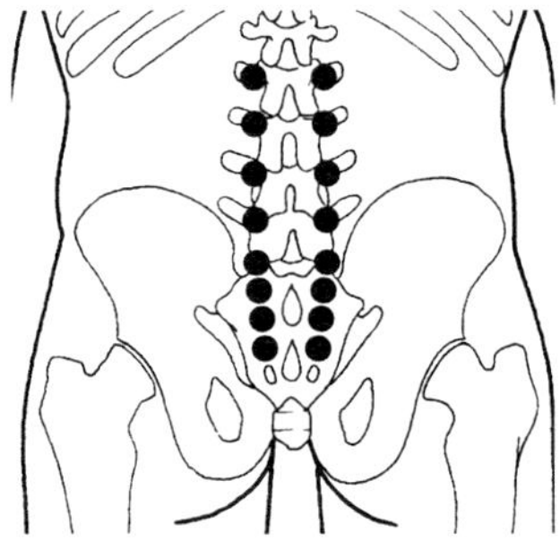

Fig. 2

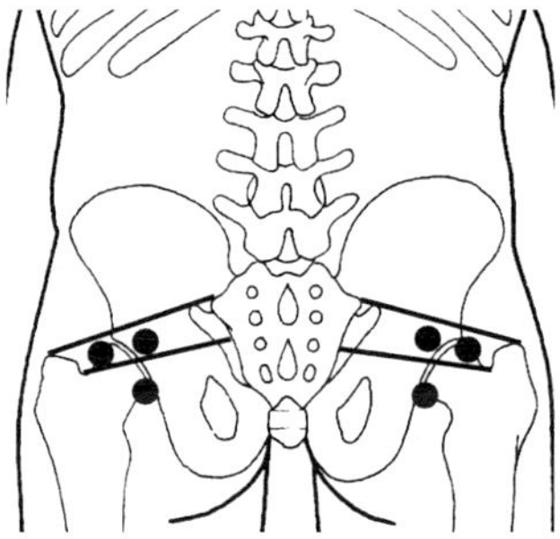

Gb 30-

Fig. 3

Gb 31-

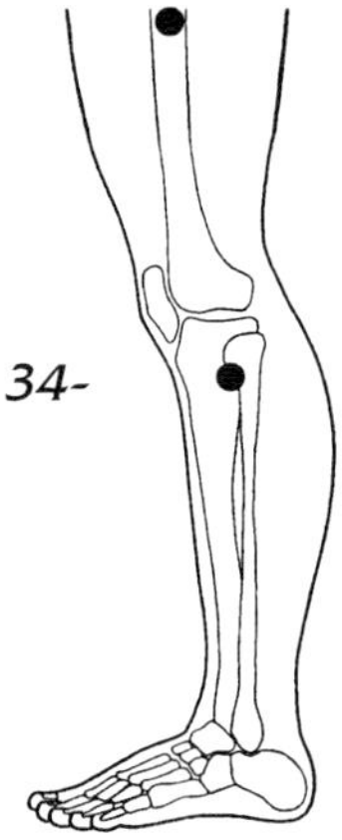

Gb 34-

Fig. 4

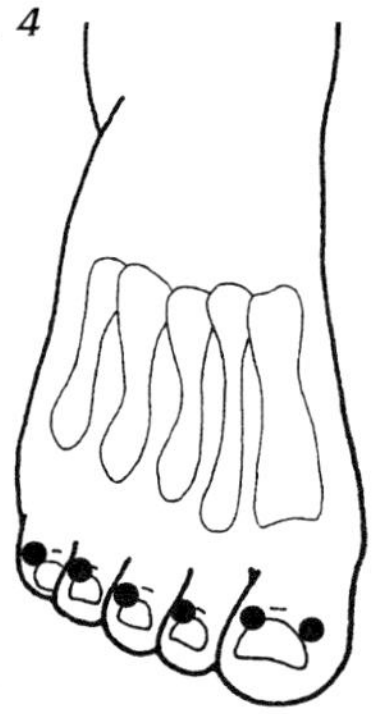

Irritable Bowel

IBS symptoms include cramping, lower abdominal pain, constipation/ diarrhoea, bloating, heartburn, fatigue, headache, faintness, back pain and weakness. Sedate the following points in addition to the parasympathetic points located on ***page 116****, for optimal relief.*

Cv 12 On the midline, midway between the belly button and the lower end of the breast bone. *Fig. 1*

St 25 2 fingers width on each side of the belly button. *Fig. 1*

Cv 6 On the midline, 2 fingers width directly ***below*** the belly button. *Fig. 1*

Cv 4 On the midline of the abdomen 4 fingers width ***below*** the belly button. *Fig. 1*

Tw 6 2 thumbs width from the middle of the transverse wrist crease. *Fig. 2*

St 34 2 thumbs width above the upper/outer border of the knee cap. *Fig. 3*

St 36 4 fingers width below the kneecap, and 1 fingers width to the outside of the shin bone. *Fig. 3*

Gb 34 Just below the bony knob outside and below the knee cap. *Fig. 3*

Sp 6 3 fingers width ***above*** the inner ankle bone and ***behind*** the prominent shin bone. *Fig. 4*

Fig. 1

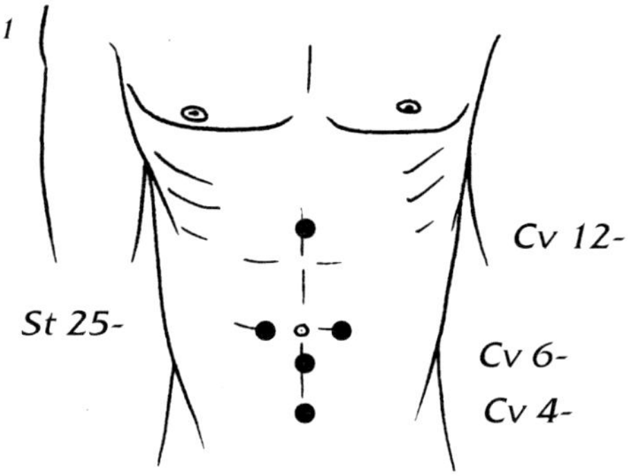

Fig. 1

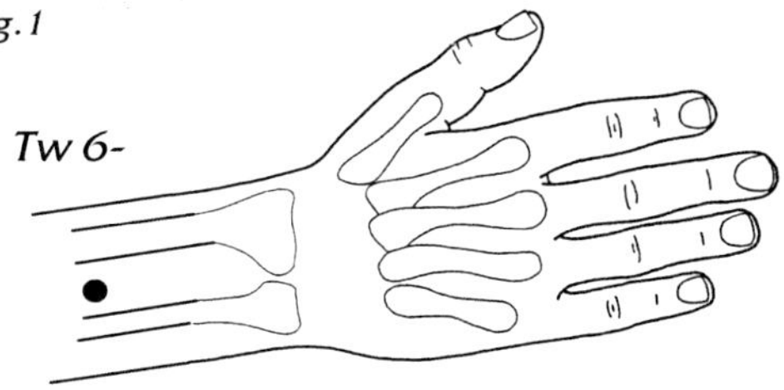

Fig. 3

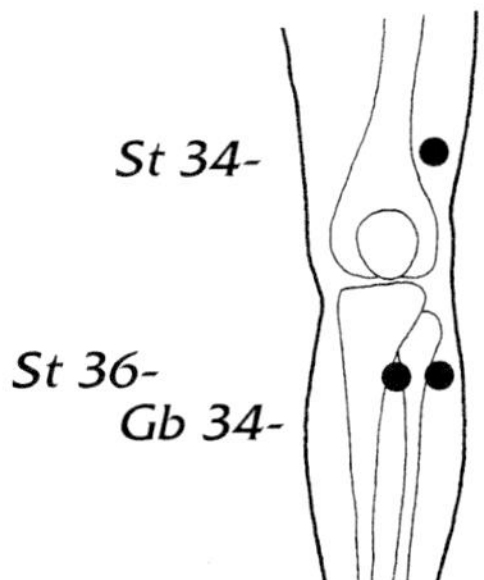

Fig. 4

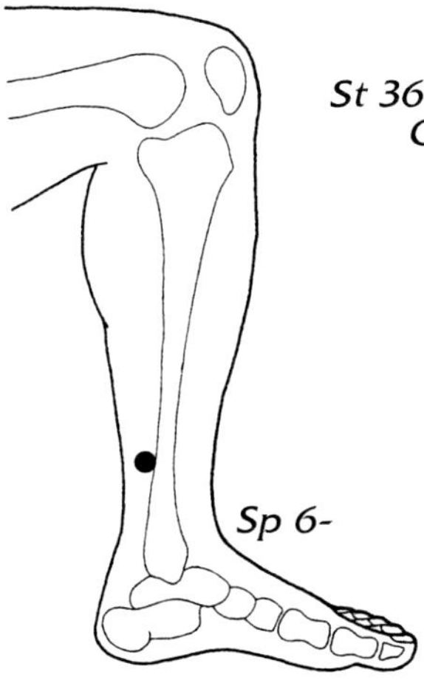

Knee - Runner's Knee

Consult a Doctor before treating any points. For chronic conditions, stimulate at the points on this page first. The distal and local points on the following page may be used after the below points. Sedate points for maximum relief.

Fig. 1

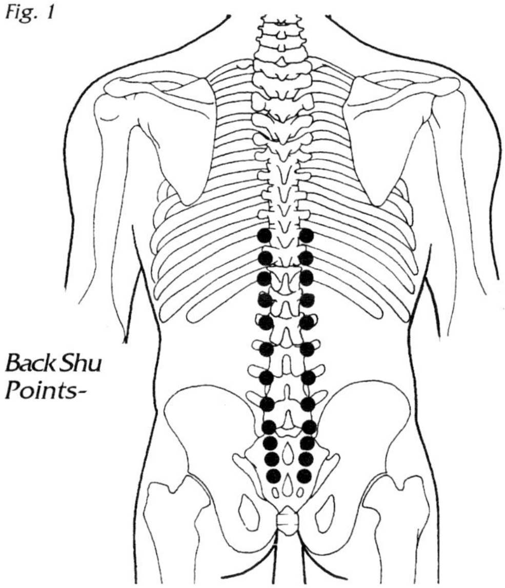

Back Shu Points:
Located 2 fingers width to each side of the spinal bones. ***Sedate these points from the middle to the lower back. Above points innervate the affected region (L 2-L5) and often provide substantial relief to knee pain.*** *Fig. 1*

Fig. 2

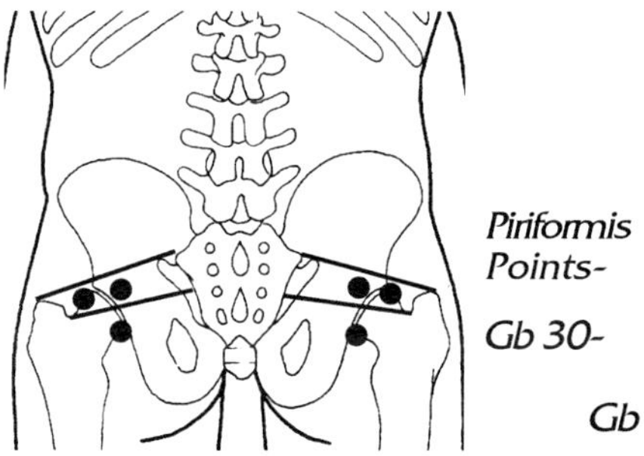

Piriformis Trigger Points:
Approximately half way between the sacrum (the triangular bone at the base of the spine) and the outside hip joint. Or, one hands width above GB 30. Press and rub (palpate) the general area until tenderness is detected. *Fig. 2*

Gb 30 This point is directly in the middle of the each buttocks half, equal distance from all sides. *Fig. 2*

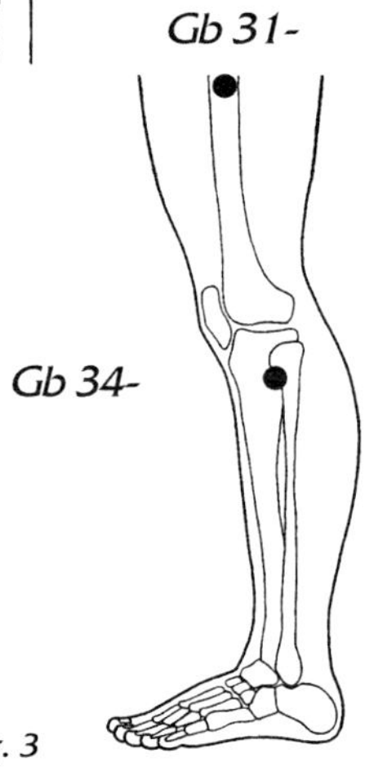

Fig. 3

Gb 31 Stand erect, hands flat along the side of the thigh. This point is at the ***tip of the middle finger***. *Fig. 3*

Gb 34 4 fingers width below the outside of the kneecap, and just in front of and below the knobby head of the fibula bone. *Fig. 3*

Knee - Runner's Knee

***R**elax the muscles above the knee by stimulating the tender points (x), before treating the local and distal points.*

B 40 On the middle of the crease behind the knee. *Fig. 1*

Extra 31 On the midpoint of the ***upper border*** of the kneecap. *Fig. 2*

Extra 32 In the depression on the ***inner*** side of the kneecap. *Fig. 2*

St 35 In the depression to the ***outer*** side of the kneecap. *Fig. 2*

St 36 4 fingers width below the kneecap, and 1 fingers width to the ***outside*** of the shinbone. *Fig. 2*

Liv 3 In the hollow between the first and second toes, where the bones merge on top of the foot. *Fig. 2*

Sp 9 On the inside of the leg 3 fingers width below the kneecap, ***in the depression between the inner knee bone and the calf muscle.*** *Fig. 3*

Liv 8 On the inner end of the knee crease, between the 2 tendons ***which become prominent when the knee is bent.*** *Fig. 3*

Sp 6 3 fingers width above the inner ankle and ***just behind the prominent shin bone.*** *Fig. 3*

B 60 This lies in the hollow midway between the tip of the outer ankle bone and the Achilles tendon. *Fig. 4*

Fig. 1

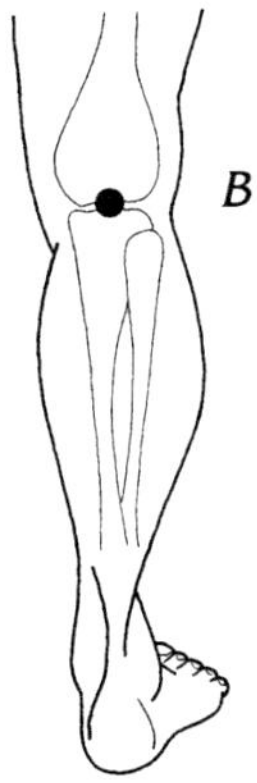

Fig. 2

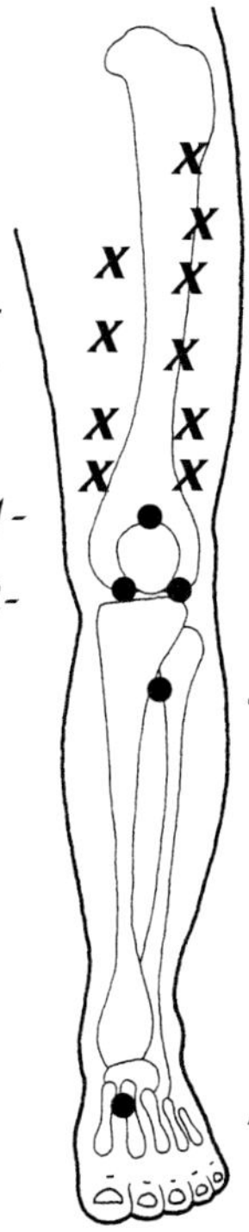

Fig. 3

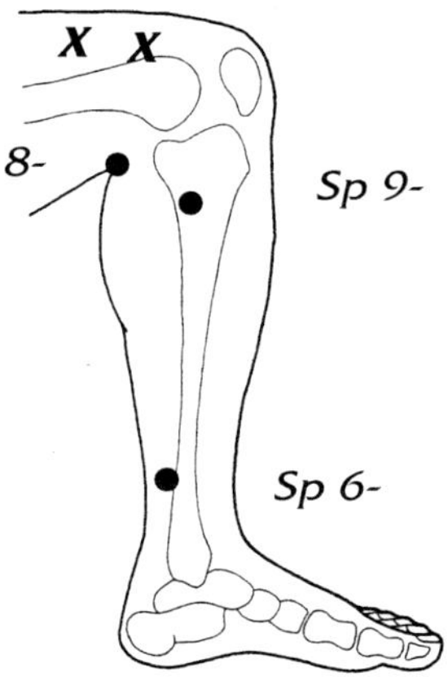

Fig. 4

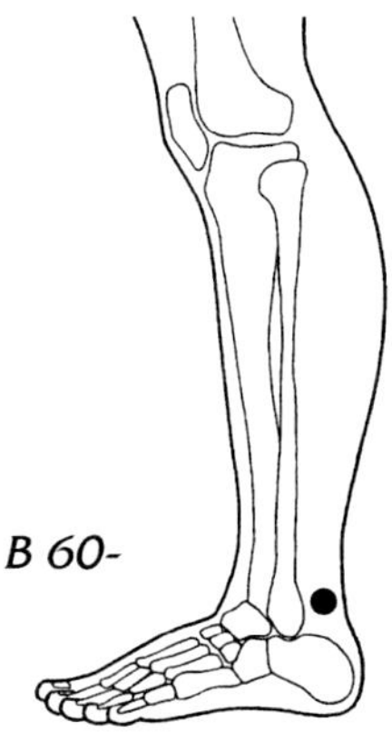

Mandibular Pain - continued next page

***T**he following points are for general pain and stiffness in the neck region. Relaxing these neck muscles often provides relief to facial pain disorders. If additional relief is required, refer to the local points on the following page.*

Gb 20 Below the base of the skull, in the hollow just outside the main spinal muscles of neck. *Fig. 1*

B 10 Located 2 fingers width from the middle of the spine at the level of the natural hairline at the back of the neck. ***In the ropy muscleson each side of the spine.*** *Fig. 1*

Gb 21 This lies halfway between the knob of bone at the base of the neck and the tip of the shoulder, in the fleshy mass of muscle. *Fig. 1*

Tw 15 1 thumbs width ***below Gb 21.*** *Fig. 1*

Si 13 4 fingers width ***below GB 21*** just on top of the spine of the shoulder blade. *Fig. 1*

Tender Points
Stimulate these tender points located in the tight muscles at the side of the neck. *Fig. 2*

Si 17 Above the prominent neck muscle, ***at the level of the corner of the jaw.*** *Fig. 2*

Li 18 4 fingers width beside the highest point of the Adam's apple in the prominent muscle at the side of the neck ***(below the corner of the jaw).*** *Fig. 2*

Si 3 On the end of the main transverse crease of the hand. ***Best located with the fist clenched.*** *Fig. 3*

Fig. 1

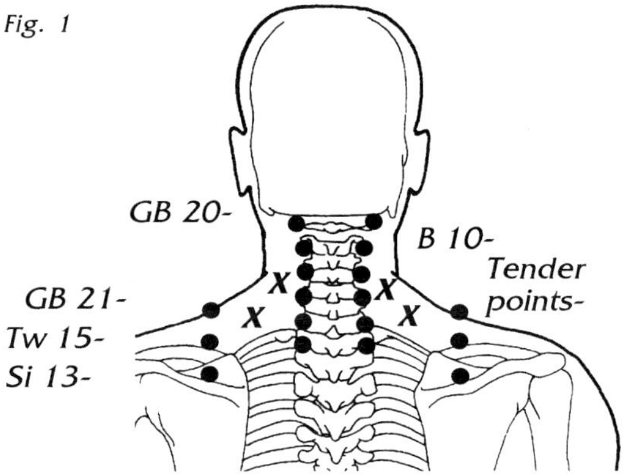

Fig. 2

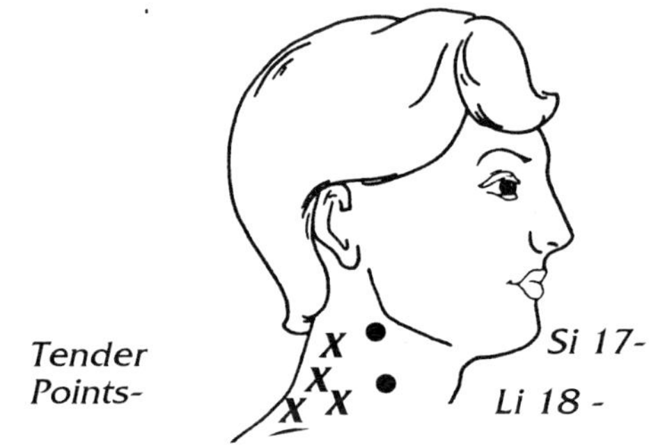

Fig. 3

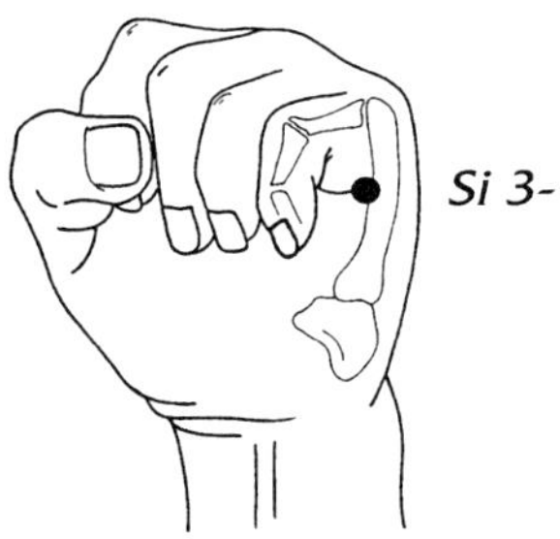

Mandibular Pain & Arthritis

***I**f additional pain relief is required in the face after treating the neck, sedate the following points. It is recommended to sedate the distal points before local points for optimal relief.*

Li 4 In the middle of the fleshy mass of muscle between the thumb and index finger, and slightly towards the index finger bone. *Fig. 1*

St 7 2 fingers width in front of the ear, in the hollow ***just below*** the upper jaw bone. *Fig. 2*

St 2 1 fingers width below the lower ridge of the eye socket, ***directly below the pupil.*** *Fig. 2*

Si 18 Below the outer corner of the eye socket, ***directly under cheek bone.*** *Figs. 2 & 3*

St 6 Over the highest point of the bulge of the muscle at the angle of the jaw ***when the jaw is clenched.*** *Fig. 2*

Tw 21 In front of the midpoint of the ear in the hollow felt ***when the mouth is opened***. *Fig. 3*

Si 19 Just in front of the upper end of the ear lobe in a hollow formed ***when the mouth is opened.*** *Fig. 3*

Gb 2 In front of lobe of the ear. *Fig. 3*

Tender Points

Stimulate these tender points located in the tight muscles in front of the ear. *Fig. 3*

Fig. 1

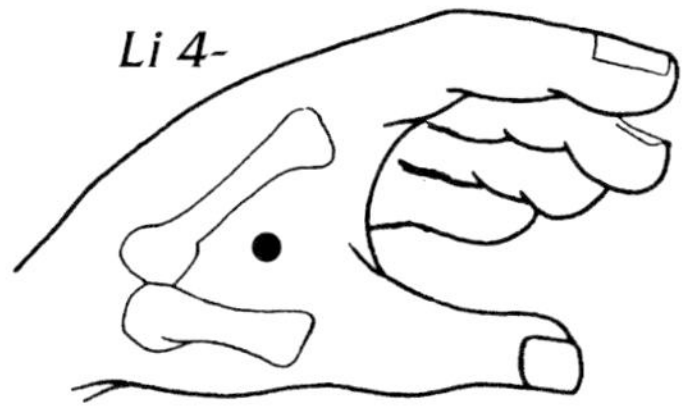

Fig. 2

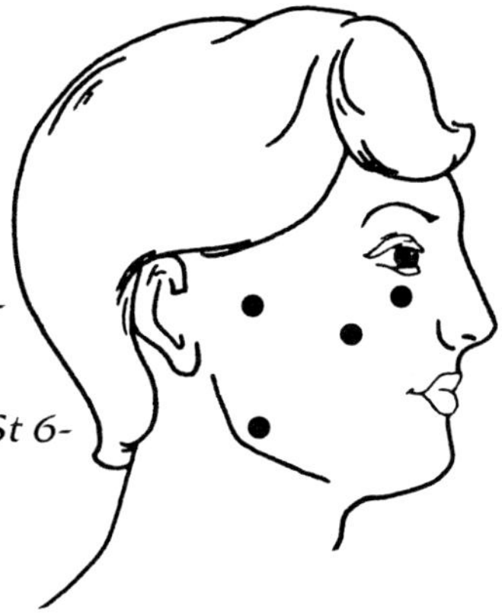

Fig. 3

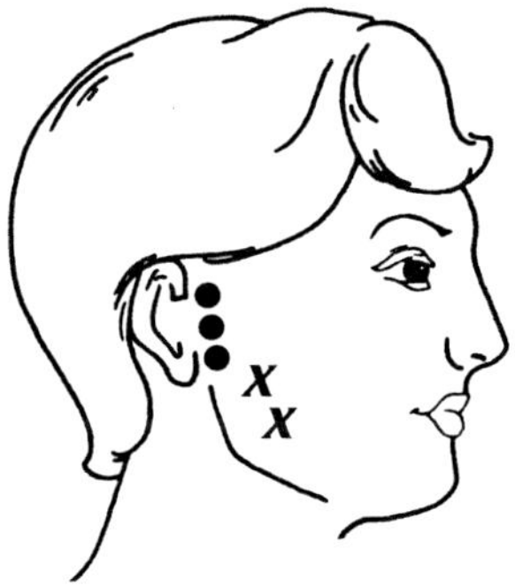

Menstrual Cramps - PMS

Consult a Doctor before treating any points. For chronic conditions, the lower back region should be treated first, followed by the jing points. For additional relief, sedate the local on the following page.

Back Shu Points:
Located 2 fingers width to each side of the spinal bones. ***Sedate these points from the lower back to the sacrum. Above points innervate the affected region(s) and often provide substantial relief to the patient.*** *Fig. 1*

Fig. 1

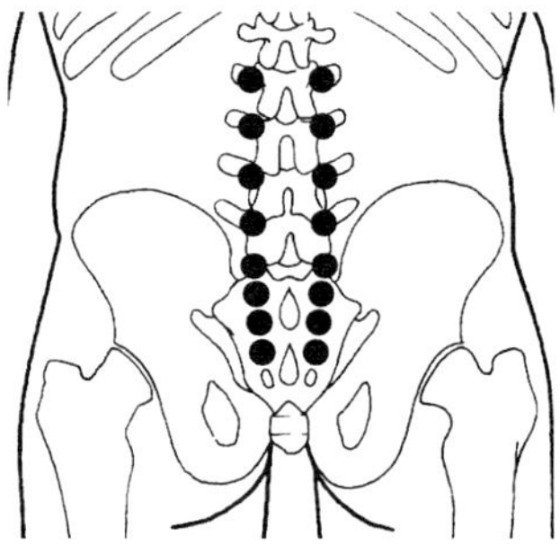

Fig. 2

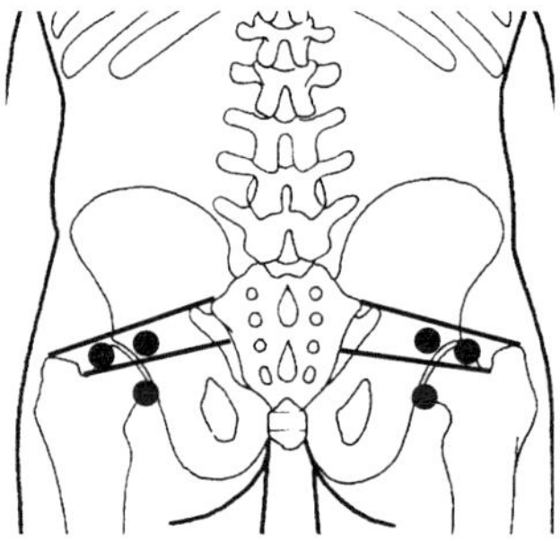

Piriformis Trigger Points:
Approximately half way between the sacrum (the triangular bone at the base of the spine) and the hip joint, or one hands width above GB 30. *Fig. 2*

Gb 30 This point is directly in the middle of the each buttocks half, equal distance from all sides. *Fig. 2*

Fig. 3

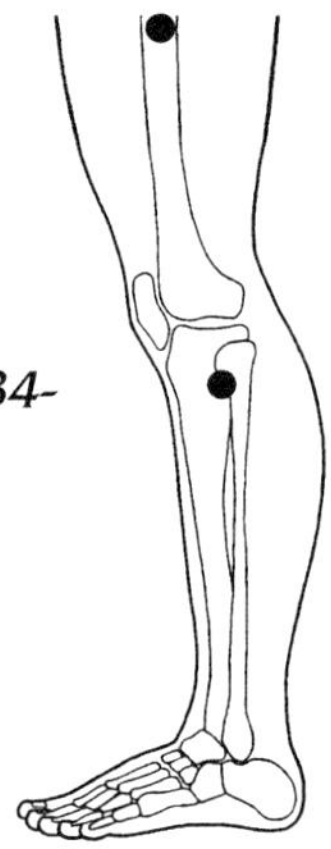

Gb 31 Standing erect with your hands laying the side of the thigh. This point is at the ***tip of the middle finger***. *Fig. 3*

Gb 34 4 fingers width below the outside of the kneecap, and just in front of and below the knobby head of the fibula bone. *Fig. 3*

Fig. 4

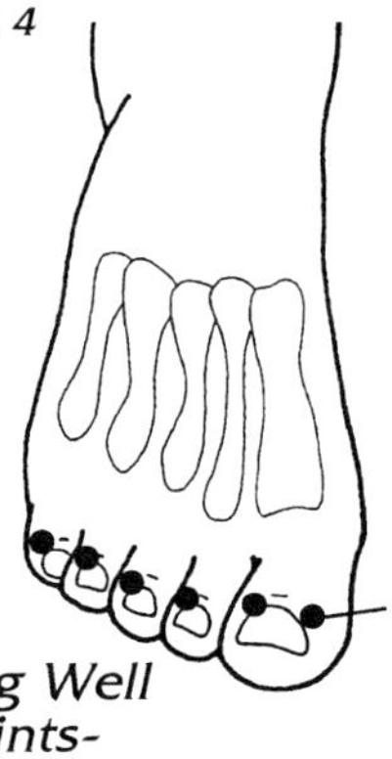

Jing Well Points
Located on outer side of the toenails at the base of the nail. *Fig. 4* *****Sp 1 - Key point***

Menstrual Cramps - PMS

For best results in treating menstrual cramps, sedate the following points once per day, 4 - 5 days prior to, and twice daily during periods. Include low back pain and jing well points on previous page for optimal relief.

Sp 6 3 fingers width above the inner ankle bone and behind the prominent shin bone. *Fig. 1*
Key point

K 3 In the hollow midway between the tip of the inner ankle bone and the Achilles tendon. *Fig. 1*

St 36 4 fingers width below the kneecap, and 1 fingers width to the outside of the shinbone. *Fig. 2*

Liv 3 On the top of the foot in the hollow between the 1st and 2nd toes, where the bones meet. *Fig. 2*

Sp 1 Located on outer side of the big toenail. (Also illustrated on previous page) . *Fig. 2*
Key point

Sp 15 4 thumbs width to ***each side*** of the belly button. *Fig. 3*

St 25 2 thumbs width to ***each side*** of the belly button. *Fig. 3*

Cv 6 On the midline, 2 fingers width directly ***below*** the belly button. *Fig. 3*

Cv 4 On the midline, 4 fingers width directly ***below*** the belly button. *Fig. 3*
Key point

Fig. 1

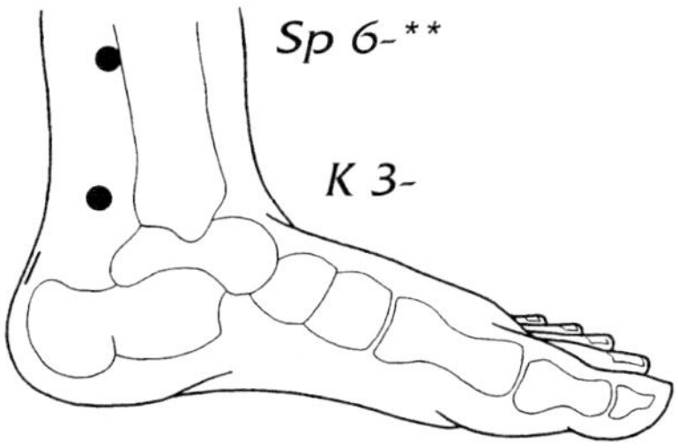

Fig. 2

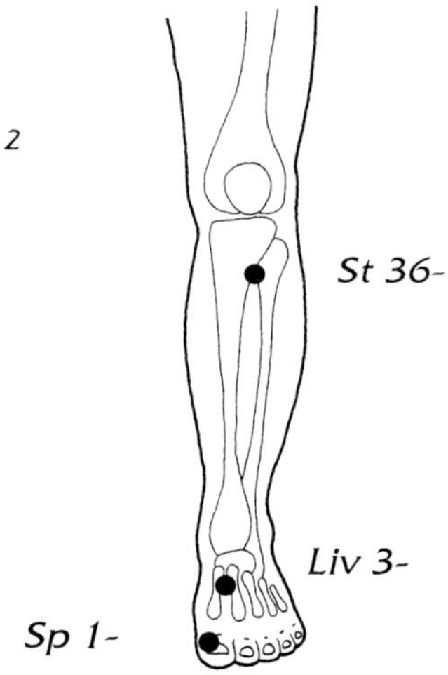

Fig. 3

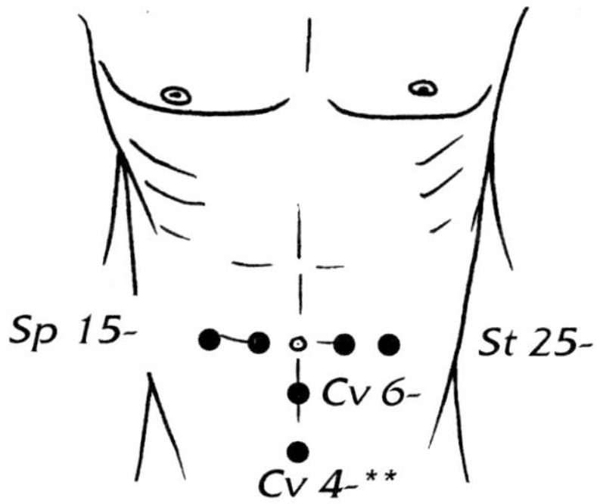

Metatarsalgia - continued next page

This is a very painful condition consisting of a burning pain under the ball of the foot. For chronic problems, sedate the lower back and calf muscles before sedating local points.

Back Shu Points:
Located 2 fingers width to each side of the spinal bones. ***Sedate these points from the lower back to the sacrum. Above points innervate the affected region(s) and often provide substantial relief to the patient.*** *Fig. 1*

Fig. 1

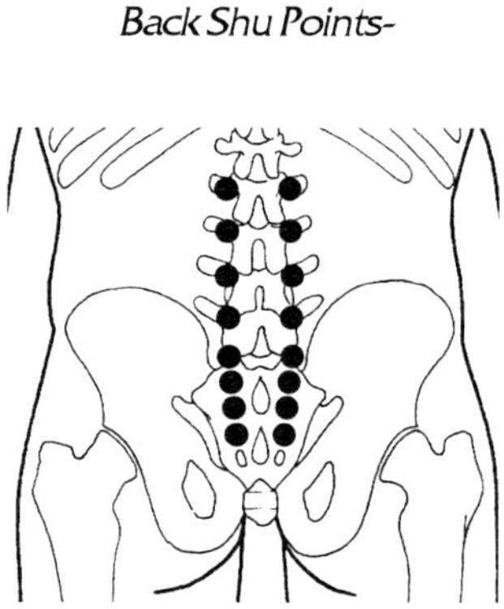

Piriformis Trigger Points:
Approximately half way between the sacrum (the triangular bone at the base of the spine) and the hip joint, or one hands width above GB 30. *Fig. 2*

Fig. 2

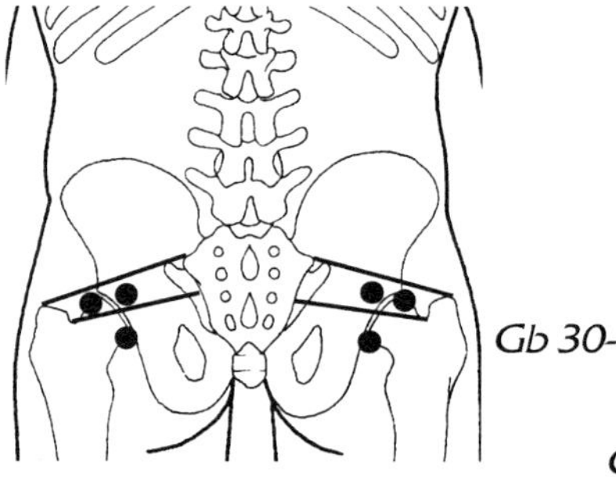

Gb 30 This point is directly in the middle of the each "cheek" equal distance from all sides. *Fig. 2*

Fig. 3

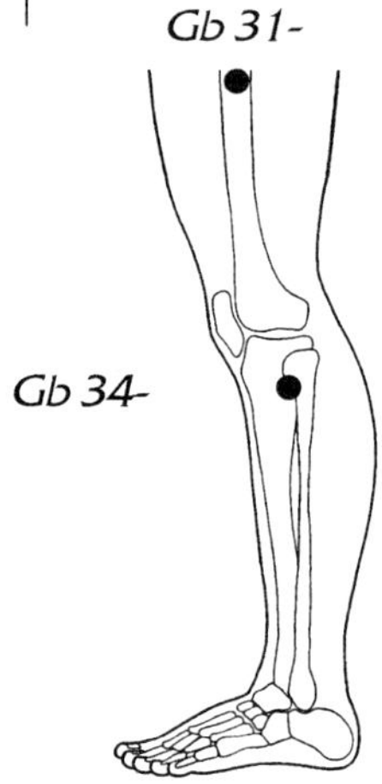

Gb 31 Standing erect with your hands laying the side of the thigh. This point is at the ***tip of the middle finger***. *Fig. 3*

Gb 34 4 fingers width below the outside of the kneecap, and just in front of and below the knobby head of the fibula bone. *Fig. 3*

Fig. 4

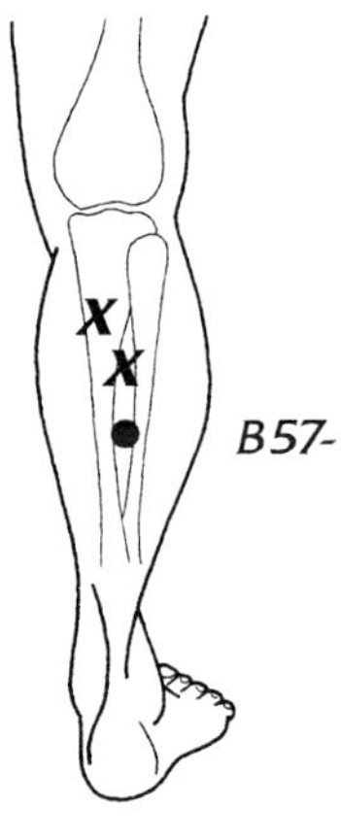

B 57 At the mid point of the calf where the calf muscle narrows to form the tendon, between the 2 calf muscles. *Fig. 4*

Metatarsalgia

***F**or enhanced relief, sedate the following points on top of the lower back and calf muscle points.*

Sp 6 3 fingers width above the inner ankle bone, located behind the prominent shin bone. ***Pressing against the shin bone will usually locate this tender point.*** *Fig. 1*

Sp 3 Just above the "Bunion" bone at the base of the big toe, ***at the junction of the red and white skin***. *Fig. 1*

Fig. 1

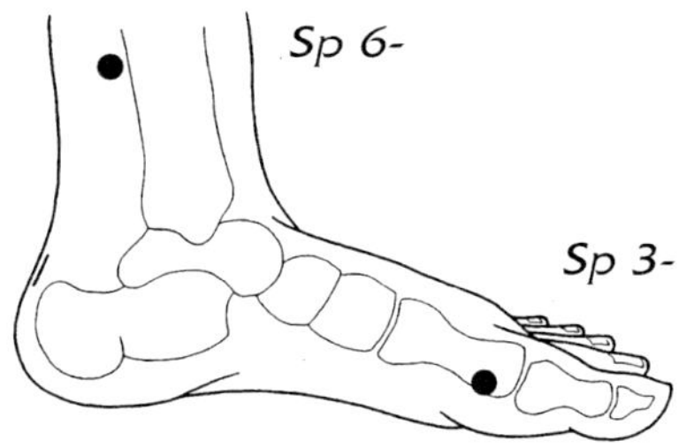

K 1 In the middle of the sole of the foot, between the ***inner and outer balls of the foot.*** *Fig. 2*

Fig. 2

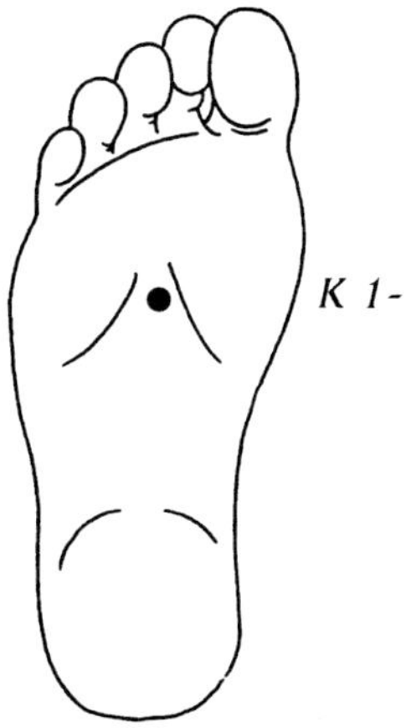

Gb 41 In the depression, immediately distal to the meeting of the bones of the 4th & 5th toes. *Fig. 3*

Liv 3 In the top of the foot, in the hollow formed where the 1st and 2nd toe bones meet. *Fig. 3*

Fig. 3

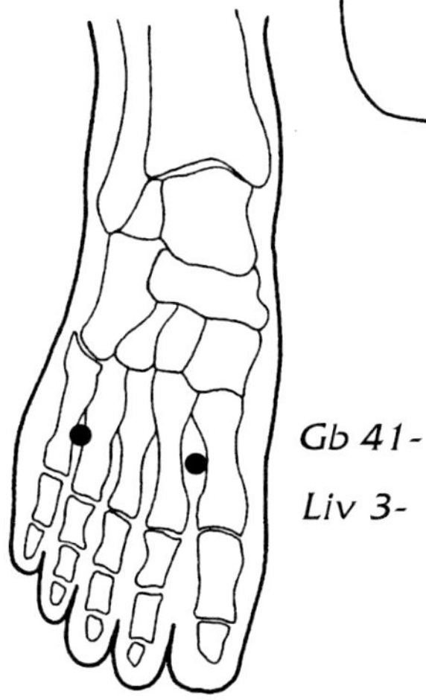

Web Points
In the web at the base of toes *Fig. 4*

Jing Well Points
At the outer base of the toe nails. Fig 4

Fig. 4

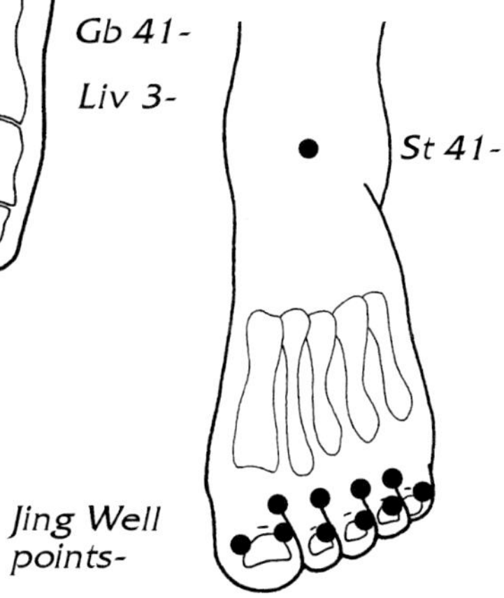

Migraine - continued next page

First, sedate H 9 & Liv 3 to calm the migraine down. Then, releasing the lower back muscles often provides relief to migraine patients. Local points next page.

H 9 At the inner/upper base of the little finger nail. *Fig. 1*
***** Key Point***

Liv 3 On the top of the foot in the hollow where the 1st and 2nd toe bones meet. *Fig. 2*
***** Key Point***

Back Shu Points:
Located 2 fingers width to each side of the spinal bones. ***Sedate from the waist level to the sacrum.*** *Fig. 3*

Piriformis Trigger Points:
Approximately half way between the sacrum (the triangular bone at the base of the spine) and the hip joint, or one hands width above GB 30. *Fig. 3*

Gb 30 This point is directly in the middle of the each buttocks half, equal distance from all sides. *Fig. 3*

Gb 31 Standing erect with your hands laying the side of the thigh. This point is at the ***tip of the middle finger***. *Fig. 4*

Gb 34 4 fingers width below the outside of the kneecap, and just in front of and below the knobby head of the fibula bone. *Fig. 4*

Gb 41 In the depression, where the 4th & 5th toe bones meet. *Fig. 5*

Fig. 1

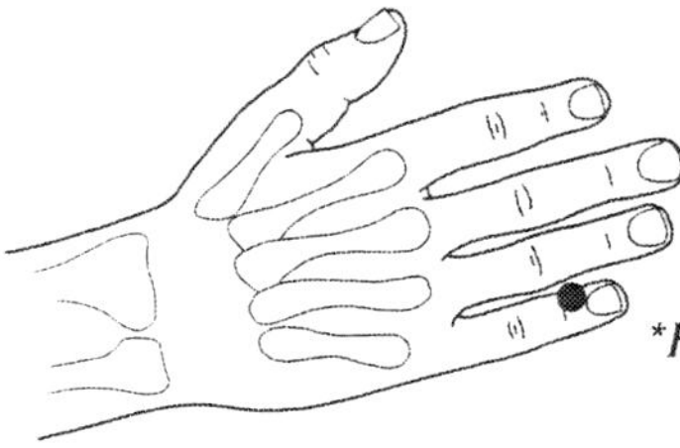

Fig. 2

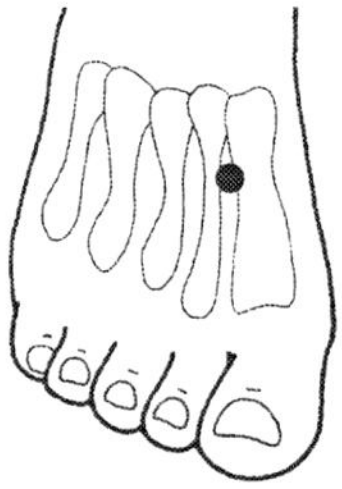

Fig. 3

Back Shu Points-

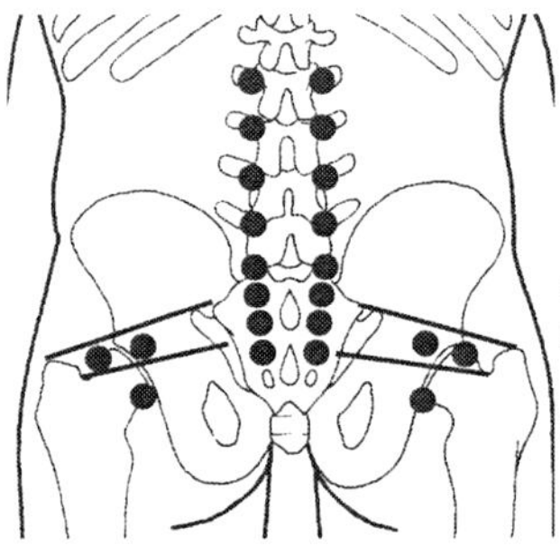

Fig. 4

Gb 31-

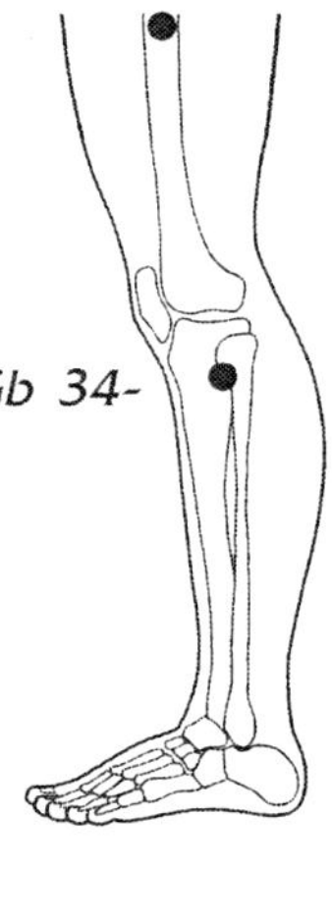

Fig. 5

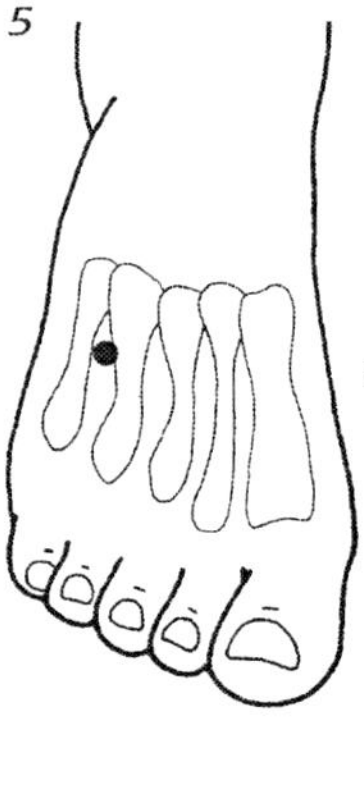

Migraine

***After sedating H 9, Liv 3** and the lower back points, assess for improvements. If required, sedate the following neck and local points for additional relief.*

Gb 20 2 fingers width outside each side of the spine below the base of the skull. Located in the hollow ***outside the muscles.*** *Fig. 1*

Gb 21 This lies halfway between the knob of bone at the base of the neck and the tip of the shoulder, in the fleshy mass of muscle. *Fig. 1*

Si 13 On the spine of the shoulder blade, half way between the outside of the shoulder and the spine. *Fig. 1*

Gv 20 Located on the midline of a line joining the tips of the ears, ***on the top of the head.*** *Fig. 2*

Extra 2

1 fingers width back from the outside of eye socket, in the hollow. *Fig. 2*

Tender Points

Stimulate these tender points located in the tight muscles at the side of the neck. *Fig. 2*

Si 17 Above the prominent neck muscle, ***at the level of the corner of the jaw.*** *Fig. 2*

Gv 14 Located 1 fingers width above the ***midpoint of the eyebrows, directly above the pupil.*** *Fig. 3*

Yintang

At the midpoint between the inner ends of the eyebrows. *Fig. 3*

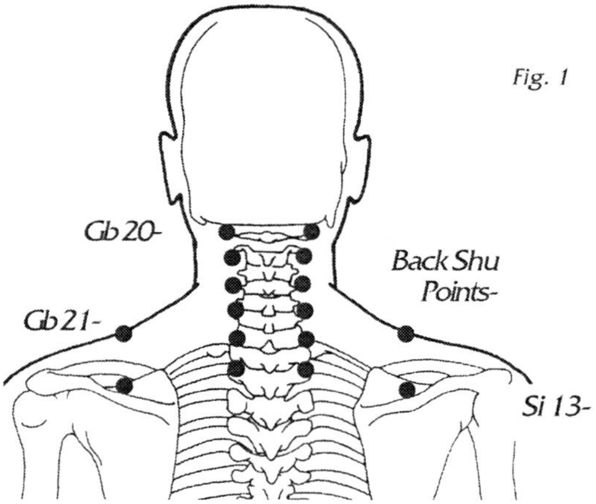

Fig. 1

Fig. 2

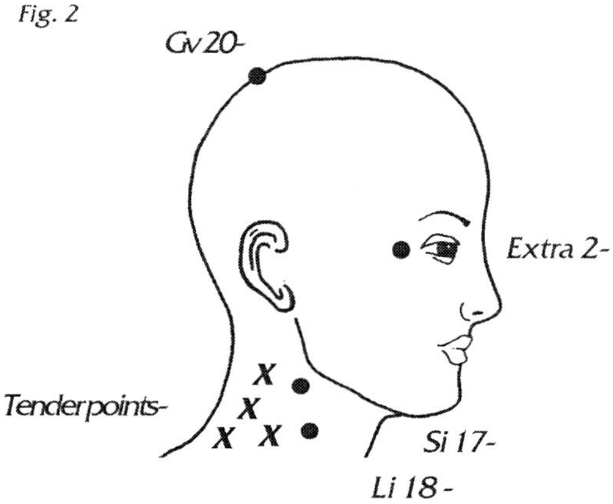

Fig. 3

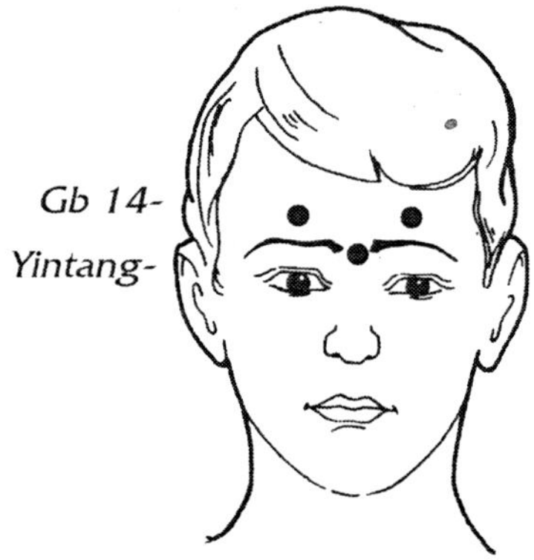

Multiple Sclerosis - continued

The following points have been successfully used to calm the autonomic nervous system (ANS). This response calms the patients, and these points have prove beneficial to Multiple Sclerosis patients.

Lu 9 In the groove at the thumb side of the wrist crease, and inside of the tendon. *Fig. 1*

H 7 On the little finger side of the wrist crease, to the inside of the tendon. *Fig. 1*

P 6 3 fingers width from the most distal wrist crease, in between the tendons. *Fig. 1*

Sp 6 3 fingers width above the inner ankle and just behind the prominent shin bone. *Fig. 2*

K 3 Halfway between the Achilles tendon and the inner ankle bone. *Fig. 2*

B 62 In the depression half a finger below the outer ankle bone. *Fig. 3*

Cv 17 On the breast bone at the heart level or the 4th rib space. Tender when pressed. *Fig. 4*

Fig. 1

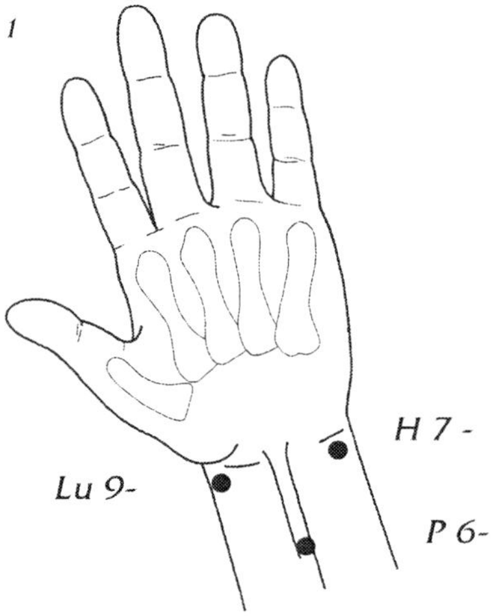

Fig. 2

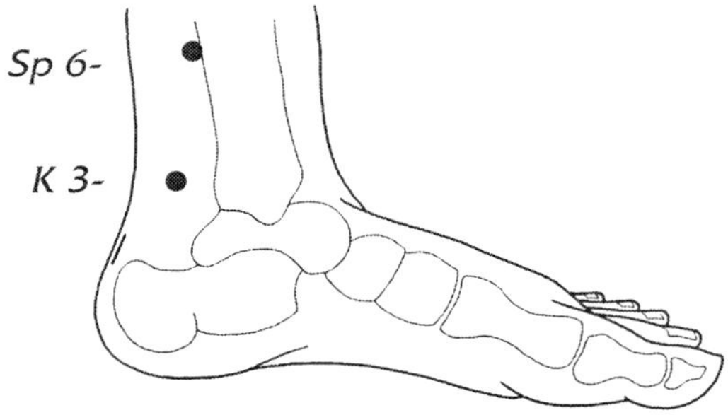

Fig. 4

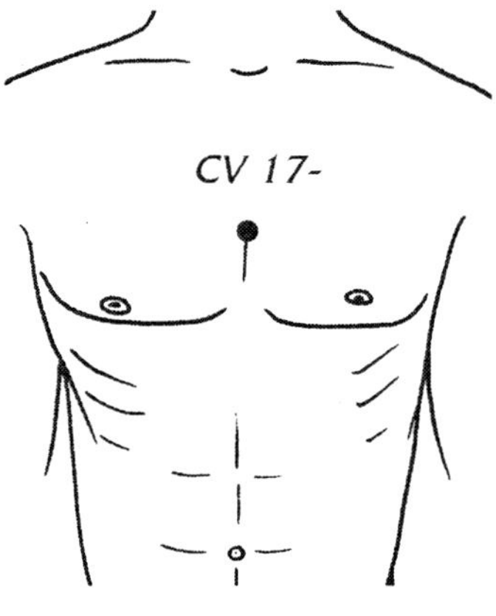

Fig. 3

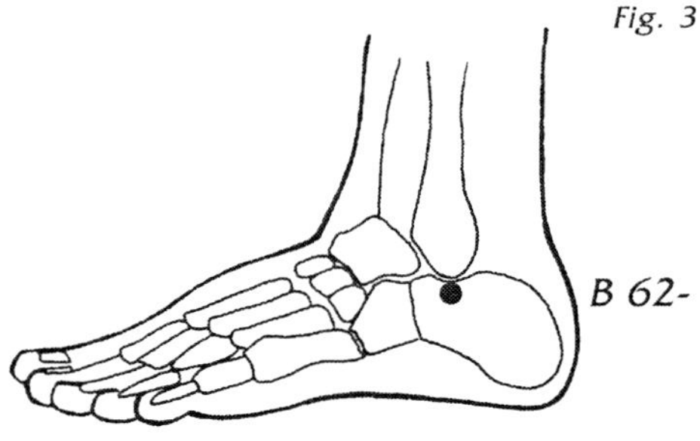

Multiple Sclerosis

***MS** is a slowly progressive neuro-degenerative disorder. Symptoms include loss of motor functions and numbness along the limbs and throughout the body. Often the eyes are targeted. After sedating the calming points, release the muscles beside the spine. For additional points, contact our toll-free number **1-(800)-567-7246** and ask for the attending therapist.*

Gb 21 This lies halfway between the bone at the base of the neck and the tip of the shoulder, directly on top of the trapezius (shoulder) muscle. *Fig. 1*

Back Shu Points:
Located 2 fingers width to each side of the spinal bones. ***Sedate these points from the lower back to the sacrum.****Fig. 1*

Gb 30 This point is directly in the middle of the each "cheek" equal distance from all sides. *Fig. 2*

Piriformis Trigger Points:
Approximately half way between the sacrum (the triangular bone at the base of the spine) and the hip joint, or one hands width above GB 30. *Fig. 1*

For MS associated eye problems

B 1 Just above the ***inner*** corner of the eye. *Fig. 2*

B 2 At the ***inner*** end of the eyebrow, in the depression. *Fig. 2*

Extra 2 1 fingers width ***behind*** the outside of the eye socket, ***in the hollow***. *Fig. 2*

Fig. 1

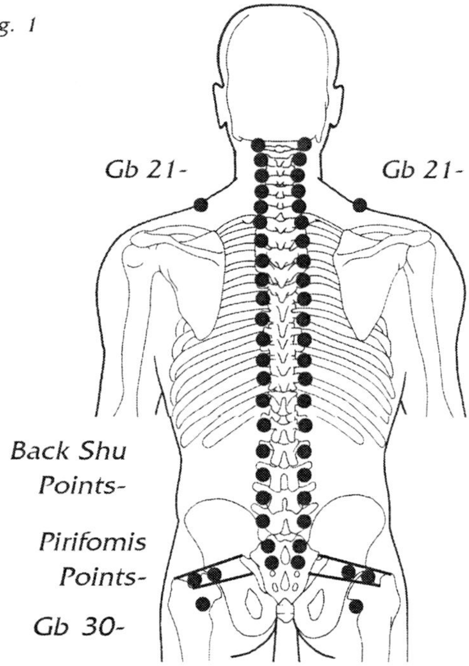

Fig. 2

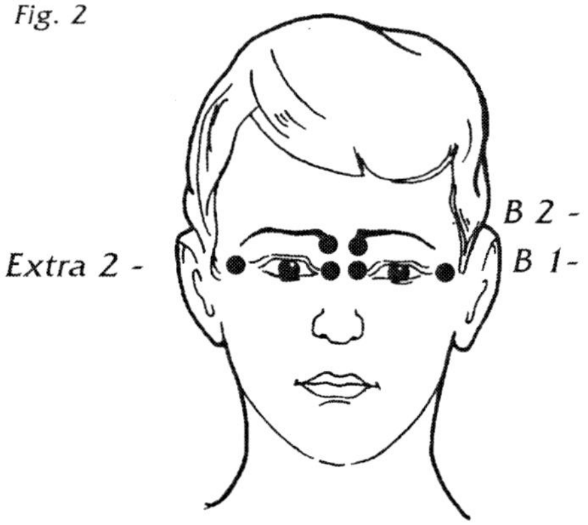

Muscle Cramps - continued next page

A cramp or, "charley horse", often produces sudden and intense pain, usually located in the calf or lower leg region. Start with the lower back region then follow up with the Jing Well Points. For additional relief, see the next page.

Back Shu Points:

Located 2 fingers width to each side of the spinal bones. ***Sedate these points from the lower back to the sacrum. Above points innervate the affected region(s) and often provide substantial relief to the patient.*** *Fig. 1*

Fig. 1

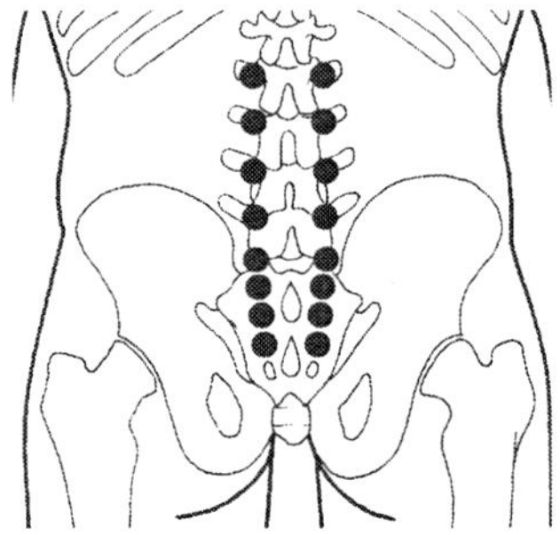

Piriformis Trigger Points:

Approximately half way between the sacrum (the triangular bone at the base of the spine) and the hip joint, or one hands width above GB 30. *Fig. 2*

Fig. 2

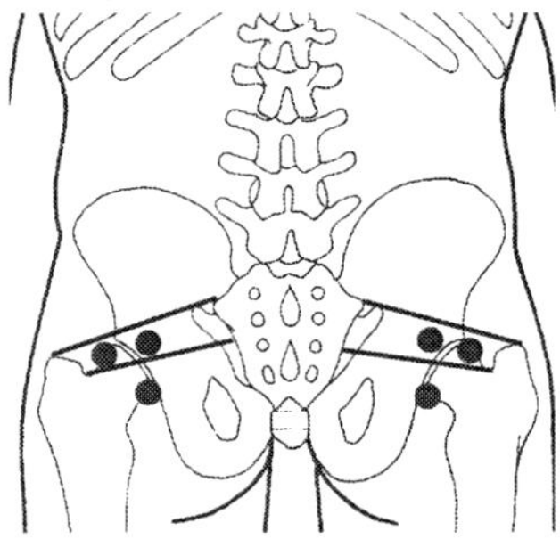

Gb 30 This point is directly in the middle of the each "cheek" equal distance from all sides. *Fig. 2*

Gb 31 Standing erect with your hands laying the side of the thigh. This point is at the ***tip of the middle finger***. *Fig. 3*

Gb 34 4 fingers width below the outside of the kneecap, and just in front of and below the knobby head of the fibula bone. *Fig. 3* ** - ***Key Point***

Fig. 3

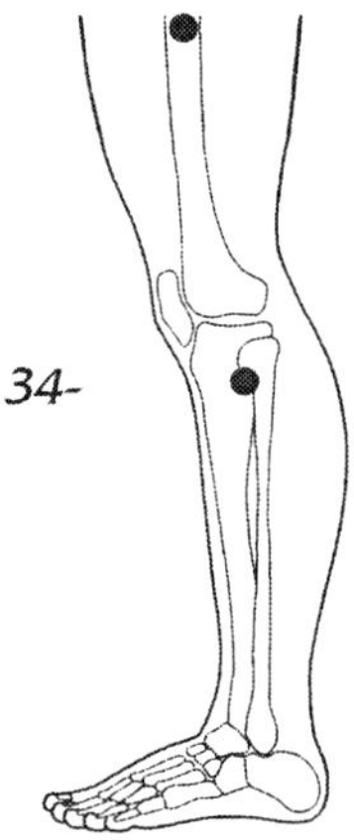

Gb 41 In the depression, where the 4th & 5th toe bones meet. *Fig. 4*

Jing Well Points

Located on each side of the toenails at the base of the nail. *Fig. 4*

Fig. 4

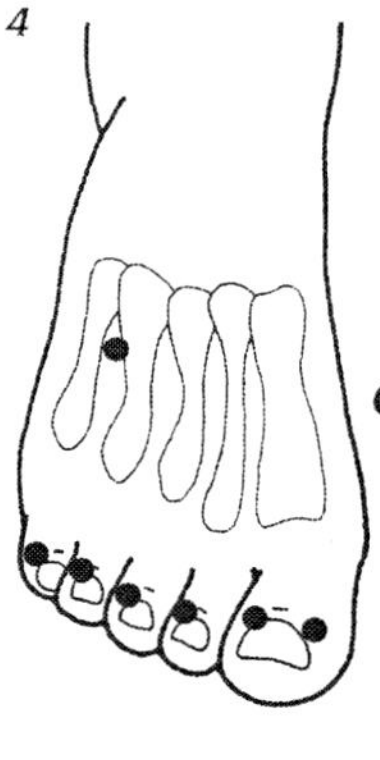

Muscle Cramps

***F**or specific muscle sprain/strains of a particular joint, refer to the index. For general muscle cramping **sedate the points illustrated on** corresponding page on top of the following points.*

Gb 31 Stand erect, hands flat along the side of the thigh. ***This point is at the tip of the middle finger***. *Fig. 1*

Gb 34 4 fingers width below the outside of the knee and just in front of and below the knobby head of the fibula bone. *Fig. 1*
** - ***Key Point***

Fig. 1

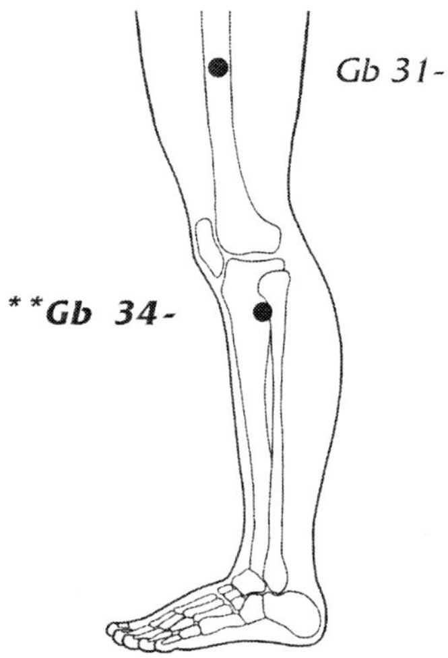

Li 11 At the outer end of the elbow crease with the arm slightly bent. *Fig. 2*

Li 4 This point is located in the fleshy mass between the thumb and index finger, closer to the index finger bone. *Fig. 2*

Fig. 2

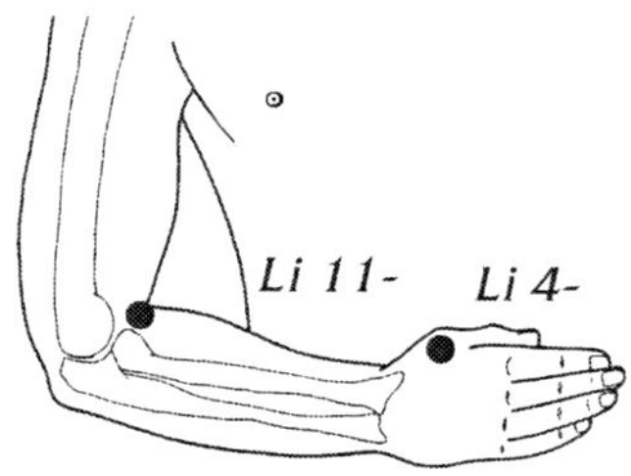

Sp 10 2 thumbs width above the upper/inner side of the knee cap. ***This tender spot is at the highest point of the inner thigh muscle***. *Fig. 3*

Sp 9 3 fingers width below the inner knee cap in the depression between the bone and the calf muscle. *Fig. 3*

Sp 6 3 fingers width above the inner ankle and behind the prominent shin bone *Fig. 3*

Fig. 3

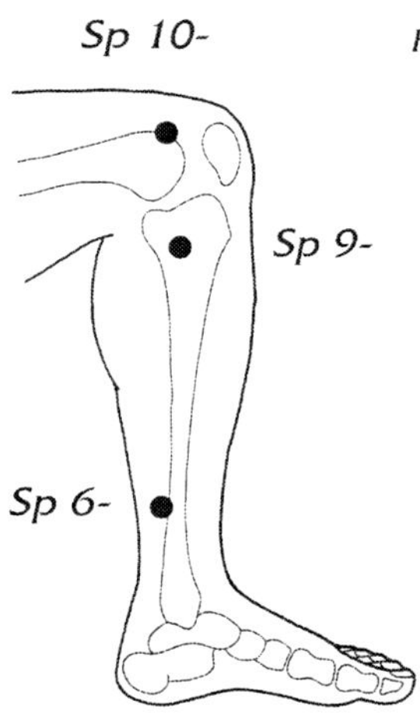

Muscle - Strain - continued next page

A cramp or, "charley horse", often produces sudden and intense pain, usually located in the calf or lower leg region. Start with the lower back region then follow up with the Jing Well Points. For additional relief, see the next page.

Back Shu Points:
Located 2 fingers width to each side of the spinal bones. ***Sedate these points from the lower back to the sacrum. Above points innervate the affected region(s) and often provide substantial relief to the patient.*** *Fig. 1*

Piriformis Trigger Points:
Approximately half way between the sacrum (the triangular bone at the base of the spine) and the hip joint, or one hands width above GB 30. *Fig. 2*

Gb 30 This point is directly in the middle of the each "cheek" equal distance from all sides. *Fig. 2*

Gb 31 Standing erect with your hands laying the side of the thigh. This point is at the ***tip of the middle finger***. *Fig. 3*

Gb 34 4 fingers width below the outside of the kneecap, and just in front of and below the knobby head of the fibula bone. *Fig. 3* ** - ***Key Point***

Gb 41 In the depression, where the 4th & 5th toe bones meet. *Fig. 4*

Jing Well Points
Located on each side of the toenails at the base of the nail. *Fig. 4*

Fig. 1

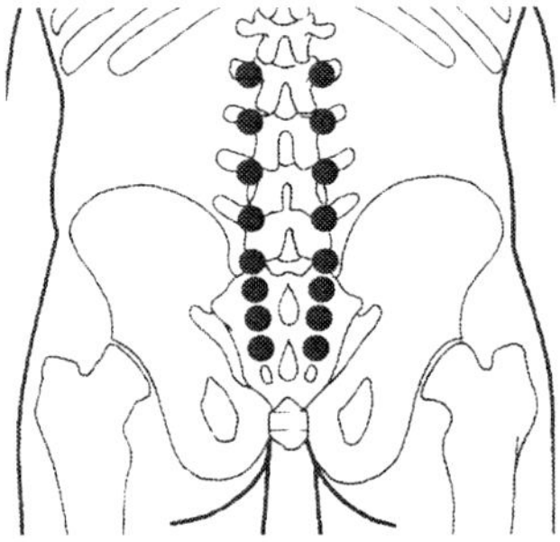

Fig. 2

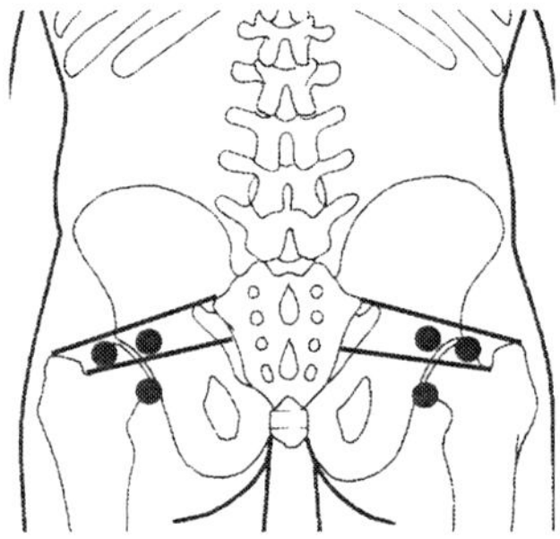

Fig. 3

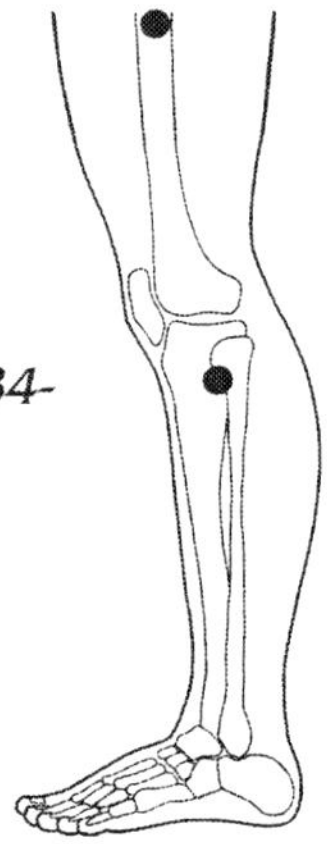

Fig. 4

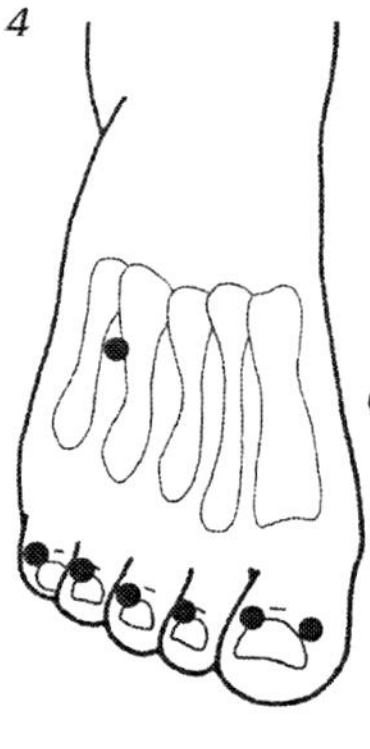

Muscle - Strain

***F**or specific muscle sprain/strains of a particular joint, refer to the index. For general muscle cramping **sedate the points illustrated on** the previous page along with the following points.*

Gb 31 Stand erect, hands flat along the side of the thigh. ***This point is at the tip of the middle finger.*** *Fig. 1*

Fig. 1

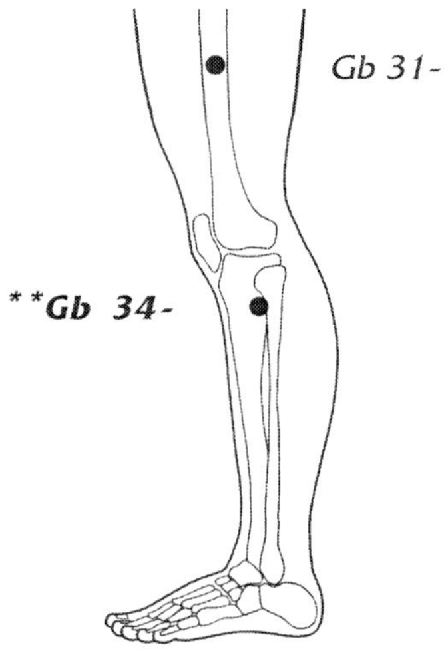

<u>Excellent post exercise point</u>

Gb 34 4 fingers width below the outside of the knee and just in front of and below the knobby head of the fibula bone. *Fig. 1*

** - ***Key Point***

Li 11 At the outer end of the elbow crease with the arm slightly bent. *Fig. 2*

Li 4 This point is located in the fleshy mass between the thumb and index finger, closer to the index finger bone. *Fig. 2*

Fig. 2

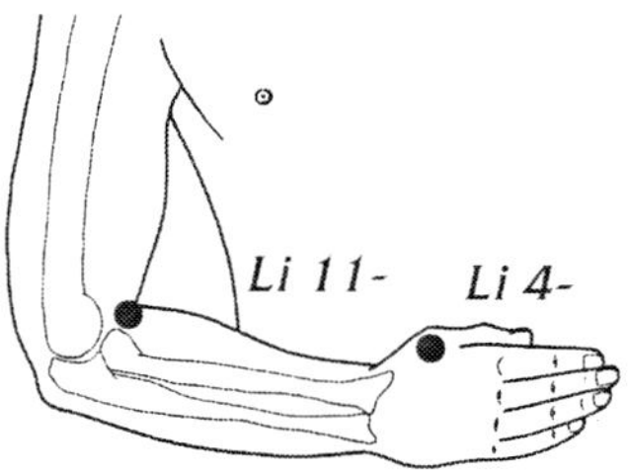

Sp 10 2 thumbs width above the upper/inner side of the knee cap. ***This tender spot is at the highest point of the inner thigh muscle.*** *Fig. 3*

Fig. 3

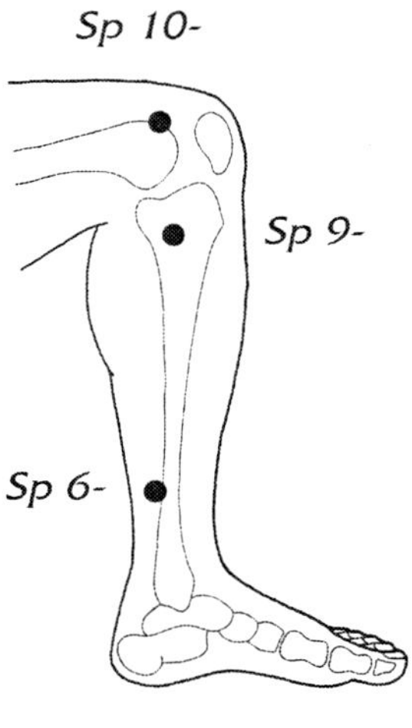

Sp 9 3 fingers width below the inner knee cap in the depression between the bone and the calf muscle. *Fig. 3*

Sp 6 3 fingers width above the inner ankle and behind the prominent shin bone *Fig. 3*

Nausea - continued next page

*It has been well documented that the following points are effective in reducing the symptoms of nausea. Sedate the following points for relief, with emphasis on **P 6.** If the condition is acute, repeat several times per day.*

<u>Key acupuncture point for nausea*</u>

P 6* 3 fingers width from the most distal wrist crease, inbetween the tendons. *Fig. 1*

Fig. 1

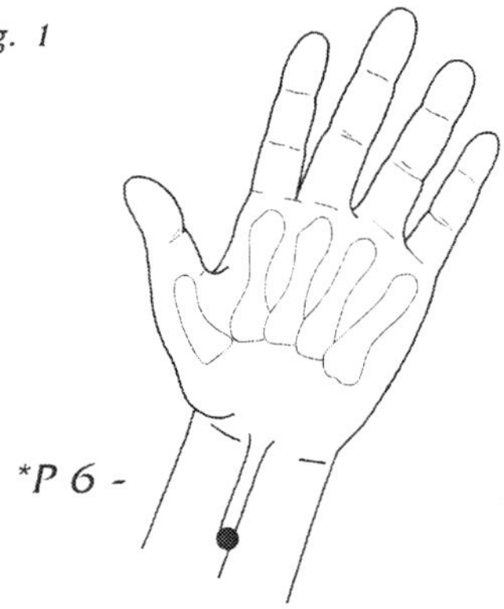

St 34 Located 2 thumbs width above the upper/outer corner of your knee cap. ***This point is usually tender when pressed.*** *Fig. 2*

St 36 4 fingers width below the kneecap and 1 fingers width to the outside of the shin bone. *Fig. 2*

St 37 4 fingers width below ***St 36*** and 1 fingers width to the outside of the shin bone. *Fig. 2*

Fig. 2

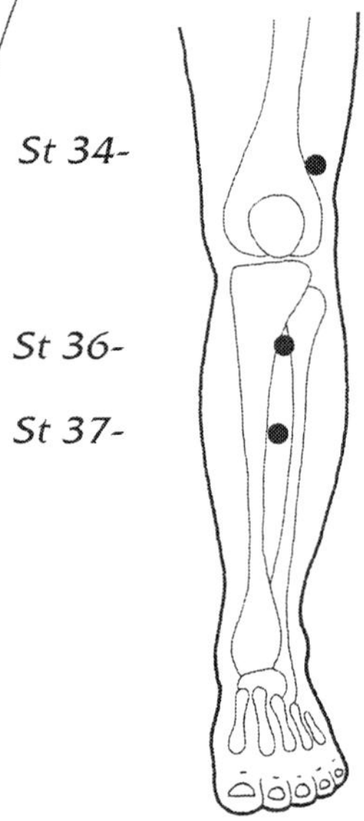

Cv 12 This lies on the midline, halfway between the lower breast bone and the belly button. *Fig. 3*

St 25 Located 2 fingers width to each side of the belly button. *Fig. 3*

Fig. 3

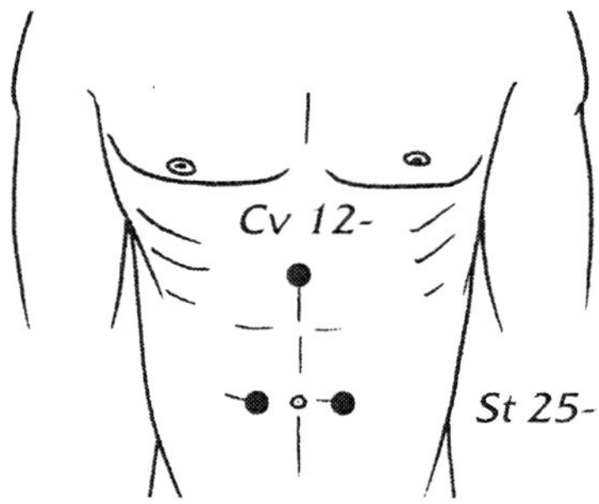

Nausea

Back Shu Points:

Located 2 fingers width to each side of the spinal bones. ***Sedate these points from the middle to the lower back. Middle of the back innervates Spleen and Stomach, and often provide substantial relief to nausea patients.*** *Fig. 1*

Fig. 1

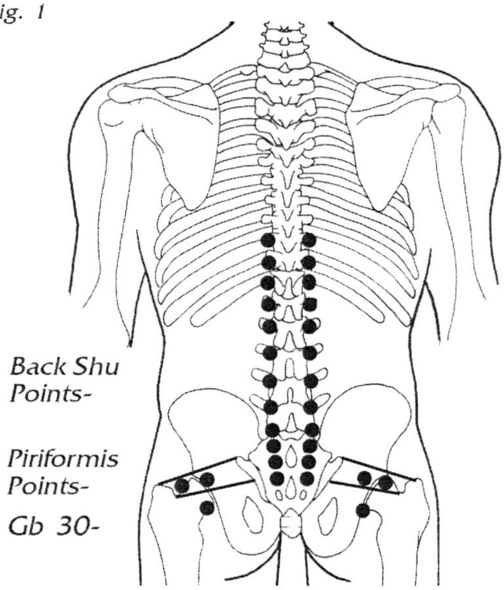

Piriformis Trigger Points:

Approximately half way between the sacrum (the triangular bone at the base of the spine) and the outside hip joint. Or, one hands width above GB 30. Press and rub (palpate) the general area until tenderness is detected. *Fig.*

Fig. 2

Sp 4 At the base of the "bunion" bone (opposite to the bunion) at the junction of the pigment change of skin. *Fig. 2*

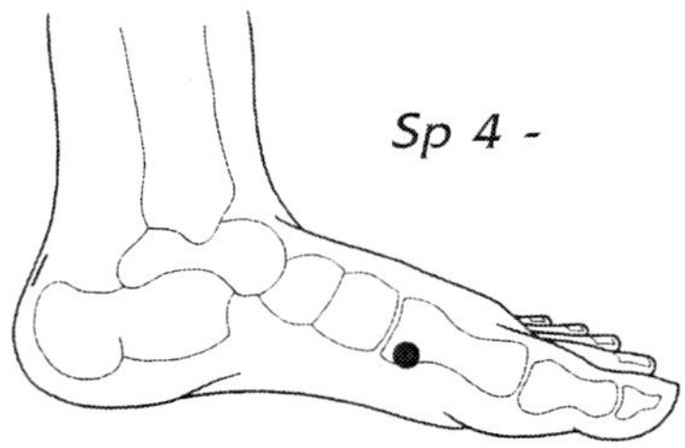

Gb 41 In the depression, where the 4th & 5th toe bones meet. *Fig. 3*

Tw 1 On the "baby" finger side base of the ring finger nail. *Fig. 4*

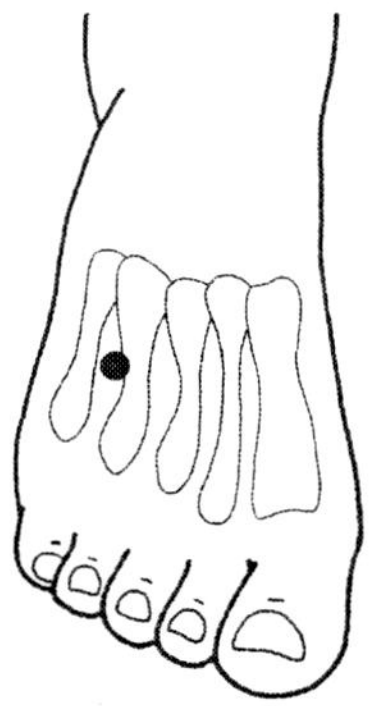

Fig. 3

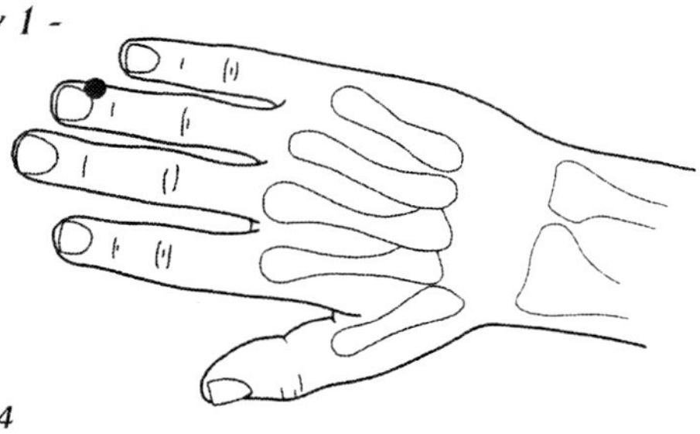

Fig. 4

Neck Pain - continued next page

***N**eck tension & pain are often caused by traumatic injury or repetitive strain for long periods of time. The following lower back points often relax tired muscles in the neck for relief. For additional points see next page.*

Si 3 On the end of the main transverse crease of the hand. ***Best located with the fist clenched***. *Fig. 1*

Fig. 1

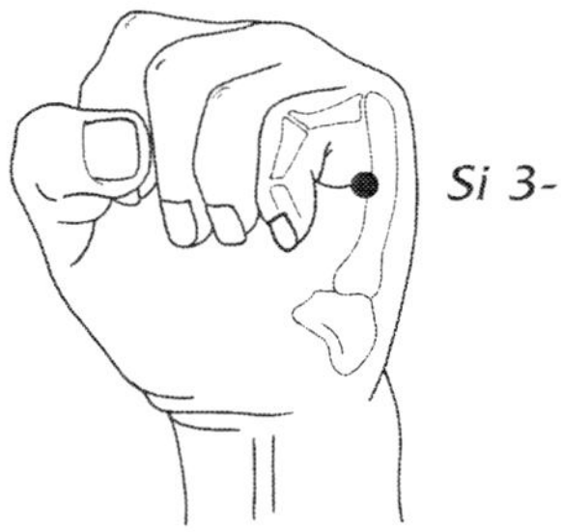

Gb 41 In the depression, where the 4th & 5th toe bones meet. *Fig.2*

Tw 3 In between the 4th and 5th carpal bones, 2 fingers proximal from the 4th and 5th knuckles. *Fig.3*

Fig. 2

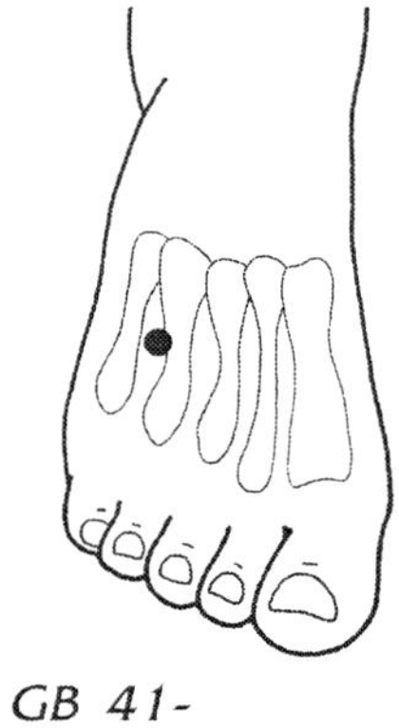

Gb 38 In front of the fibula bone, 4 fingers and 1 thumb width above the outer ankle bone. *Fig.2*

Fig. 4

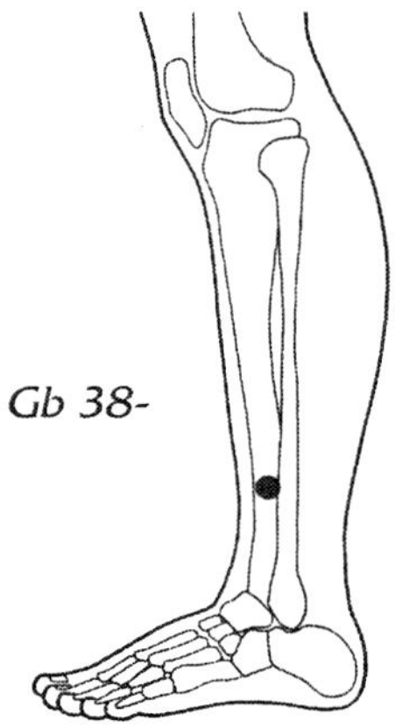

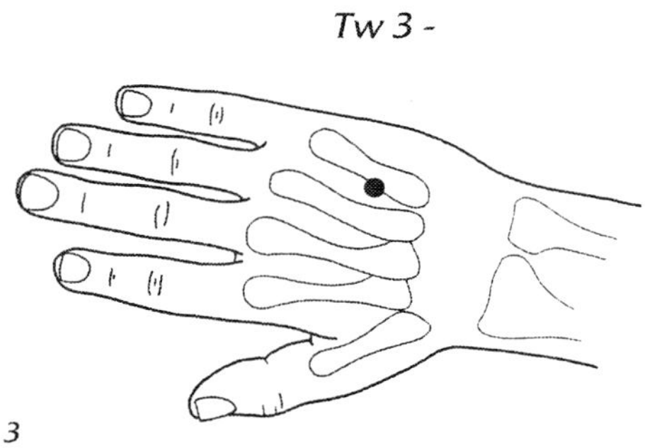

Fig. 3

Neck Pain

The following local points should release combined with the lower back points should provide relief to neck pain patients.

Gb 20 Below the base of the skull, in the hollow just outside the main spinal muscles of neck. *Fig. 1*

B 10 Located 2 fingers width from the middle of the spine at the level of the natural hairline at the back of the neck. ***In the middle of the ropy muscles on each side of the spine.*** *Fig. 1*

Gb 21 This lies halfway between the bone at the base of the neck and the tip of the shoulder, directly on top of the trapezius (shoulder) muscle. *Fig. 1*

Tw 15 1 thumbs width ***below Gb 21.*** *Fig. 1*

Si 13 4 fingers width ***below GB 21*** just on top of the spine of the shoulder blade. *Fig. 1*

Tender Points
Stimulate these tender points located in the tight muscles at the side of the neck. *Fig. 2*

Si 17 Above the prominent neck muscle, ***at the level of the corner of the jaw.*** *Fig. 2*

Li 18 4 fingers width beside the highest point of the Adam's apple in the prominent muscle at the side of the neck ***(below the corner of the jaw).*** *Fig. 2*

Fig. 1

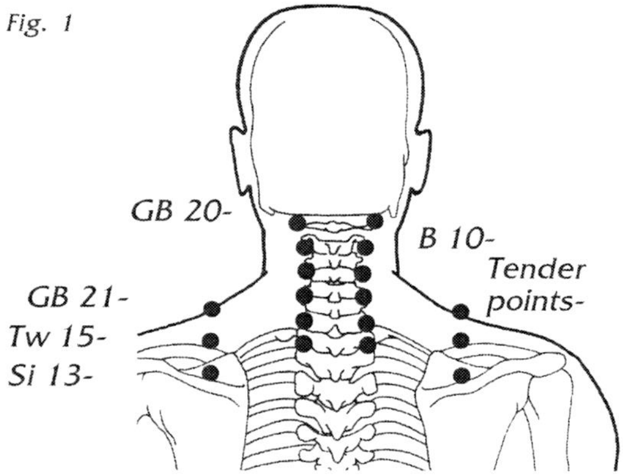

Fig. 2

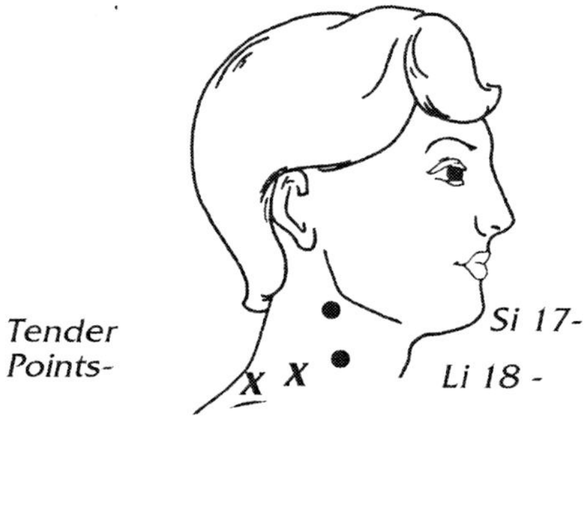

Fig. 3

Osteoarthritis - Knee

Consult a Doctor before treating any points. For chronic conditions, stimulate at the points on this page first. The distal and local points on the following page may be used after the below points. Sedate points for maximum relief.

Back Shu Points:

Located 2 fingers width to each side of the spinal bones. ***Sedate these points from the middle to the lower back. Above points innervate the affected region and often provide substantial relief.*** *Fig. 1*

Fig. 1

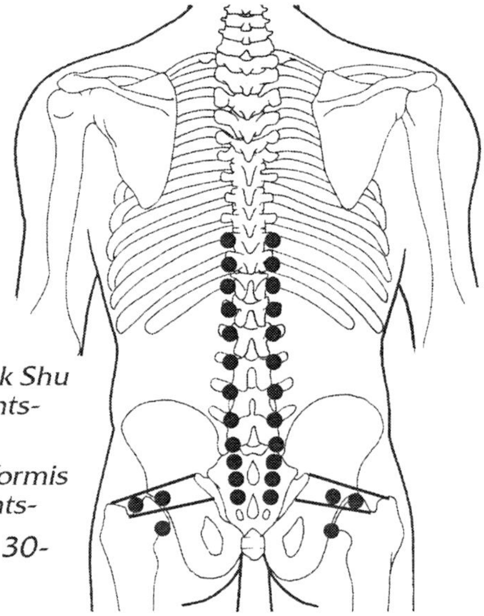

Piriformis Trigger Points:

Approximately half way between the sacrum (the triangular bone at the base of the spine) and the outside hip joint. Or, one hands width above GB 30. Press and rub (palpate) the general area until tenderness is detected. *Fig. 2*

Gb 30 This point is directly in the middle of the each buttocks half, equal distance from all sides. *Fig. 2*

Fig. 2

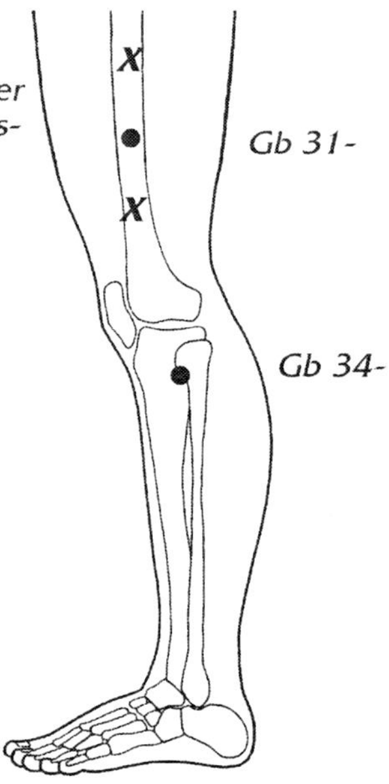

Tender Points

Stimulate these tender points located in the tight muscles at the side of the leg. *Fig. 2*

Gb 31 Stand erect, hands flat along the side of the thigh. This point is at the ***tip of the middle finger***. *Fig. 3*

Gb 34 4 fingers width below the outside of the kneecap, and just in front of and below the knobby head of the fibula bone. *Fig. 3*

Osteoarthritis Knee

***R**elax the muscles above the knee by stimulating the tender points (x), before treating the local and distal points.*

B 40 On the middle of the crease behind the knee. *Fig. 1*

Sp 10 In the belly of the muscle 2 fingers from the upper/inner border of the knee cap. *Fig. 2*

St 34 In the belly of the muscle 2 fingers from the upper/outer border of the knee cap. *Fig. 2*

Extra 31
On the midpoint of the ***upper border*** of the kneecap. *Fig. 2*

Extra 32
On the depression on the ***inner*** side of the kneecap. *Fig. 2*

St 35 In the depression to the ***outer*** side of the kneecap. *Fig. 2*

St 36 4 fingers width below the kneecap, and 1 fingers width to the ***outside*** of the shinbone. *Fig. 2*

Liv 3 In the hollow between the first and second toes, where the bones merge on top of the foot. *Fig. 2*

Liv 8 On the inner end of the knee crease, between the 2 tendons ***which become prominent when the knee is bent.*** *Fig. 3*

Sp 9 On the inside of the leg 3 fingers width below the kneecap, ***in the depression of the inner knee bone.*** *Fig. 3*

Sp 6 3 fingers width above the inner ankle and ***just behind the prominent shin bone.*** *Fig. 3*

Fig. 1

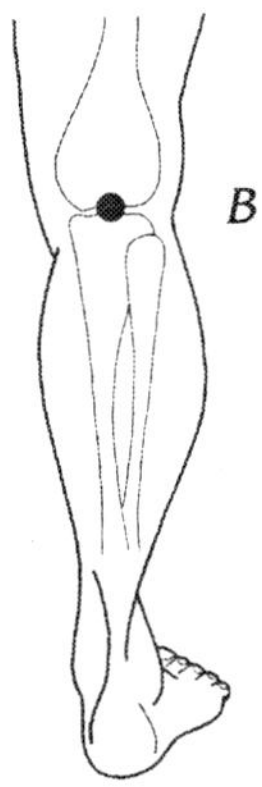

Fig. 2

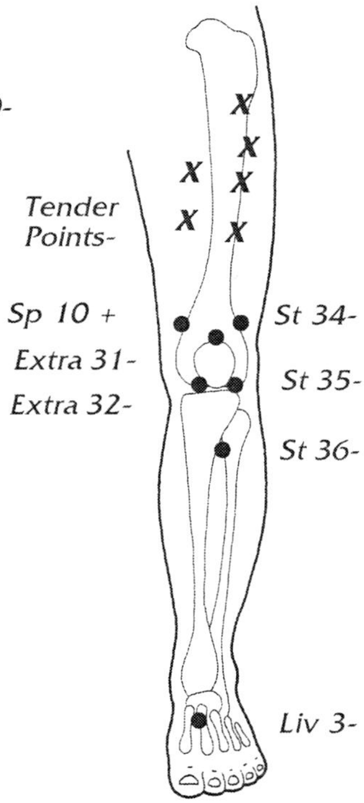

Fig. 3

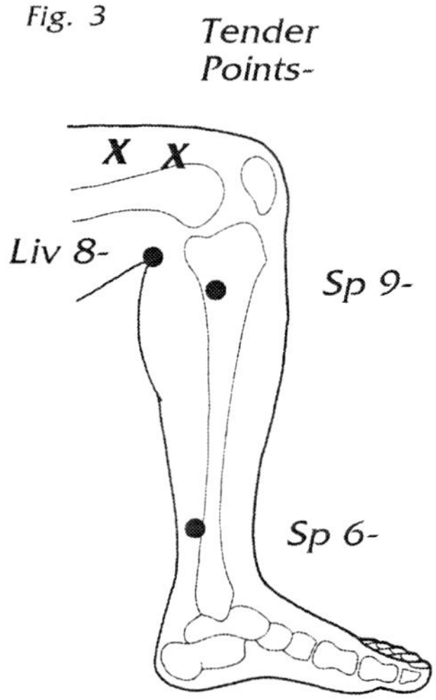

Parasympathetic - Calming

The following points have been successfully used to calm the autonomic nervous system (ANS). This response calms the patients, and these points are often sedated prior to the use of any other points throughout the book.

Lu 9 In the groove at the thumb side of the wrist crease, and inside of the tendon. *Fig. 1*

H 7 On the little finger side of the wrist crease, to the inside of the tendon. *Fig. 1*

P 6 3 fingers width from the most distal wrist crease, in between the tendons. *Fig. 1*

Sp 6 3 fingers width above the inner ankle and just behind the prominent shin bone. *Fig. 2*

K 3 Halfway between the Achilles tendon and the inner ankle bone. *Fig. 2*

Gv 20 In the middle of the top of the head, halfway between the ears. *Fig. 3*

B 62 In the depression half a finger below the outer ankle bone. *Fig. 4*

Cv 17 On the breast bone at the heart level or the 4th rib space. Tender when pressed. *Fig. 5*

Fig. 1

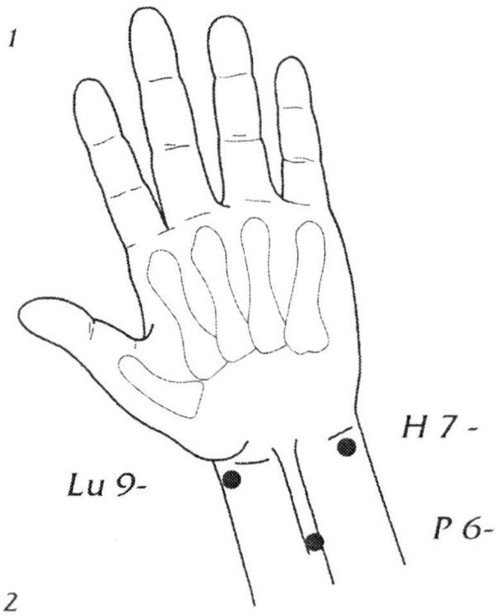

Fig. 2

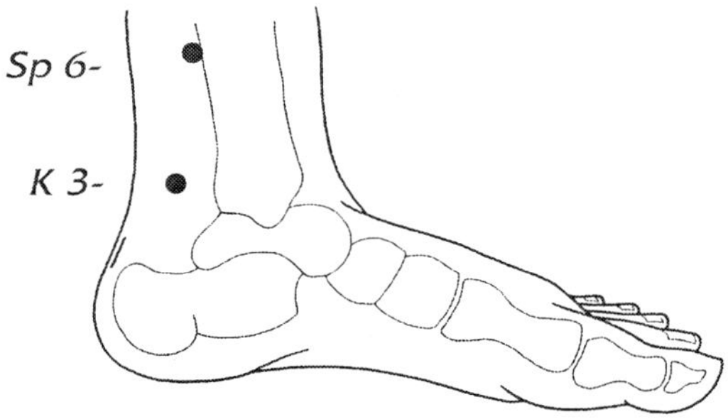

Fig. 3

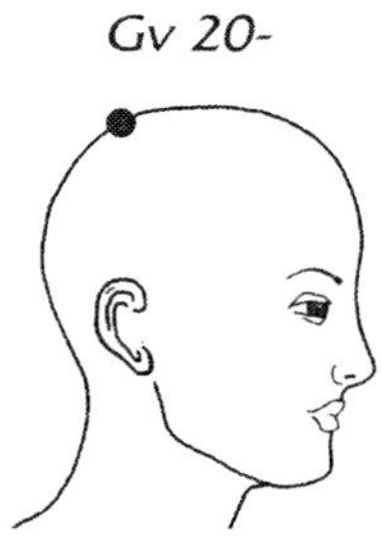

Fig. 4

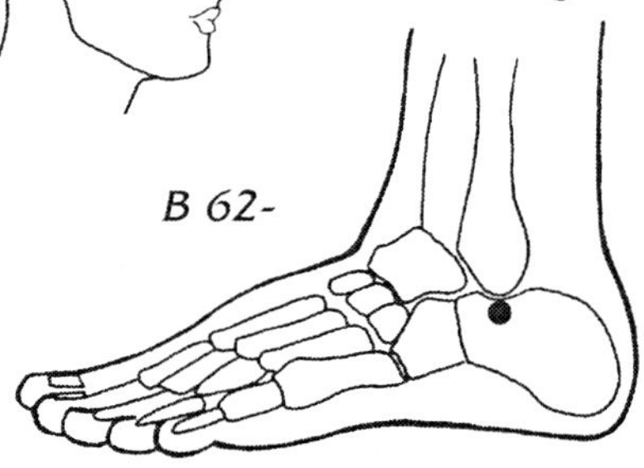

Fig. 5

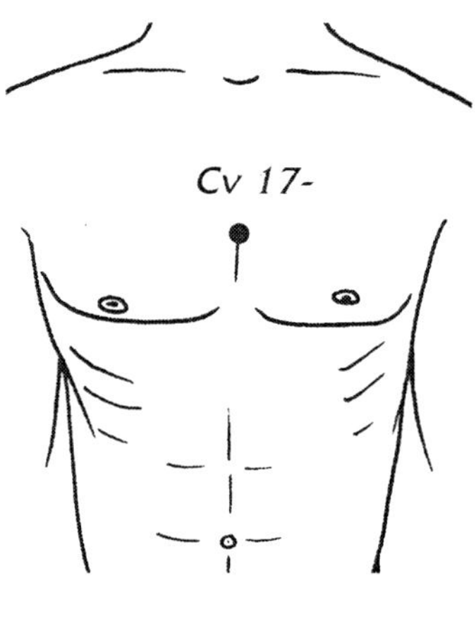

Pelvic Pain

***C**onsult a Doctor before initiating treatment to ensure proper diagnosis. For optimal relief, sedate the distal points in the feet and legs before sedating points in the abdomen.*

Cv 12 On the midline, midway between the belly button and the lower end of the breast bone. *Fig. 1*

St 25 2 thumbs width ***to each side*** of the belly button. *Fig. 1*

Sp 15 4 thumbs width ***to each side*** of the belly button. *Fig. 1*

Cv 6 In the midline, 2 fingers width directly below the belly button. *Fig. 1*

St 36 4 fingers width below the kneecap, and 1fingers width to the outside of the shin bone. *Fig. 2*

Liv 3 On the top of the foot in the hollow between the 1st and 2nd toes, where the bones meet. *Fig. 3*

Jing Well Points
At the outer base of the finger nails. *Fig. 3*

St 44 At meeting of the base of 2nd and 3rd toes in between the web. *Fig. 3*

Sp 6 3 fingers width above the inner ankle and just behind the prominent leg bone. ***Pressing firmly in this area will locate this tender point.*** *Fig. 4*

Fig. 1

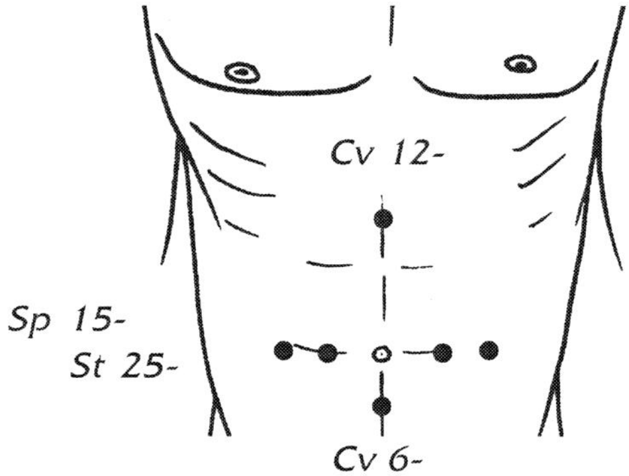

Fig. 2

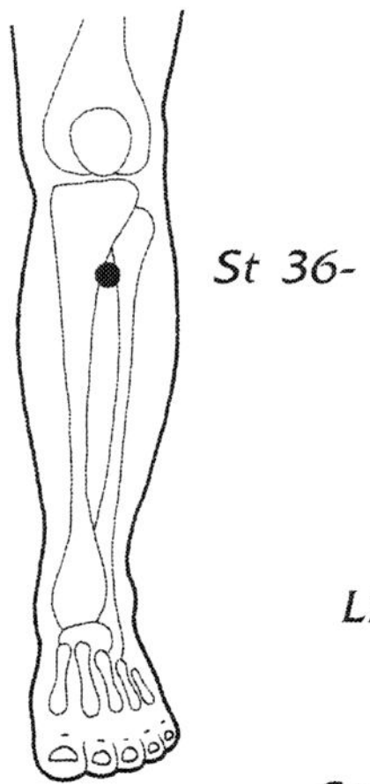

Fig. 3

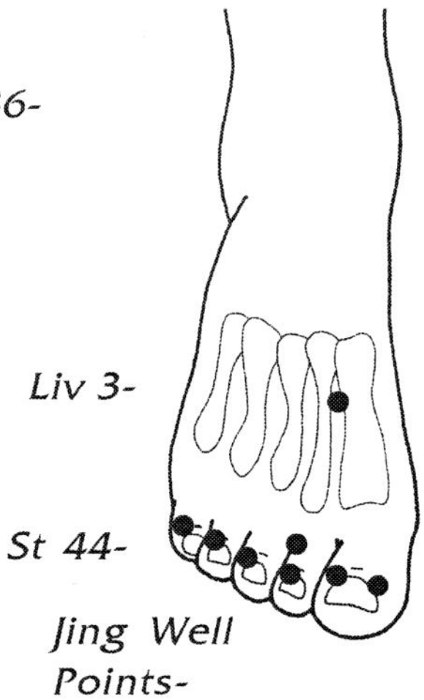

Fig. 4

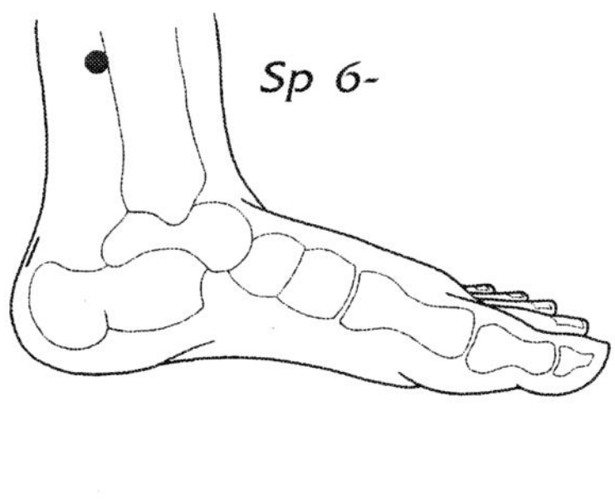

Peripheral Neuropathy (feet)

Peripheral Neuropathy is a lifestyle disorder causing pain, swelling, burning, and temperature changes of the extremities. For relief of this condition, sedate the following points. Also sedate parasymapthic points on ***page 116.***

Back Shu Points

Located 2 fingers width to each side of the spinal bones. ***Sedate these points from the lower back to the sacrum. Above points often provide substantial relief to the patient.*** *Fig. 1*

Piriformis Trigger Points

Approximately half way between the sacrum (the triangular bone at the base of the spine) and the hip joint, or one hands width above GB 30. *Fig. 2*

Gb 30 This point is directly in the middle of the each buttocks half, equal distance from all sides. *Fig. 2*

Gb 31 Standing erect with your hands laying the side of the thigh. This point is at the ***tip of the middle finger***. *Fig. 3*

Gb 34 4 fingers width below the outside of the kneecap, and just in front of and below the knobby head of the fibula bone. *Fig. 3* ** - ***Key Point***

Gb 41 In the depression, where the 4th & 5th toe bones meet. *Fig. 4*

Jing Well Points

Located on each side of the toenails at the base of the nail. *Fig. 4*

Sp 6 3 fingers width above the inside ankle bone and behind the shin bone. *Fig. 5*

Fig. 1

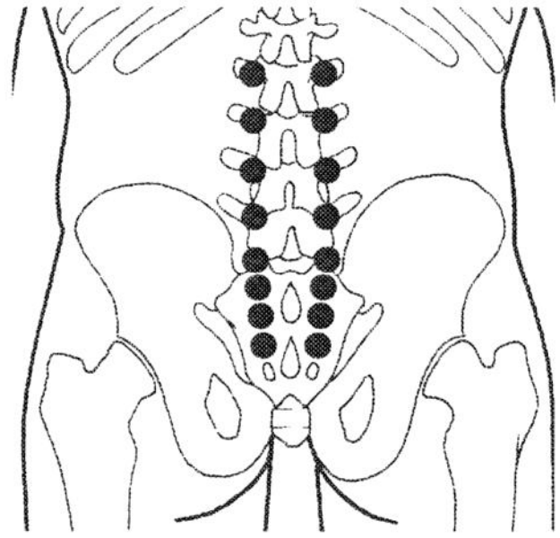

Fig. 2

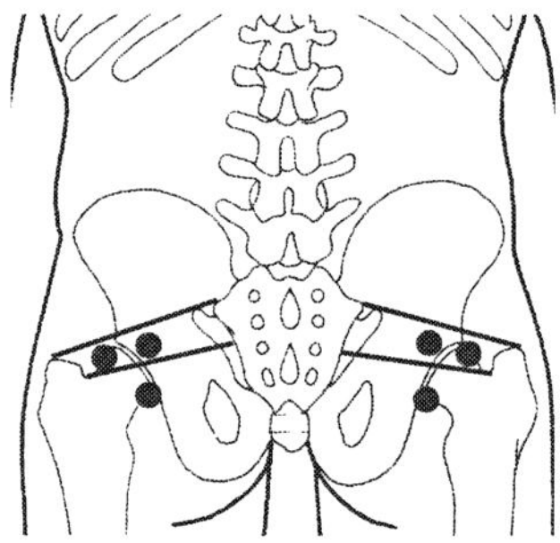

Fig. 3

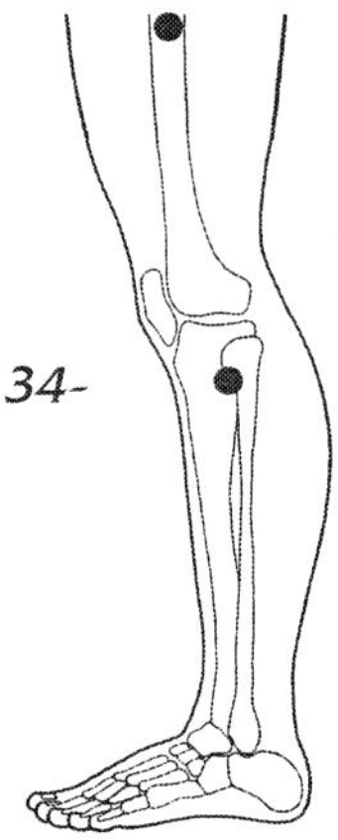

Fig. 4

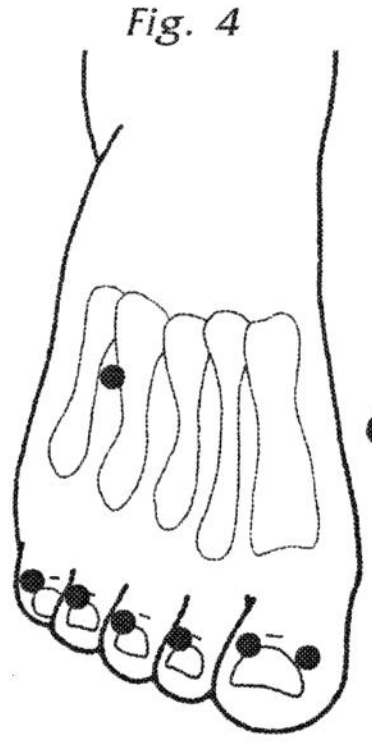

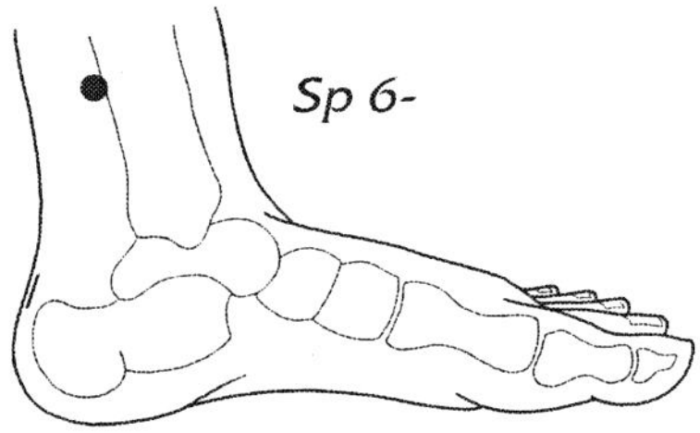

Fig. 5

Peripheral Neuropathy (hands)

Peripheral Neuropathy is a lifestyle disorder causing pain, swelling, burning, and temperature changes of the extremities. For relief of this condition, sedate the following points. Also sedate parasymapthic points on ***page 116.***

Gb 20 Below the base of the skull, in the hollow just outside the main spinal muscles of neck. *Fig. 1*

Back Shu Points
Located 2 fingers width from the middle of the spine at the level of the natural hairline at the back of the neck. ***In the middle of the ropy muscles*** *Fig. 1*

Gb 21 This lies halfway between the bone at the base of the neck and the tip of the shoulder, directly on top of the trapezius (shoulder) muscle. *Fig. 1*

Tw 15 1 thumbs width ***below Gb 21.*** *Fig. 1*

Si 13 4 fingers width ***below GB 21*** just on top of the spine of the shoulder blade. *Fig. 1*

Tender Points
Stimulate these tender points located in the tight muscles at the side of the neck. *Fig. 2*

Li 18 4 fingers width beside the highest point of the Adam's apple in the prominent muscle at the side of the neck ***(below the corner of the jaw).*** *Fig. 2*

Jing Well Points
Located on each side of the finger nails at the base of the nail. *Fig. 3*

Sp 6 3 fingers width above the inside ankle bone and behind the shin bone. *Fig. 4*

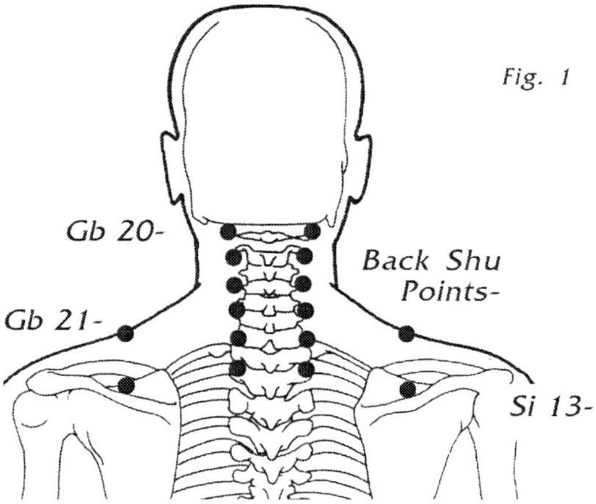

Fig. 1

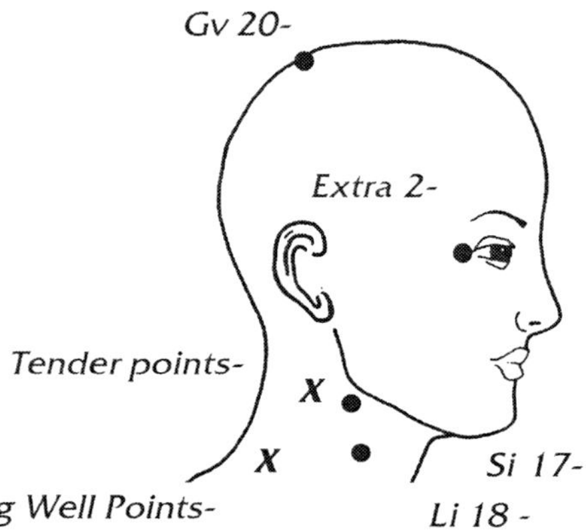

Fig. 2

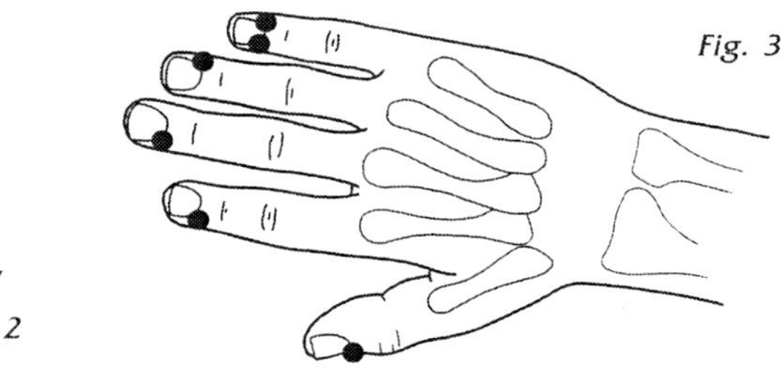

Fig. 3

Fig. 4

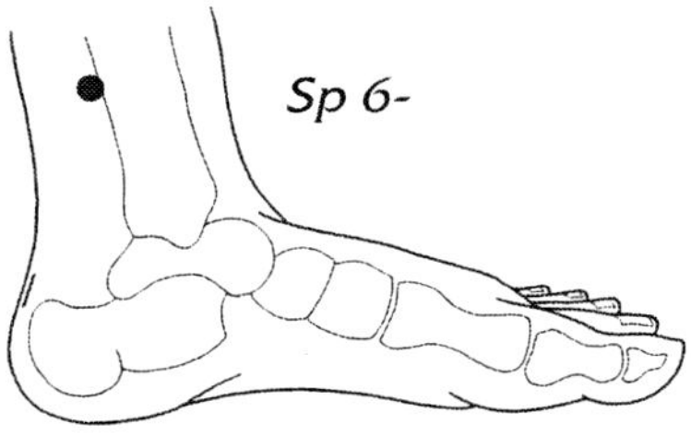

Post Operative Pain

***S**timulation of the following points has been reported to substantially reduce the pain associated with an operation. For more specific points which may relate to your operation, refer to index for the anatomical region of your operation, & stimulate the points illustrated.*

B 23 2 fingers width on each side of the spine, ***at waist level.*** *Fig. 1* ***(tonify +)***

Li 11 This is located at the outer end of the elbow crease, with the elbow slightly bent. *Fig. 2*

Li 4 This lies in middle of the fleshly mass of muscle seen between the thumb and index finger. *Fig. 2*

Gb 34 4 fingers width below the outside of the knee. Just in front of and below the knobby head of the fibula bone. *Fig. 3*

B 60 This lies in the hollow midway between the tip of the outer ankle bone and Achilles tendon. *Fig. 3*

Gv 20 In the middle of the top of the head, halfway between the ears. *Fig. 4*

Sp 6 3 fingers width above the inner ankle bone and behind the prominent shin bone. ***Pressing in this area will locate this tender point.*** *Fig. 5*

Fig. 1

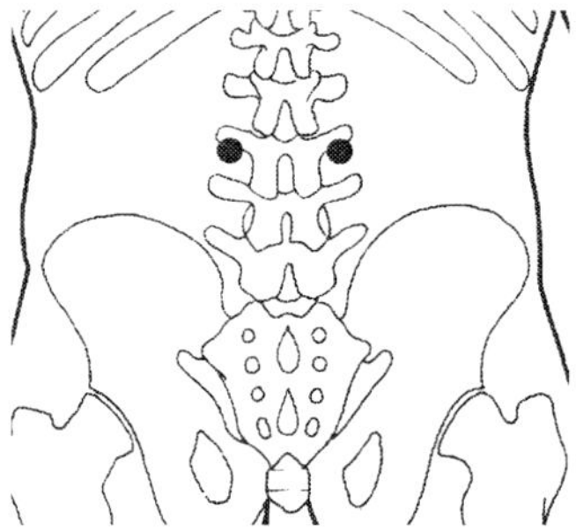

Fig. 2

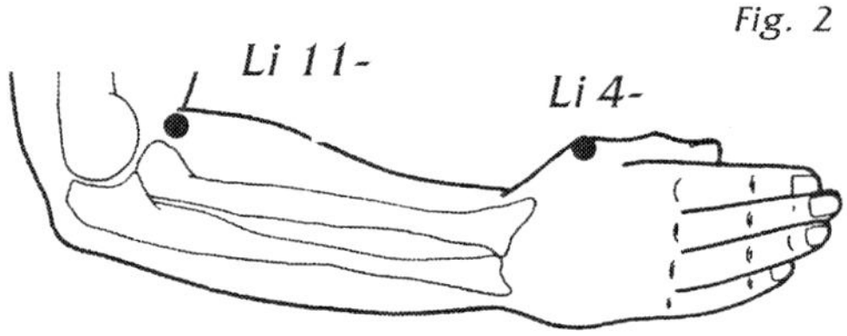

Fig. 3

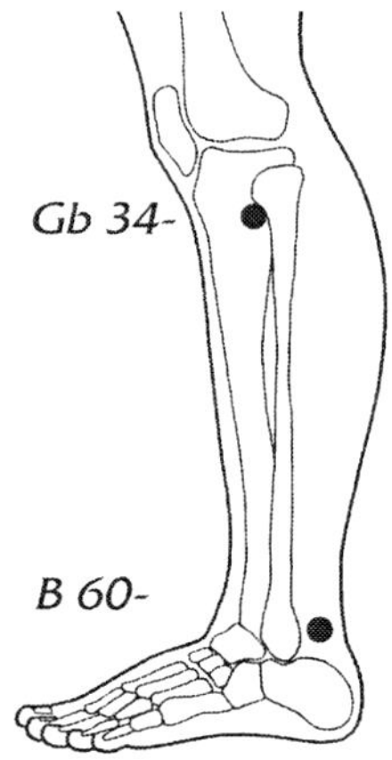

Fig. 4

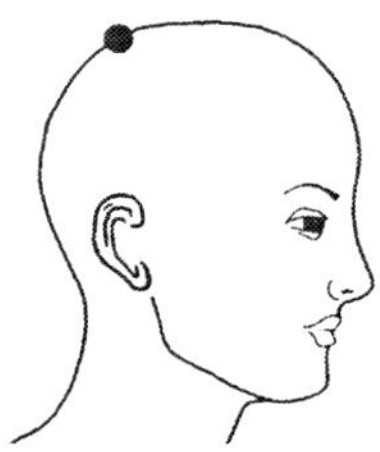

Fig. 5

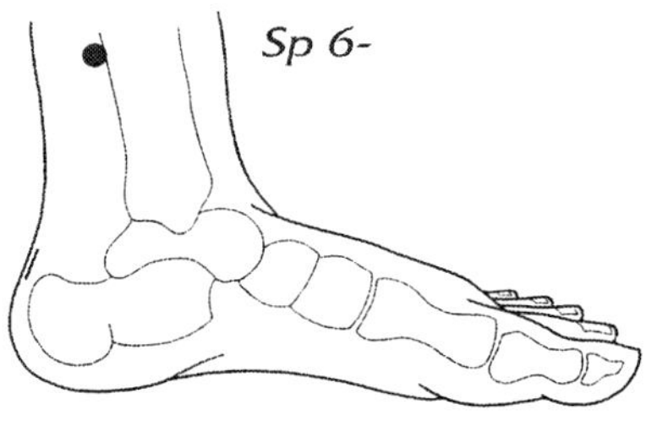

Prolapsed Disc (Low Back)

Most commonly the prolapsed disc is in the lower back. Numbness or weakness may occur in the buttocks, legs, or feet. Sedate the following points to help alleviate the pain.

Back Shu Points:

Located 2 fingers width to each side of the spinal bones. ***Sedate these points from the lower back to the sacrum. Above points innervate the affected region(s) and often provide substantial relief to the patient.*** *Fig. 1*

Fig. 1

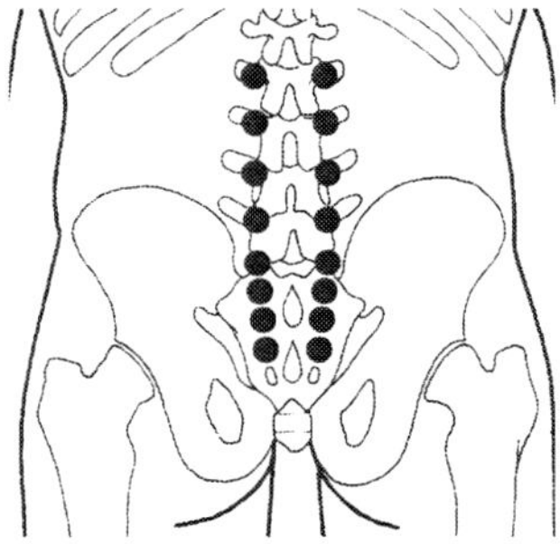

Piriformis Trigger Points:

Approximately half way between the sacrum (the triangular bone at the base of the spine) and the hip joint, or one hands width above GB 30. *Fig. 2*

Gb 30 This point is directly in the middle of the each "cheek" equal distance from all sides. *Fig. 2*

Fig. 2

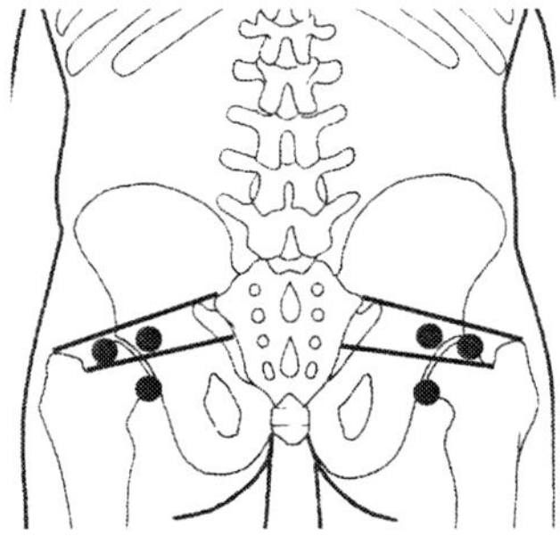

Gb 31 Standing erect with your hands laying the side of the thigh. This point is at the ***tip of the middle finger***. *Fig. 3*

Gb 34 4 fingers width below the outside of the kneecap, and just in front of and below the knobby head of the fibula bone. *Fig. 3*

Fig. 3

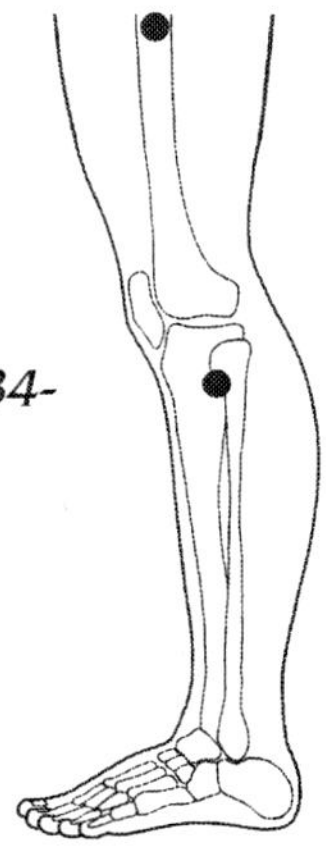

Jing Well Points

Located on each side of the toenails at the base of the nail. *Fig. 4*

Fig. 4

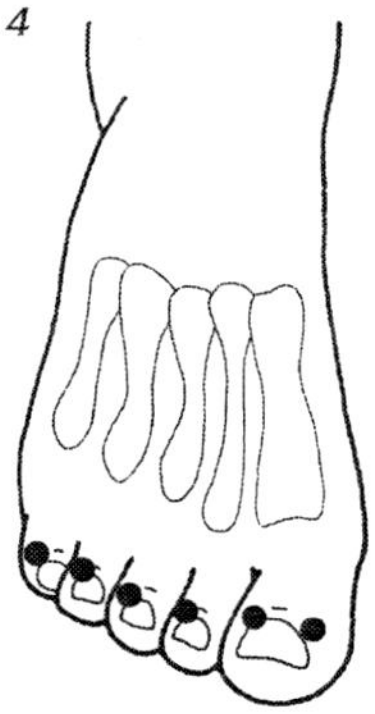

Renal (Kidney) Disorders

*This encompasses all disorders of the kidneys which cause abnormal or insufficient functioning. To increase kidney functioning & health, **TONIFY (+)** the following points. **PLEASE NOTE: For Kidney Stones, SEDATE (-) the following points to assist in pain management.***

Sp 15 4 thumbs width ***to each side*** of the belly button.

St 25 2 fingers width ***to each side*** of the belly button.

St 26 1 thumbs width below **St 25.**

Sp 14 1 thumbs width below **Sp15.**

St 27 1 thumbs width below **St 26.**

Gb 25 At the tip of the free end of the ***12th*** rib.

K 3 In the hollow midway between the tip of the inner ankle bone and the Achilles tendon.

B 23 This lies 2 fingers width to each side of the second lumbar vertebra. ***Located at waist level,*** at the lower border of the rib cage.

Gv 4 On the back midline, between the spinal bones of the ***2nd and 3rd lumbar vertebrae, located at waist level.***

K 1 In the middle of the sole of the foot, between and the ***inner and outer balls of the foot.***

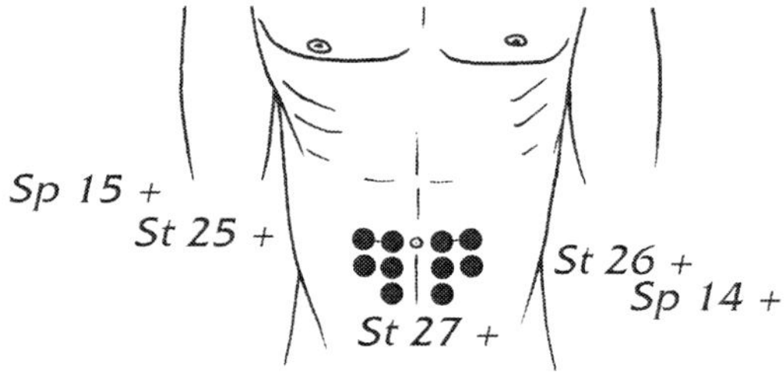

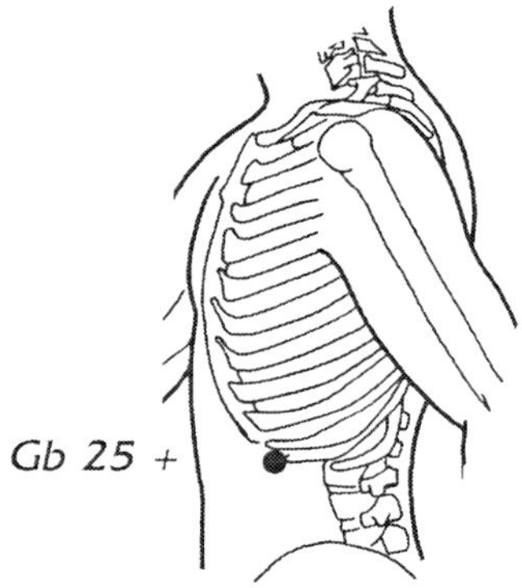

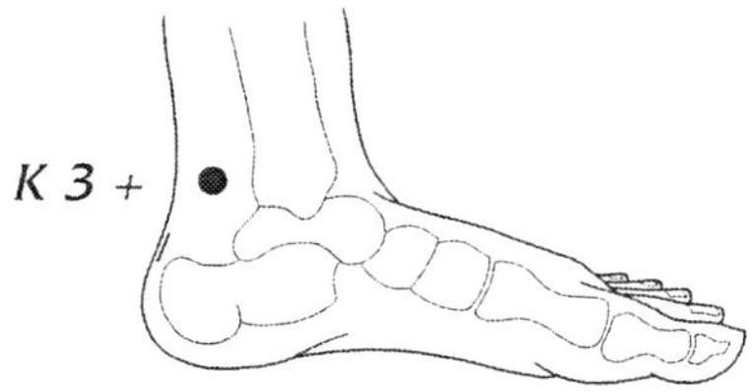

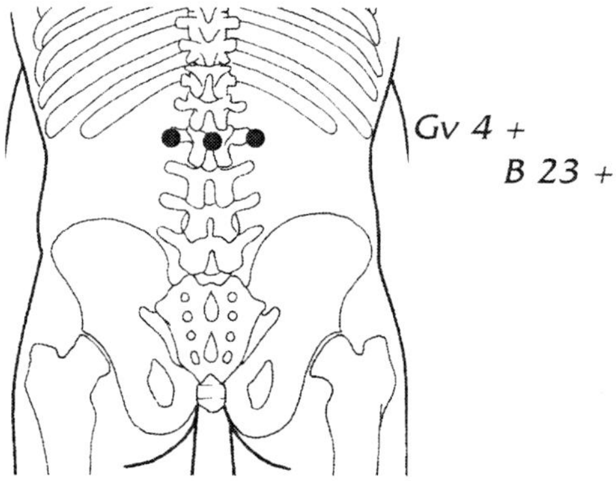

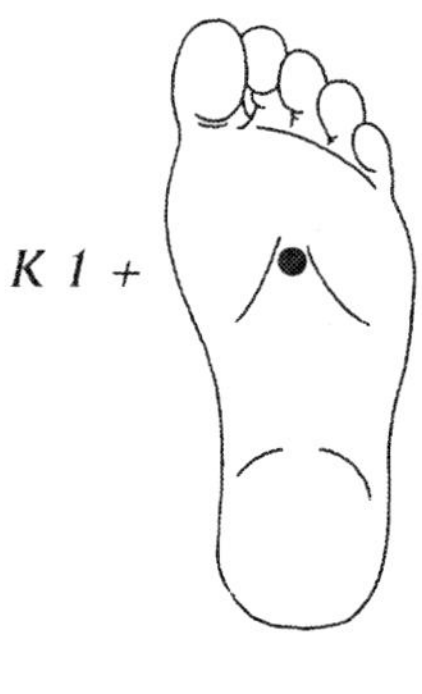

Rheumatoid Arthritis- continued

The following points are suggested to provide enhancement to the immune system if stimulated on a regular basis. Patients with immune deficient disorders should stimulate these points regularly for enhanced benefits. RA patients should tonify the immune points prior to sedating the neck or local points.

Gv 14 Just below the most prominent bone at the base of the neck, easily located with the ***chin pressed towards chest.*** *Fig. 1*

B 11 2 fingers width to each side of Gv 14. *Fig. 1*

Fig. 1

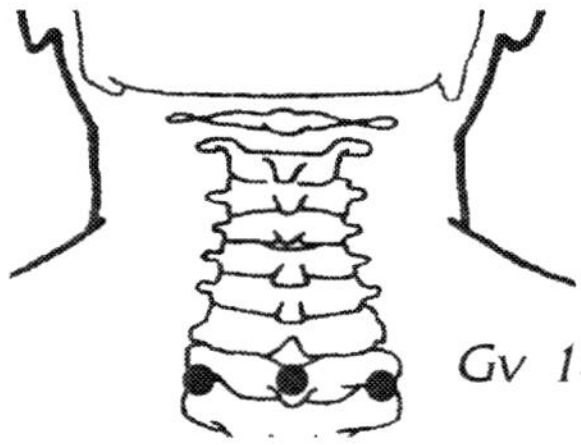

Li 11 This lies at the outer end of the elbow crease, with the ***arm slightly bent.*** *Fig. 2*

Fig. 2

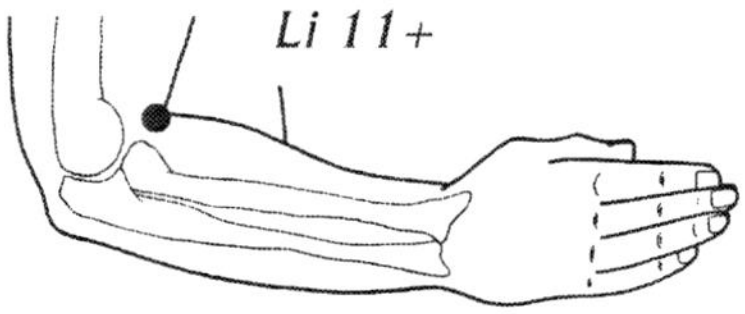

St 36 4 fingers width below the kneecap and 1 fingers width to the outside of the shin bone. *Fig. 3*

Sp 9 On the inside of the leg, 3 fingers width below the kneecap, in the depression between the bone and the calf muscle. *Fig. 3*

Sp 10 2 thumbs width above the upper/inner border of the kneecap. ***This tender spot is at the highest spot of the inner thigh muscle.*** *Fig. 3*

Sp 6 This point lies 3 fingers width above the inner ankle bone and is located behind the prominent shin bone. ***Usually very tender when pressed.*** *Fig. 4*

Fig. 3

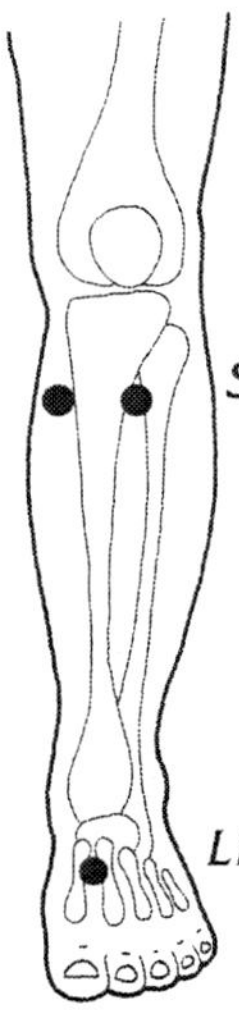

Fig. 4

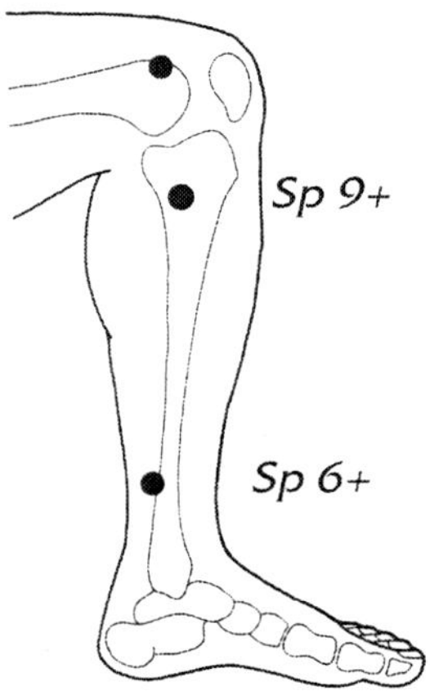

Rheumatoid Arthritis

This type of arthritis is auto-immune related, often with pain and swelling in the smaller joints of the hands and feet. For best results tonify the immunity points and sedate the neck points. Knuckle and extra points may be tonified or sedated depending on patient preference.

Gb 20 Below the base of the skull, in the hollow just outside the main spinal muscles of neck. *Fig. 1*

Back Shu Points
These lie 2 fingers width to each side of the spinal bones. *Fig. 1*

Gb 21 This lies halfway between the bone at the base of the neck and the tip of the shoulder, directly on top of the trapezius (shoulder) muscle. *Fig. 1*

Si 13 4 fingers width ***below GB 21*** just on top of the spine of the shoulder blade. *Fig. 1*

Tender Points
Stimulate these tender points located in the tight muscles at the side of the neck. *Fig. 2*

Si 17 Above the prominent neck muscle, ***at the level of the corner of the jaw***. *Fig. 2*

Li 4 In the middle of the fleshy mass between the thumb and index finger. *Fig. 4*

Knuckle Points
Sedate these tender points located between the knuckles. *Fig. 4*

Extra Points
Close the fist. These are located on the end of the crease where the fingers meet *Fig. 4*

Fig. 1

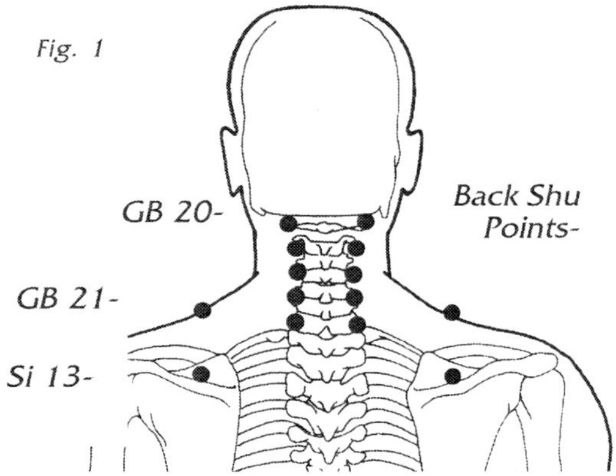

Fig. 2

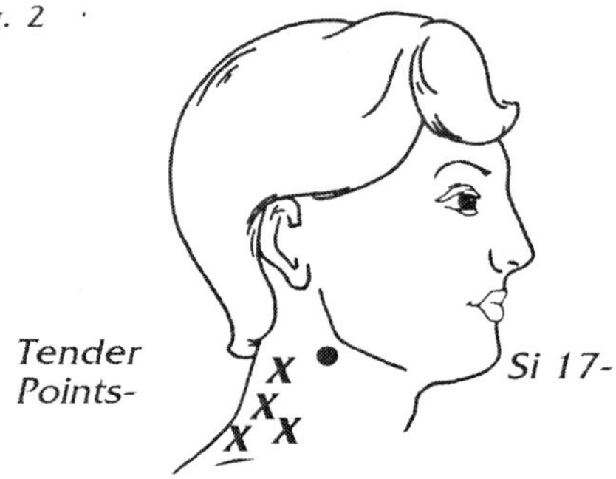

Fig. 3

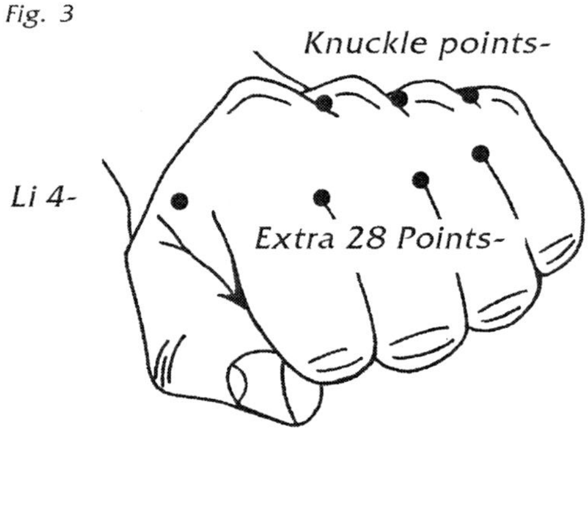

Sciatica - continued next page

***U**sually caused by soft tissue muscle strain due to repetitive overuse, postural imbalances or just poor lifestyle. For relief, sedate the following points to relax muscles and calm the nervous system.*

Back Shu Points:
Located 2 fingers width to each side of the spinal bones. *Fig. 1*

Gv 4 Below the spinal bone of the 4th lumbar vertabrae. *Fig. 1*

Piriformis Trigger Points:
Half way between the sacrum and the hip joint. *Fig. 1*

Gb 30 This point is directly in the middle of the each "cheek" equal distance from all sides. *Fig. 1*

Gb 31 Standing erect with your hands laying the side of the thigh. This point is at the ***tip of the middle finger***. *Fig. 2*

Gb 34 4 fingers width below the outside of the kneecap, and just in front of and below the knobby head of the bone. *Fig. 2*

B 60 This lies in the hollow midway between the tip of the outer ankle bone and the Achilles tendon. *Fig. 2*

Jing Well Points
Located on each side of the toenails at the base of the nail. *Fig. 3*

Fig. 1

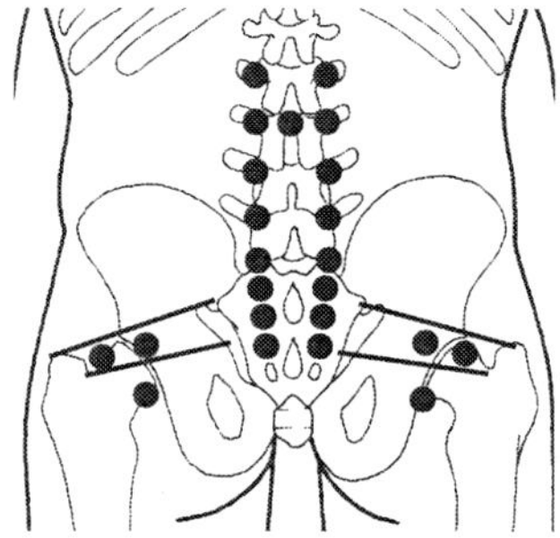

Fig. 2

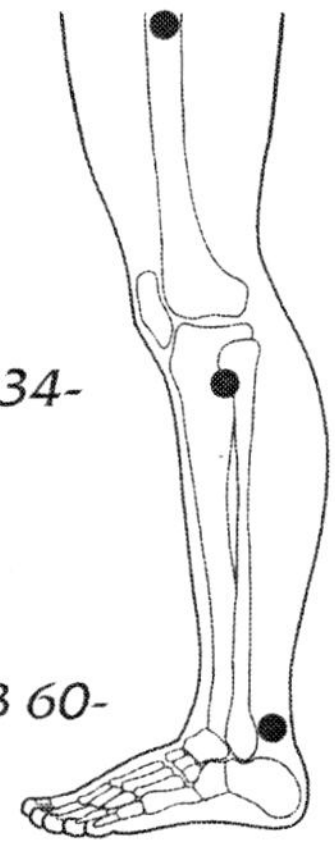

Fig. 3

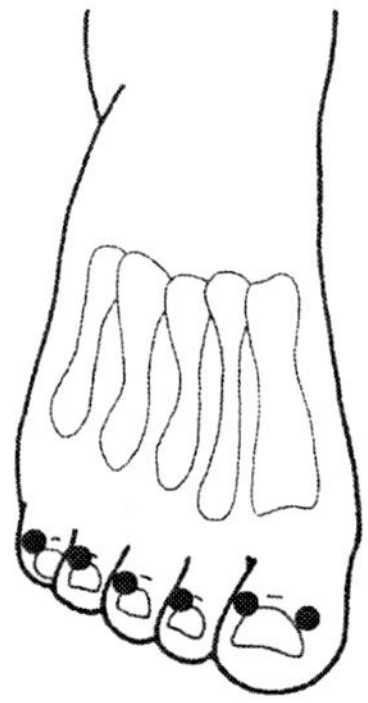

Sciatica

***F**or additional relief for sciatica, sedate the following Huotao points and points down the legs. Parasymapthetic points on **pages 35-36,** also provide relief.*

Huatao Points:
Located 1 fingers width to each side of the spinal bones. *Fig. 1*

Tender Points
*Sedate any tender points that are located in the buttocks, **marked with an "X".*** *Fig. 1*

B 31 This lies at the top of the sacral bone and ***2 fingers width away from the midline.*** *Fig. 1*

B 32 This lies 1 thumbs width ***below B 31.*** *Fig. 1*

B 34 At the ***highest level of the upper leg bone***, this point lies 1 thumbs width to each side of the midline. *Fig. 1*

B 36 At the midpoint, just below the gluteal fold. *Fig. 2*

B 37 At the midpoint in the back of the thigh. *Fig. 2*

B 40 On the middle of the crease behind the knee. *Fig. 2*

B 57 At the mid point of the calf where the calf muscle narrows to form the tendon, between the 2 calf muscles. *Fig. 2*

B 60 This lies in the hollow midway between the tip of the outer ankle bone and the Achilles tendon. *Figs. 2*

St 44 At meeting of the base of 2nd and 3rd toes in between the web. *Fig. 3*

Fig. 2

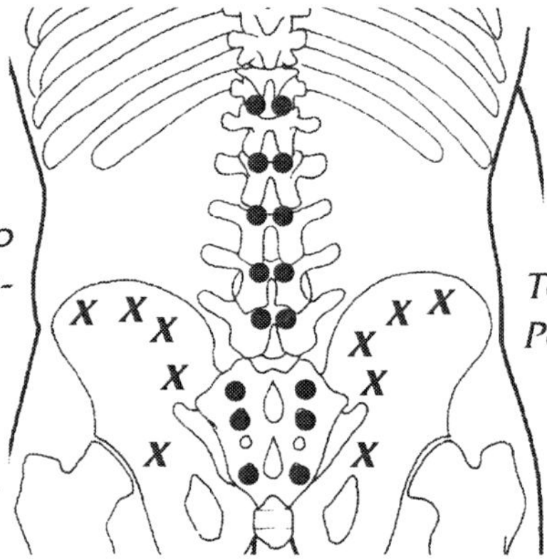

Fig. 2

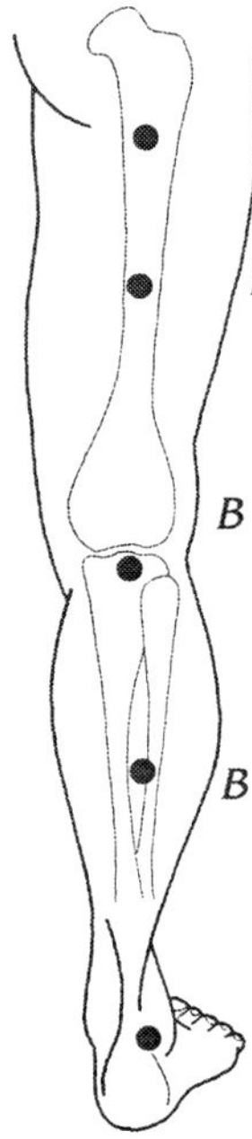

Fig. 3

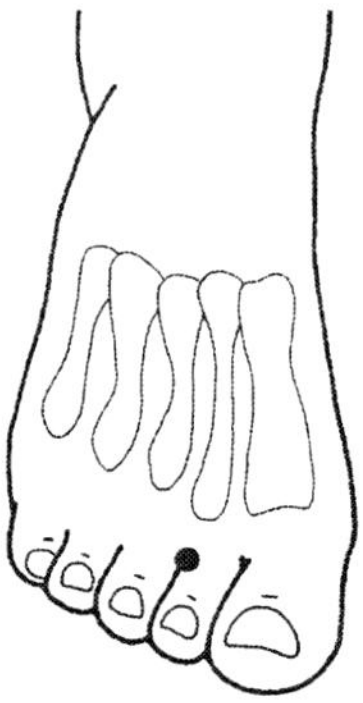

Scoliosis

S**coliosis is an abnormal curvature of the spine, usually to one side. Sedating these points will relax the spinal muscles, allowing for pain relief and greater flexibility. For additional relief, see Parasymapthetic points,* ***pages 35-36.

Back Shu Points:
Located 2 fingers width to each side of the spinal bones. ***Sedate these points the entire length of spine or in the region(s) where the scoliosis occurs.*** *Fig. 1*

B 52 4 fingers width to each side of the spine ***at waist level.*** *Fig. 1*

Piriformis Trigger Points:
Approximately half way between the sacrum (the triangular bone at the base of the spine) and the hip joint, or one hands width above GB 30. *Fig. 1*

Gb 30 This point is directly in the middle of the each "cheek" equal distance from all sides. *Fig. 1*

Gb 31 Standing erect with your hands laying the side of the thigh. This point is at the ***tip of the middle finger***. *Fig. 2*

Gb 34 4 fingers width below the outside of the kneecap, and just in front of and below the knobby head of the fibula bone. *Fig. 2*

Jing Well Points
Located on each side of the toenails at the base of the nail.. *Fig. 3*

Fig. 1

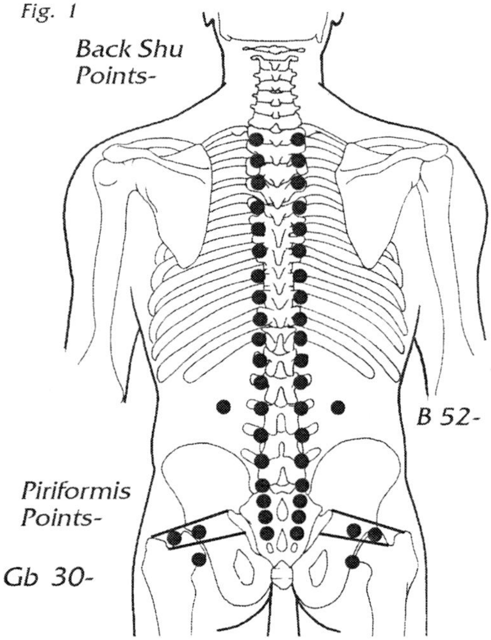

Fig. 2

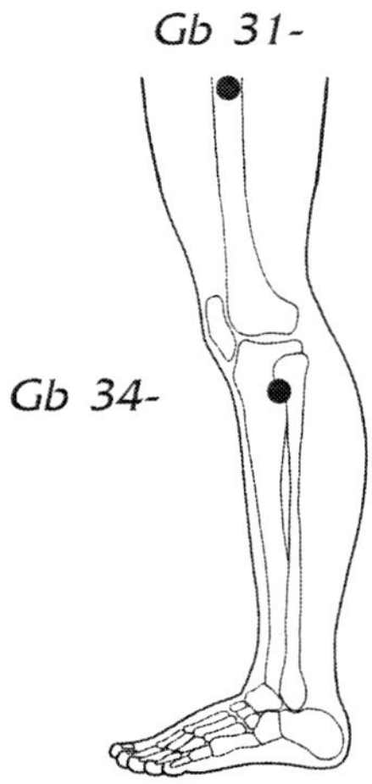

Fig. 3

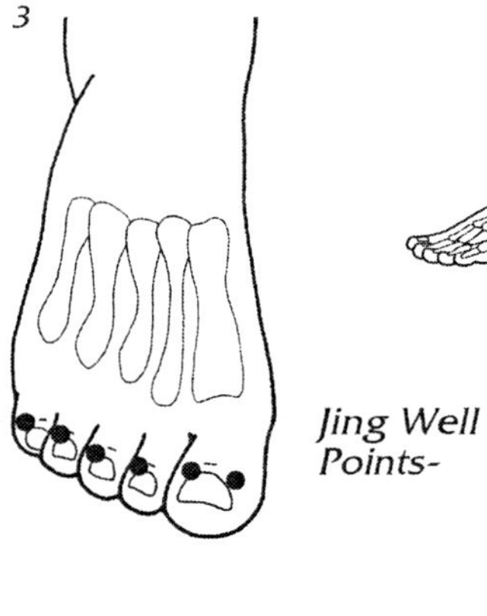

Shin Splints - continued next page

***C**onsult a Doctor before treating any points. For chronic conditions, the lower back region should be treated first, followed by the jing points. For additional relief, sedate the local on the following page.*

Back Shu Points:
Located 2 fingers width to each side of the spinal bones. ***Sedate these points from the lower back to the sacrum. Above points innervate the affected region(s) and often provide substantial relief to the patient.*** *Fig. 1*

Fig. 1

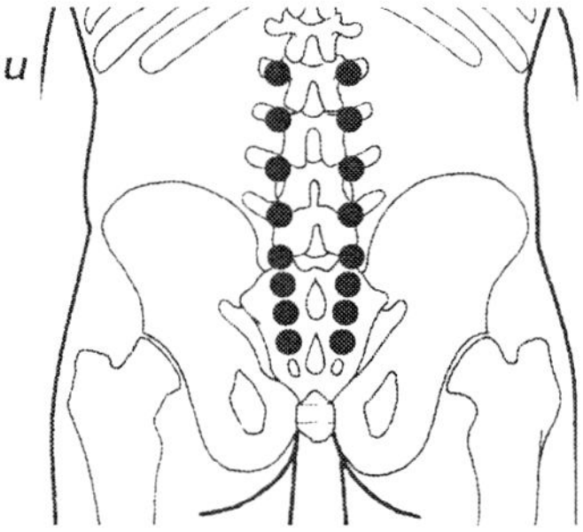

Fig. 2

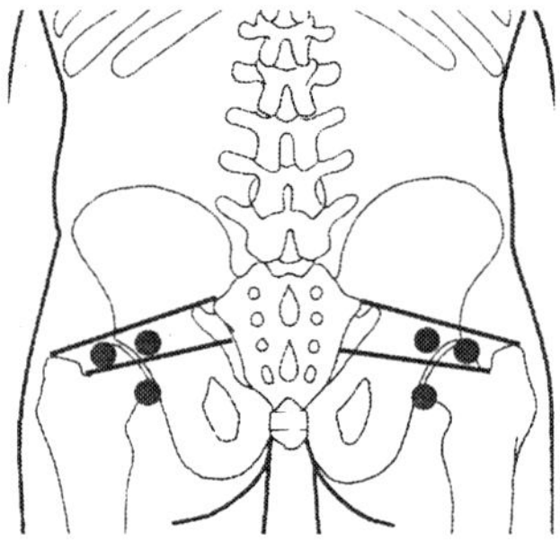

Piriformis Trigger Points:
Approximately half way between the sacrum (the triangular bone at the base of the spine) and the hip joint, or one hands width above GB 30. *Fig. 2*

Gb 30 This point is directly in the middle of the each "cheek" equal distance from all sides. *Fig. 2*

Fig. 3

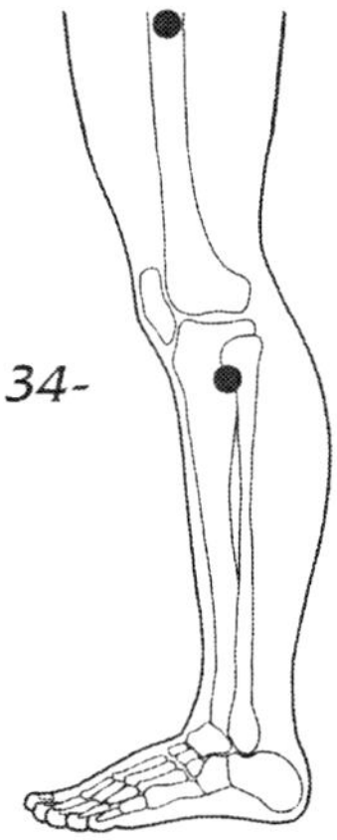

Gb 31 Standing erect with your hands laying the side of the thigh. This point is at the ***tip of the middle finger***. *Fig. 3*

Gb 34 4 fingers width below the outside of the kneecap, and just in front of and below the knobby head of the fibula bone. *Fig. 3*

Fig. 4

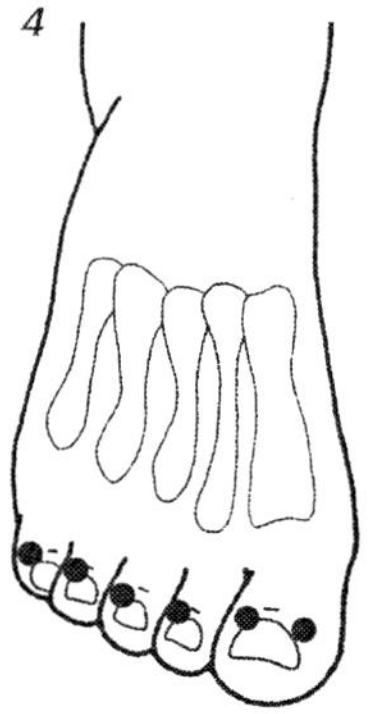

Jing Well Points
Located on each side of the toenails at the base of the nail. *Fig. 4*

Shin Splints

***S**hin splints are a pain on the shin, due to irritation often caused by repetitive motion, such as jogging. Frequently sedate the following points and rest. Be sure to concentrate on the points in **Fig. 3** (St 36, St 38, St 41).*

Sp 6 3 fingers width above the inner ankle bone and behind the prominent shin bone. *Fig. 1*

K 3 In the hollow midway between the tip of the inner ankle bone and the Achilles tendon. *Fig. 1*

Gb 34 4 fingers width below the outside of the knee. In front of and below the knobby head of the fibula bone. *Fig. 2*

Gb 39 4 fingers width above the tip of the outer ankle bone and just behind the fibula bone. *Fig. 2*

B 60 This point lies in the hollow midway between the tip of the outer ankle bone and the Achilles tendon. *Fig. 2*

St 36 4 fingers width below the kneecap and 1 finger width to the ***outside*** of the shinbone. *Fig. 3*

St 38 This lies halfway between the knee and ankle, and 1 fingers width ***to the outside*** the shin bone. *Fig. 3*

St 41 This lies halfway between the ankle bones, between the tendons. *Fig. 3*

B 40 On the middle of the crease behind the knee. *Fig. 4*

B 57 At the midpoint of the calf where the calf muscle narrows to form the tendon. *Fig. 4*

Fig. 1

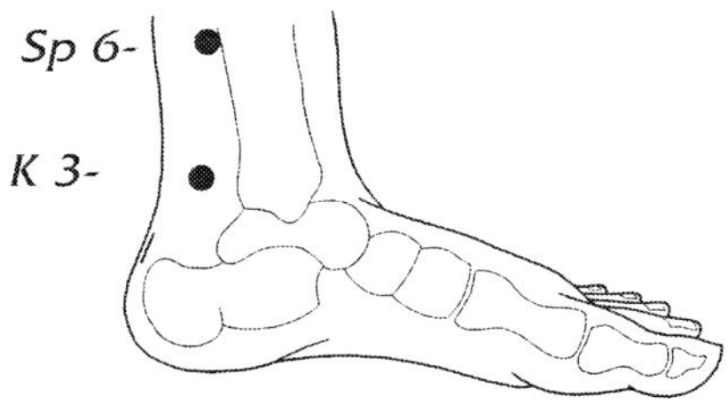

Fig. 2

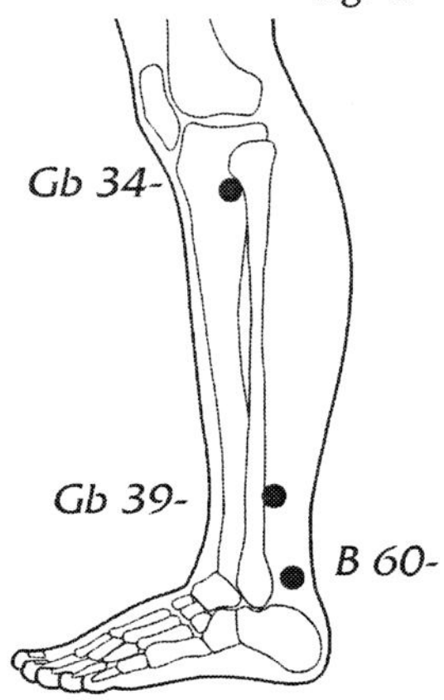

Fig. 3

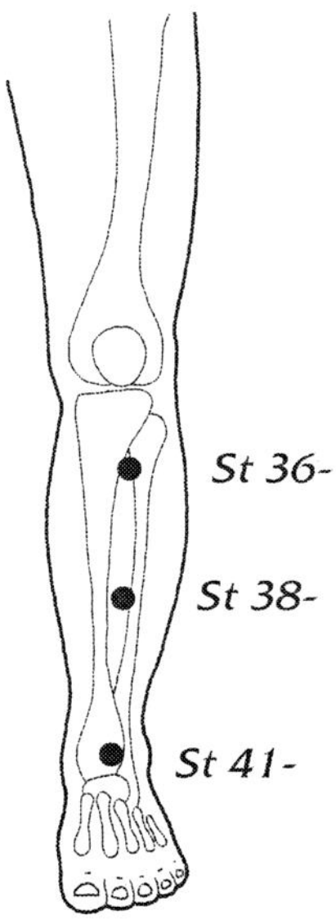

Fig. 4

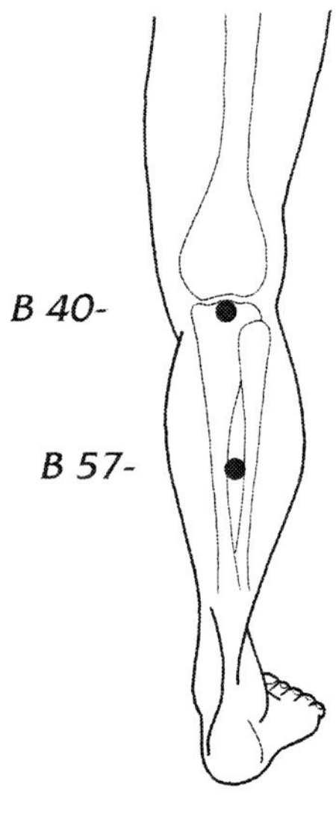

Shingles (Herpes Zoster) - continued

***S**hingles is a viral inflammation of the nerve root which causes a painful blistering rash and intense pain along the course of a nerve. The following nerve calming points often provide substantial relief to some patients.*

Lu 9 In the groove at the thumb side of the wrist crease, and inside of the tendon. *Fig. 1*

H 7 On the little finger side of the wrist crease, to the inside of the tendon. *Fig. 1*

P 6 3 fingers width from the most distal wrist crease, in between the tendons. *Fig. 1*

Sp 6 3 fingers width above the inner ankle and just behind the prominent shin bone. *Fig. 2*

K 3 Halfway between the Achilles tendon and the inner ankle bone. *Fig. 2*

B 62 In the depression half a finger below the outer ankle bone. *Fig. 3*

Cv 17 On the breast bone at the heart level or the 4th rib space. Tender when pressed. *Fig. 4*

Fig. 1

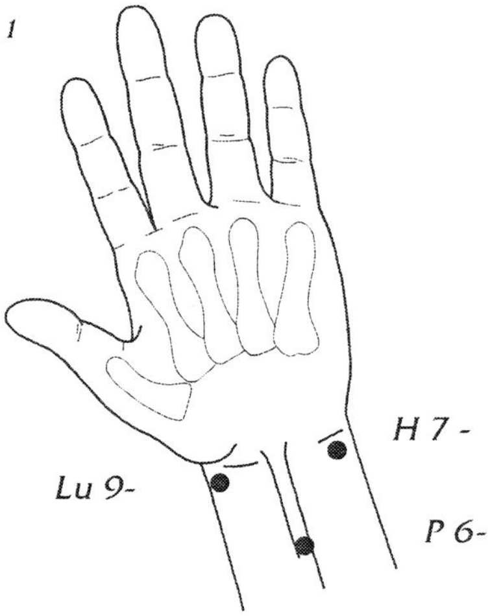

Fig. 2

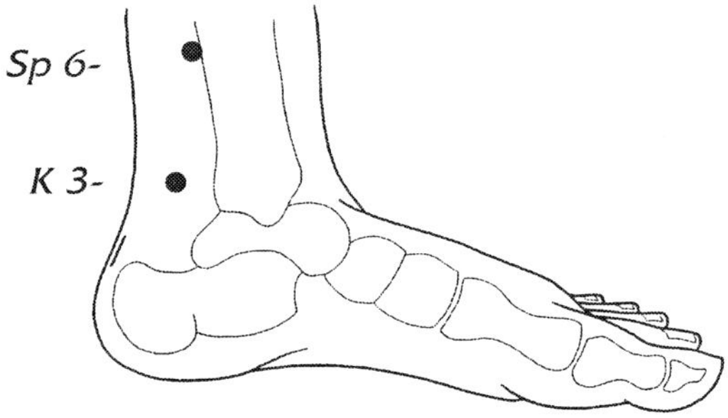

Fig. 3

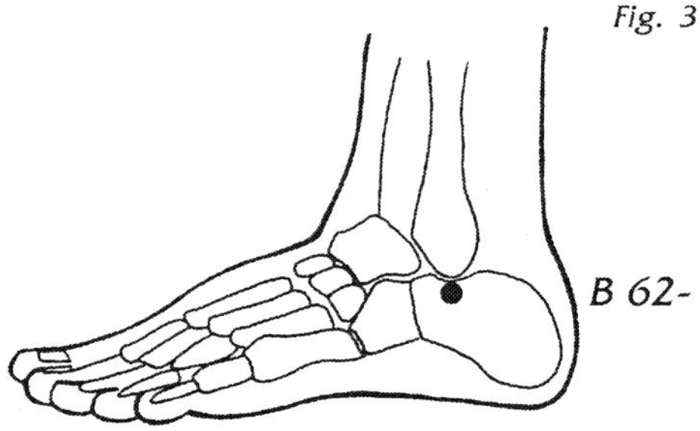

Fig. 4

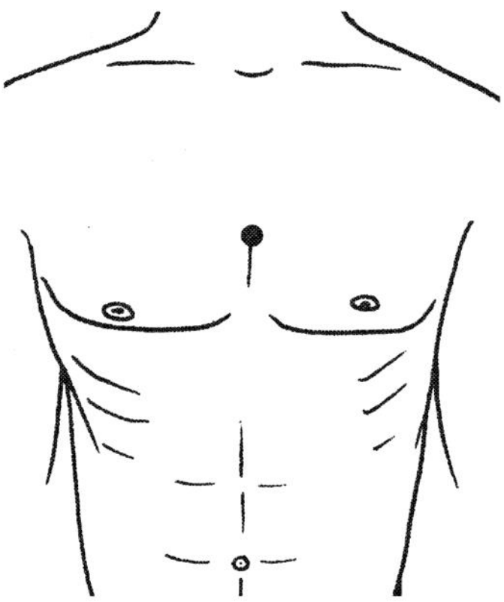

Shingles - continued next page

***A**fter the parasympathetic points have been sedated, sedate the following points. Apply to fingers for neck and arm, and feet for legs and back. Apply in short bursts until the pain subsides.*

Si 3 On the outer side of the hand at the end of the main (distal) palm crease ***at the junction of the pigment change in the skin.*** *Fig. 1*

For Lower Extremities

Jing Well Points
At the outer base of the toe nails. *Fig. 2*

St 44 On top of the foot in the web at the base of the 2nd and 3rd toes. *Fig. 2*

Gb 41 In the depression, where the 4th & 5th toe bones meet. *Fig. 2 & 4*

For Upper Extremities

Jing Well Points
At the outer base of the finger nails. *Fig. 3*

Gb 41 In the depression, where the 4th & 5th toe bones meet. *Fig. 2 & 4*

Fig. 1

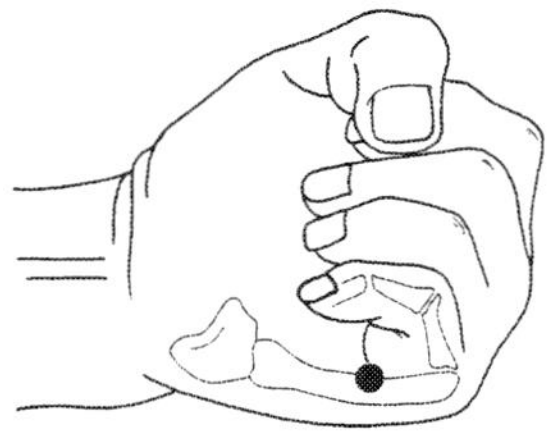

Fig. 2

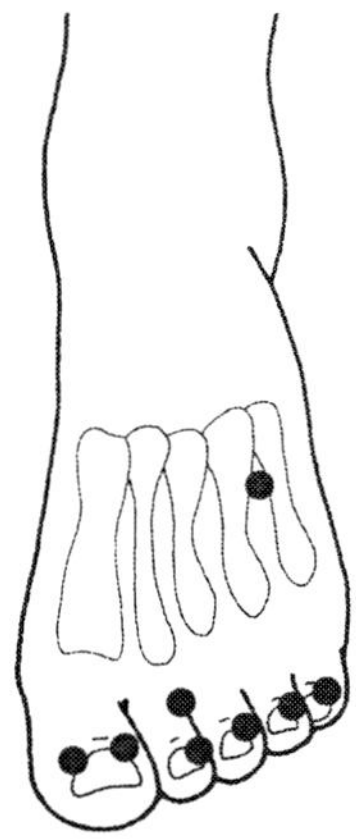

Fig. 3

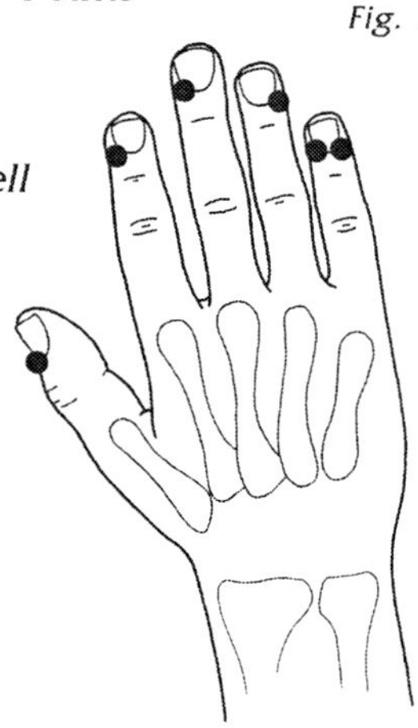

Fig. 4

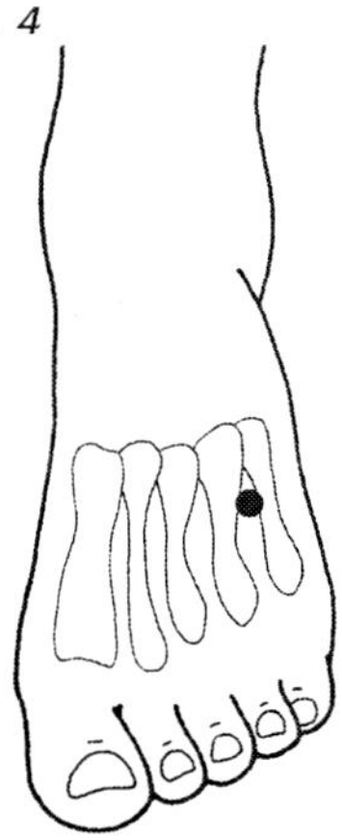

Shingles - continued next page

Shingles is a viral inflammation of the nerve root which causes a painful blistering rash appearing along the final fibres of the nerve, and intense neuralgic pain along the course of the nerve. Start by treating the spine at the origin of the nerve root. Follow by sedating the following points in short bursts until the pain subsides. For questions, ***call 1-800-567-7246.***

Back Shu Points

Trace the pain back to the spine (site of segmental innervation) and sedate 2 fingers width to each side of the spinal bone. *Fig. 1*

Si 13 On the spine of the shoulder blade, half way between the outside of the shoulder and the middle of the spine. *Fig. 1*

Piriformis Trigger Points:
Approximately half way between the sacrum (the triangular bone at the base of the spine) and the hip joint, or one hands width above GB 30. *Fig. 1*

Gb 30 This point is directly in the middle of the each buttocks half, equal distance from all sides. *Fig. 1*

Gb 34 4 fingers width below the outside of the kneecap and just in front and below the knobby head of the fibula bone. *Fig. 2*

B 60 This lies in the hollow midway between the tip of the outer ankle bone and the Achilles tendon. *Fig. 2*

Fig. 1

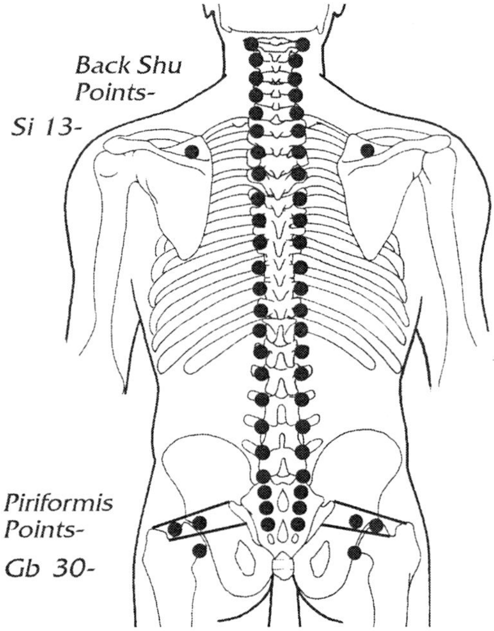

Fig. 2

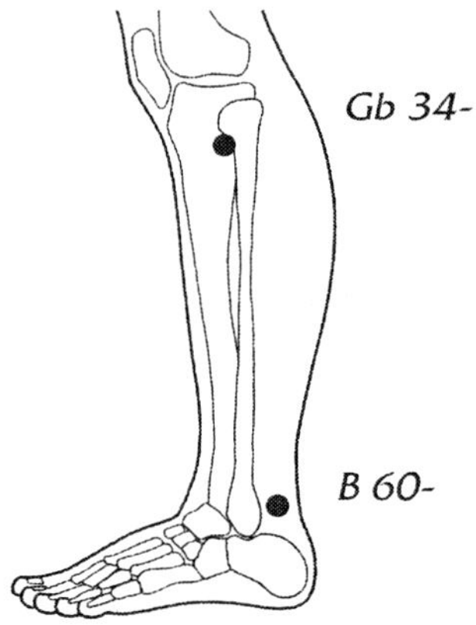

Shingles

***T**he following points are generally sedated after treating the spine. They are reported to balance the bodies energetic and nervous systems.*

Li 11 This lies on the end of the outerelbow crease ***with the arm bent***. *Fig. 1*

Li 4 In the middle of the fleshy mass between the thumb and index finger. ***Slightlytowards the index finger bone.*** *Fig. 1*

Fig. 1

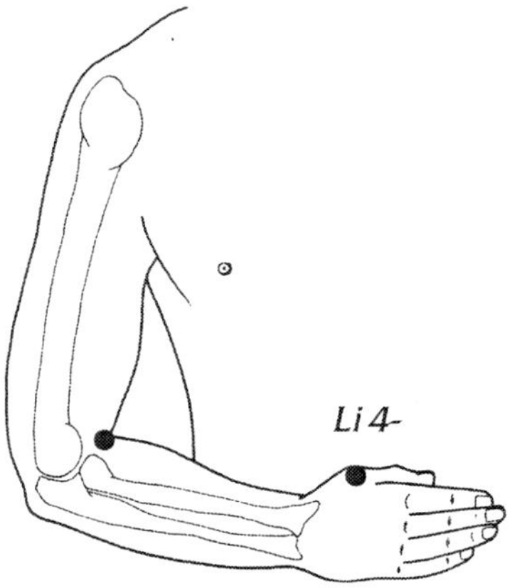

Sp 10 2 thumbs width above the upper/inner border of the kneecap. ***This tender spot is at the highest point of the inner thigh muscle.*** *Fig. 2*

Sp 9 4 fingers width below the inner knee joint in the depression between the bone and the calf muscle. *Fig. 2*

Sp 6 3 fingers width above the inner ankle bone and behind the prominent shin bone. ***Pressing against this bone will locate this tender oint.*** *Fig. 2*

Fig. 2

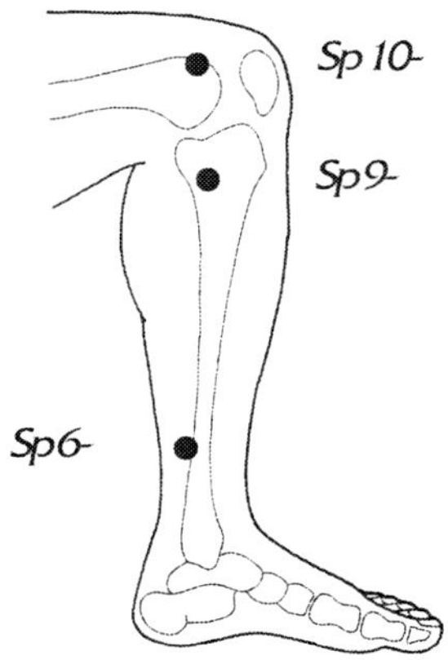

Shingles (Post) - Immunity

The following points are suggested to provide enhancement to the immune system when stimulated. Recommended for a Post Shingles patient.

Fig. 1

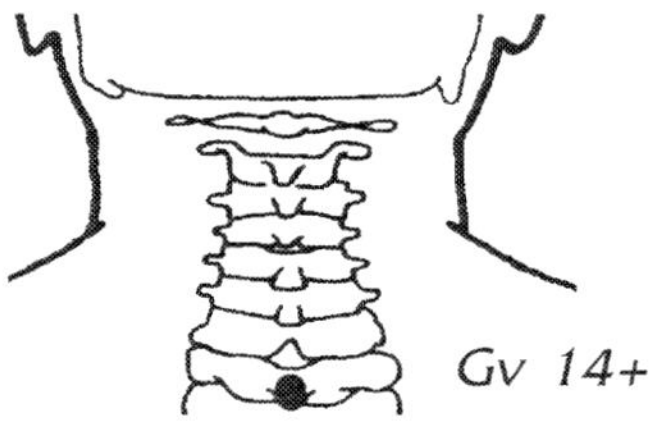

GV 14 Just below the most prominent bone at the base of the neck, easily located with the ***chin pressed towards chest.*** *Fig. 1*

Li 11 This lies at the outer end of the elbow crease, with the ***arm slightly bent.*** *Fig. 2*

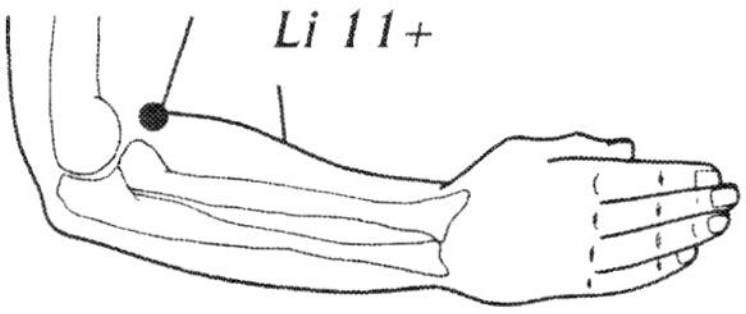

Fig. 2

St 36 4 fingers width below the kneecap and 1 fingers width to the outside of the shin bone. *Fig. 3*

Fig. 3

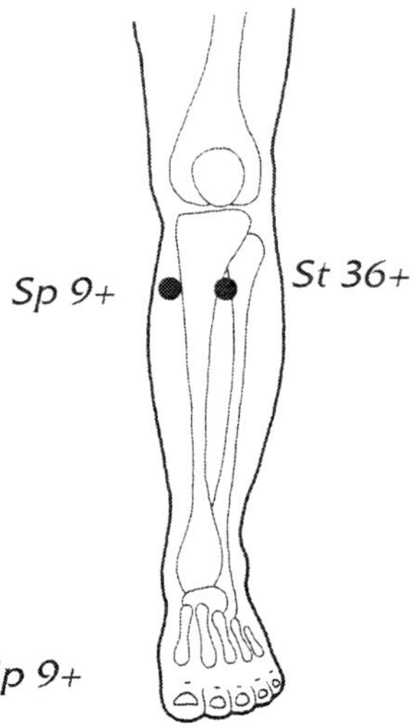

Sp 10 2 thumbs width above the upper/inner border of the kneecap. ***This tender spot is at the highest spot of the inner thigh muscle.*** *Fig. 4*

Fig. 4

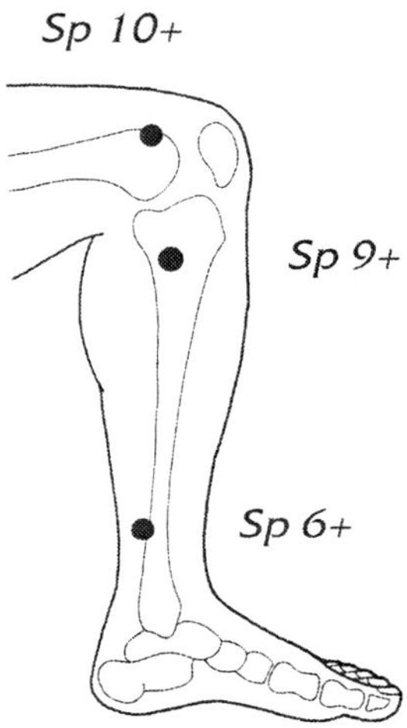

Sp 9 On the inside of the leg, 3 fingers width below the kneecap, in the depression between the bone and the calf muscle. *Fig. 3*

Sp 6 This point lies 3 fingers width above the inner ankle bone and is located behind the prominent shin bone. ***Usually very tender when pressed.*** *Fig. 4*

Shoulder Pain - Frozen

***S**edate the following points for relief of general shoulder pain and stiffness. For optimal relief, start with the points in the legs and feet. Neck points and local points may be added if required.*

Gb 34 4 fingers width below the outside of the kneecap, and just in front of and below the knobby head of the fibula bone. *Fig. 1*

St 38 Halfway between the kneecap and ankle, and 1 fingers width to the outside of the shin bone. *Fig. 1*

Gb 41 On top of the foot. In the hollow formed where the 4th and 5th toes bones meet. *Fig.2*

GB 20 Below the base of the skull, in the hollow just outside the spinal muscles of neck. *Fig. 3*

Back Shu Points:
Located 2 fingers width to each side of the spinal bones. *Fig. 3*

Gb 21 This lies halfway between the bone at the base of the neck and the tip of the shoulder, directly on top of the trapezius (shoulder) muscle. *Fig. 3*

Tw 15 1 thumbs width ***below Gb 21.*** *Fig. 3*

Si 13 4 fingers width below GB 21 just above the boney portion of the shoulder blade. *Fig. 3*

Li 18 4 fingers width beside the highest point of the Adam's apple in the prominent muscle at the side of the neck. *Fig. 3*

Tender Points
Stimulate tender points located in the tight muscles at the side of the neck. *Fig. 3*

Fig. 1

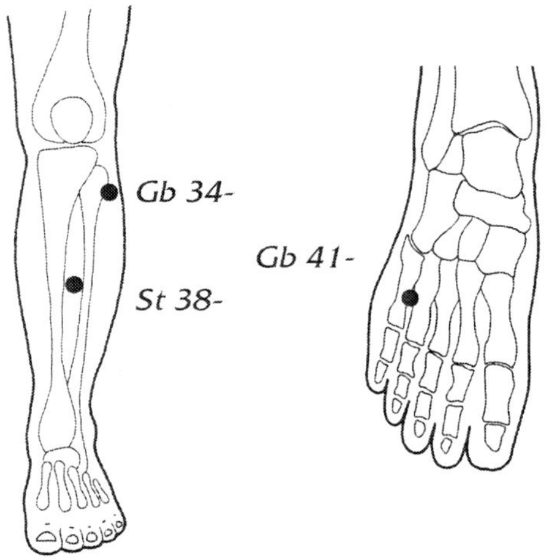

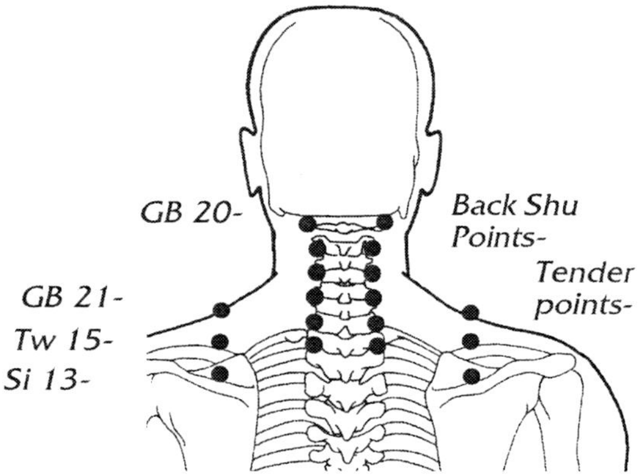

Fig. 3

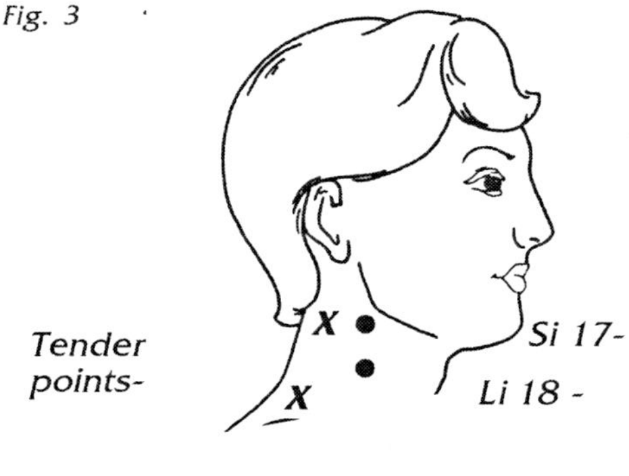

Shoulder Pain

For additional relief to the points on the previous page, sedate the following local points.

Tw 15 This point is located in the ***hollow formed in the deltoid muscle crease in the back of the shoulder. Opposite position to Li 15.*** Located with arm raised. *Fig. 1*

Li 15 This point is located in the ***hollow formed in the deltoid muscle in front of the shoulder*** *Fig. 1*

Jianqian
Midway between ***Li 15*** and the armpit fold. *Fig. 1*

Li 14 On the ***lower border*** of the deltoid muscle, on the outside of the arm. *Fig. 1*

Gb 21 Halfway between the most prominent bone at the bottom of the neck and the outside tip of the shoulder bone. *Fig. 2*

Si 13 Located on the spine of the shoulder blade, ***4 fingers width below Gb 21.*** *Fig. 2*

Si 10 Directly in the middle of the shoulder blade, very tender when pressed. *Fig. 2*

Si 9 With an arm at the side, this point is located 1 thumbs width above the fold. *Fig. 2*

Tender Points
Stimulate tender points located in the tight muscles in the shoulder & outer chest. *Fig. 3*

Cv 17 On the breast bone at the heart level or the 4th rib space. Tender when pressed. *Fig. 3*

Fig. 1

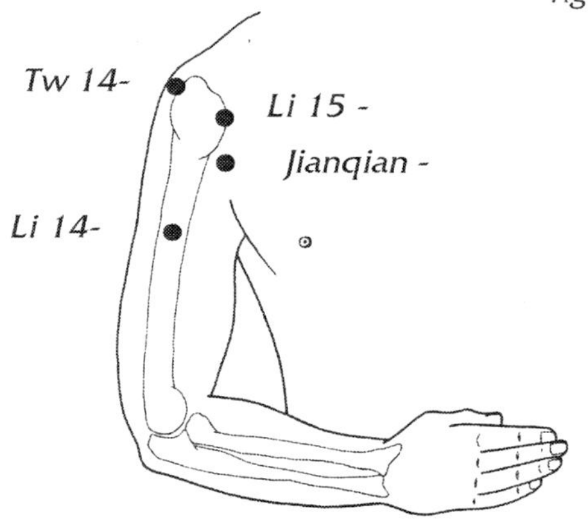

Fig. 2

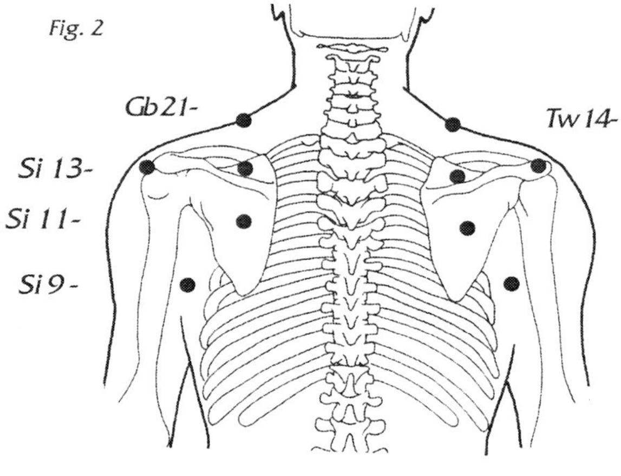

Fig. 3

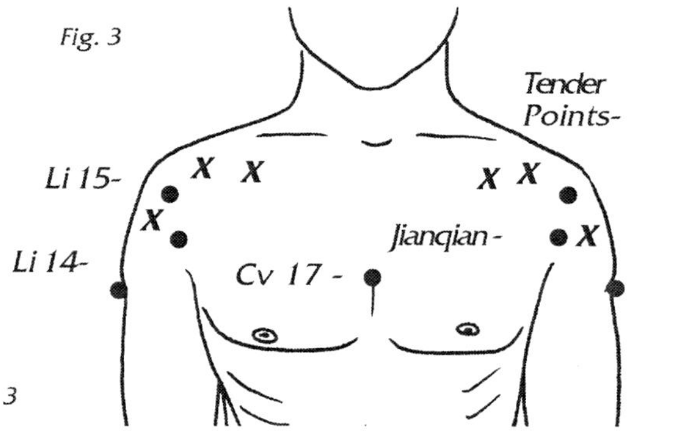

Sinus Problems - continued next page

***S**edate the following points to relieve stuffiness and pain relating to sinus problems. If allergies are responsible or the condition is chronic, include tonifying the immune points on following page.*

Gb 14 Located 1 fingers width above the ***midpoint*** of the eyebrows, directly ***above*** the pupils. *Fig. 1*

Extra 1 (Yintang)

At the midpoint between the inner ends of the eyebrows. *Fig. 1*

St 2 1 fingers width below the lower ridge of the eye socket, ***directly below the pupil with the eyes straight.*** *Fig. 1*

Liv 3 On the top of the foot in the hollow formed between the 1st and 2nd toes, where the toe bones meet. *Fig. 2*

St 44 In the web at the base of the 2nd and 3rd toes. *Fig. 2*

Sp 6 3 fingers width above the inner ankle bone and just ***behind*** the shin bone. ***Tonify to help improve immune system.*** *Fig. 3*

Li 4 Located approximately in the middle of the fleshy mass of muscle between the thumb and index finger, and slightly towards the index finger bone. *Fig. 4*

Fig. 1

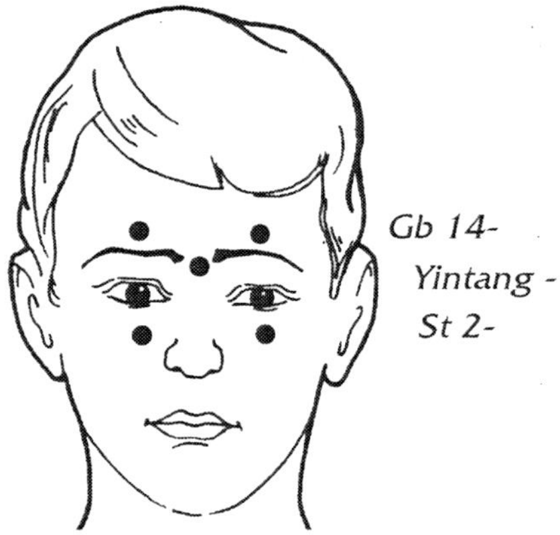

Fig. 2

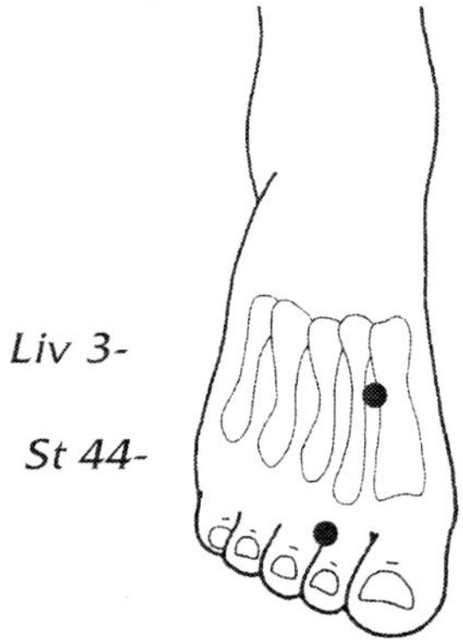

Fig. 3

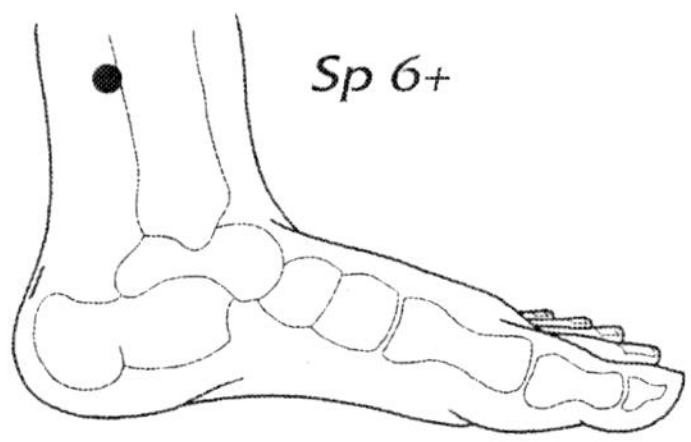

Fig. 4

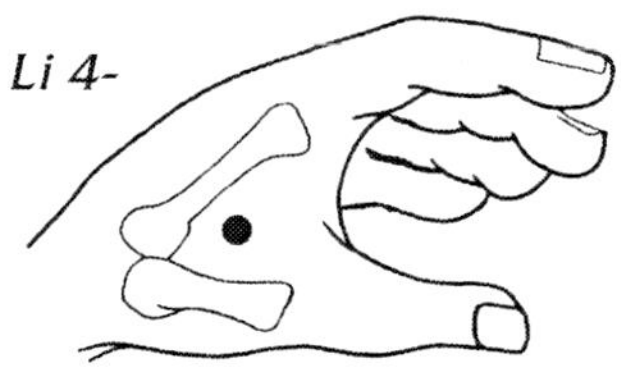

Sinus - Immunity

For chronic sinus conditions, tonify the following immune points are suggested to provide enhancement to the immune system.

GV 14 Just below the most prominent bone at the base of the neck, easily located with the ***chin pressed towards chest.*** *Fig 1*

Fig. 1

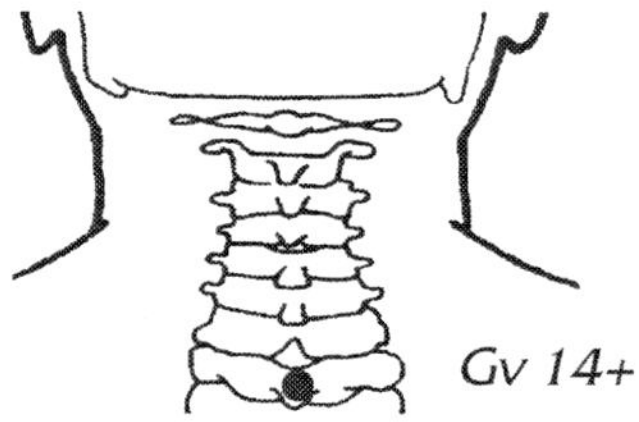

Li 11 This lies at the outer end of the elbow crease, with ***the arm slightly bent.*** *Fig. 2*

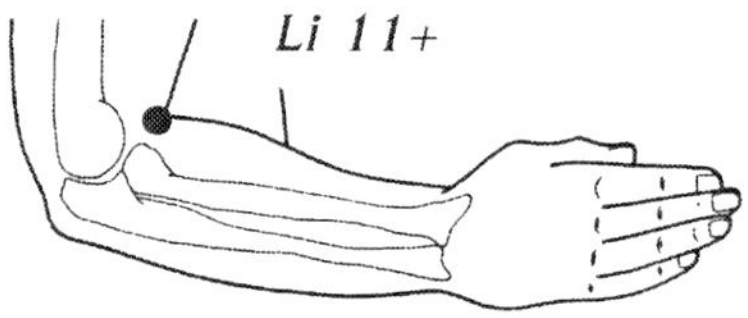

Fig. 2

St 36 4 fingers width below the kneecap and 1 fingers width to the outside of the shin bone. *Fig. 3*

Fig. 3

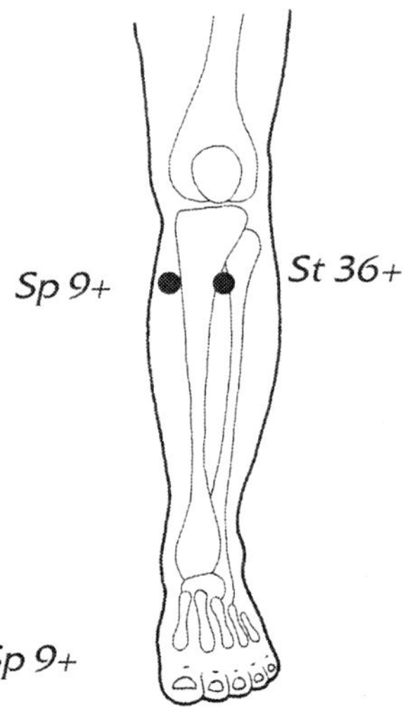

Sp 9 On the inside of the leg, 3 fingers width below the kneecap, in the depression between the bone and the calf muscle. *Fig. 4*

Sp 10 2 thumbs width above the upper/inner border of the kneecap. ***This tender point is at the highest spot of the inner thigh muscle.*** *Fig. 4*

Sp 6 This point lies 3 fingers width above the inner ankle bone and is located behind the prominent shin bone. ***Usually very tender when pressed.*** *Fig. 4*

Fig. 4

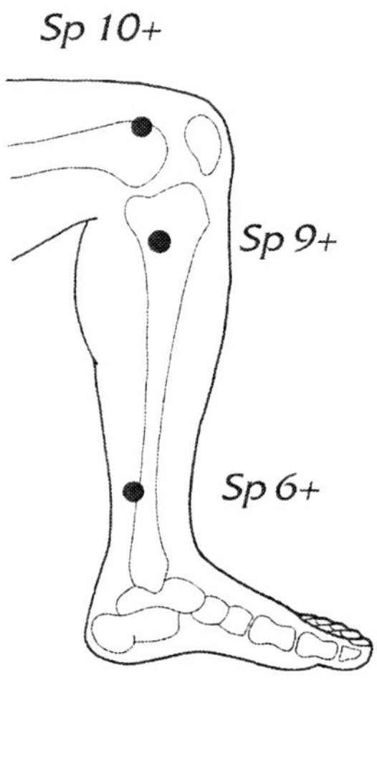

Snoring & Sleep Apnea

***C**onsult a Doctor before treating any points. For chronic conditions, sedate regularly until the condition subsides, then follow up with occasional maintainence.*

Lu 9 In the groove at the thumb side of the wrist crease, and inside of the tendon. *Fig. 1*

H 7 On the little finger side of the wrist crease, to the inside of the tendon. *Fig. 1*

P 6 3 fingers width from the most distal wrist crease, in between the tendons. *Fig. 1*

Sp 6 3 fingers width above the inner ankle and just behind the prominent shin bone. *Fig. 2*

K 6 1 thumbs width below the inner ankle bone. *Fig. 2*

B 62 In the depression half a finger below the outer ankle bone. *Fig. 3*

Cv 22 In the notch on top of the sternum. *Fig. 4*

Cv 17 On the breast bone at the heart level or the 4th rib space. Tender when pressed. *Fig. 4*

Fig. 1

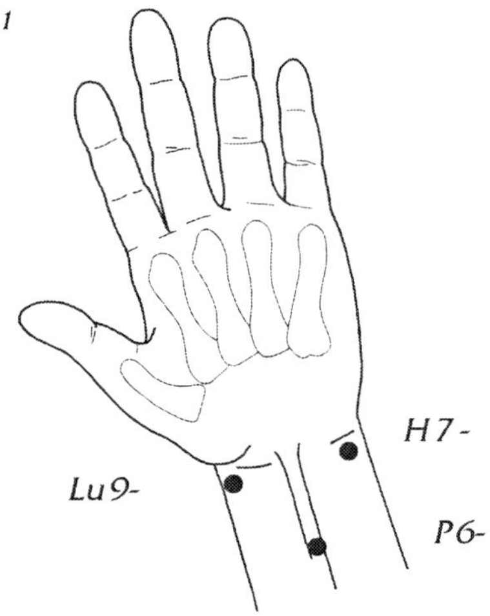

Fig. 2

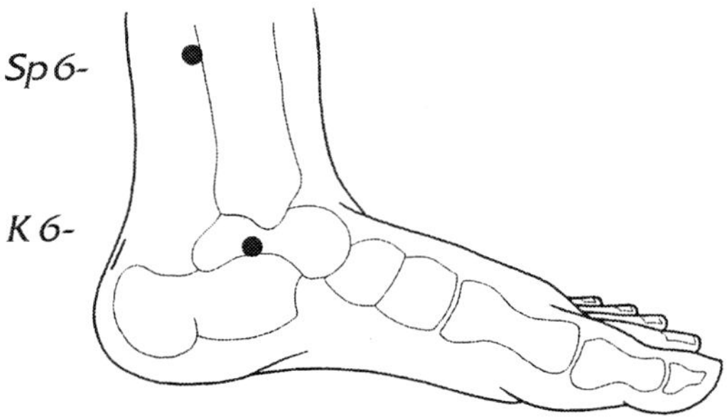

Fig. 4

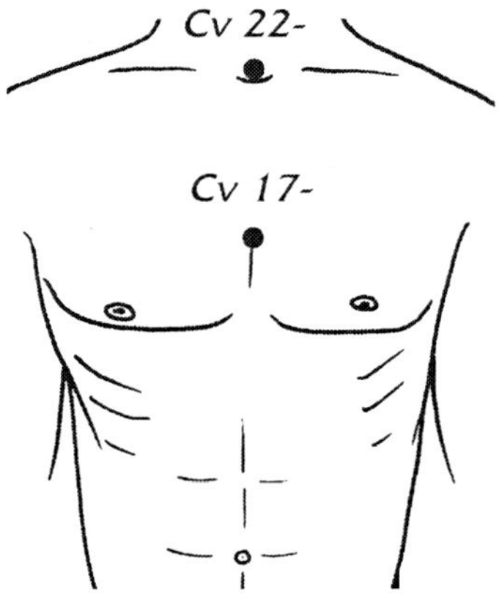

Fig. 3

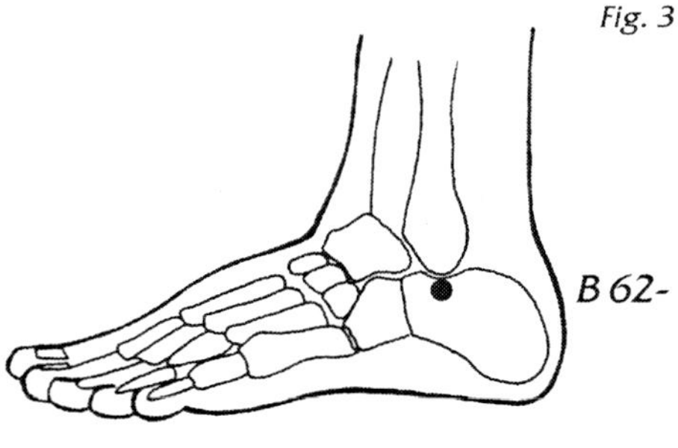

Spondylosis

S**pondylosis is characterized by local pain, tenderness and difficulty in moving the back. For pain relief and greater flexibility, sedate the following points on a regular basis.* ***It is recommended to release the entire spine as well as the distal points in the limbs.

Gv14 This lies just below the ***most prominent bone*** at the base of the neck in the midline. *Fig. 1*

Back Shu Points
Trace the pain back to the spine (site of segmental innervation) and sedate 2 fingers width to each side of the spinal bone. *Fig. 1*

Piriformis Trigger Points:
Approximately half way between the sacrum and the hip joint, (1hands width above GB 30). Press and rub (palpate) the general area until tenderness is detected. *Fig. 1*

Gb 30 This point is directly in the middle of the each "cheek" equal distance from all sides. *Fig. 1*

Gb 34 4 fingers width below the outside of the kneecap and just in front and below the knobby head of the fibula bone. *Fig. 2*

B 60 This lies in the hollow midway between the tip of the outer ankle bone and the Achilles tendon. *Fig. 2*

Lu 7 2 fingers width above the wrist crease from the base of thumb. ***In the slight hollow of the wrist bone.*** *Fig. 3*

Fig. 1

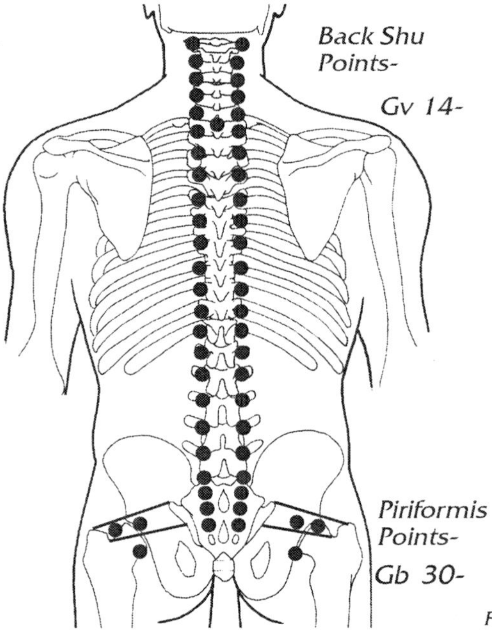

Fig. 2

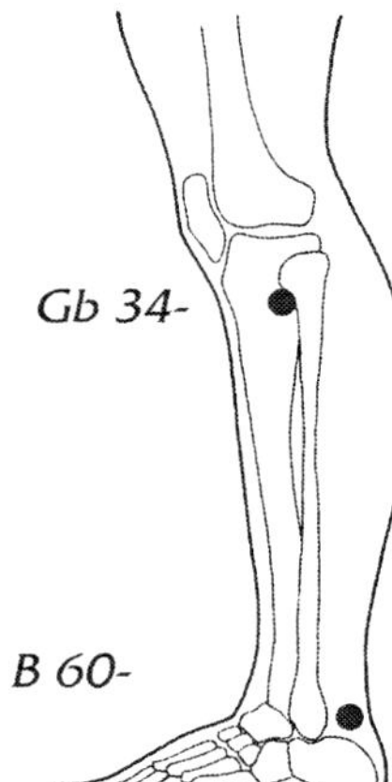

Fig. 3

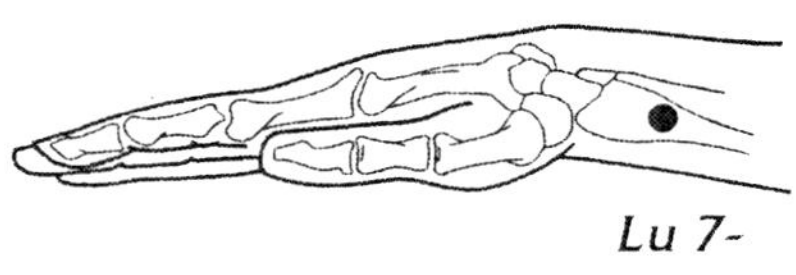

Temporo-Mandibular Pain

*This condition **(TMD or TMJ)** causes pain and clicking in the jaw just in front of the ear. Sedate the following points in the lower back and test for improvement. For additional points, see the following 2 pages.*

Back Shu Points:

Located 2 fingers width to each side of the spinal bones. ***Sedate these points from the middle to the lower back. Above points innervate the affected region and often provide substantial relief.*** *Fig. 1*

Piriformis Trigger Points:

Approximately half way between the sacrum (the triangular bone at the base of the spine) and the outside hip joint. Or, one hands width above GB 30. Press and rub (palpate) the general area until tenderness is detected. *Fig. 2*

Gb 30 This point is directly in the middle of the each "cheek" equal distance from all sides. *Fig. 1*

Gb 31 Stand erect, hands flat along the side of the thigh. This point is at the ***tip of the middle finger***. *Fig. 3*

Gb 34 4 fingers width below the outside of the kneecap, and just in front of and below the knobby head of the fibula bone. *Fig. 3*

Fig. 1

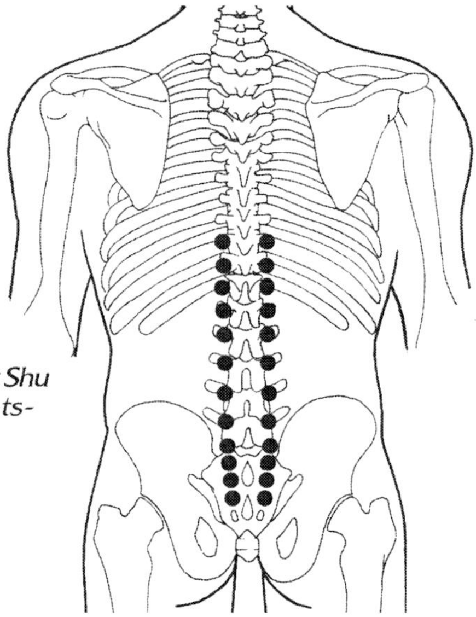

Back Shu Points-

Fig. 2

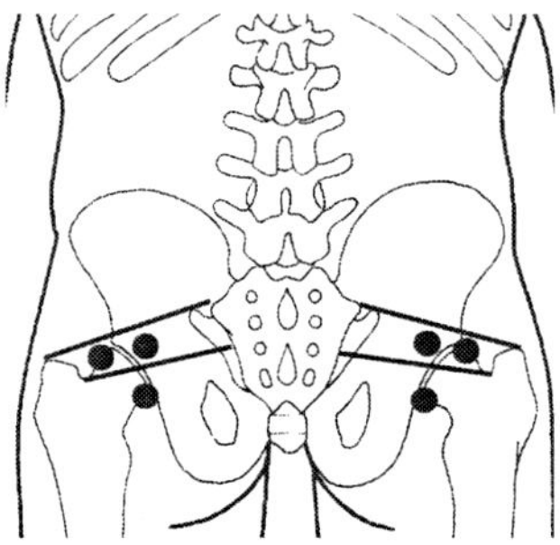

Piriformis Points-

Gb 30-

Gb 31-

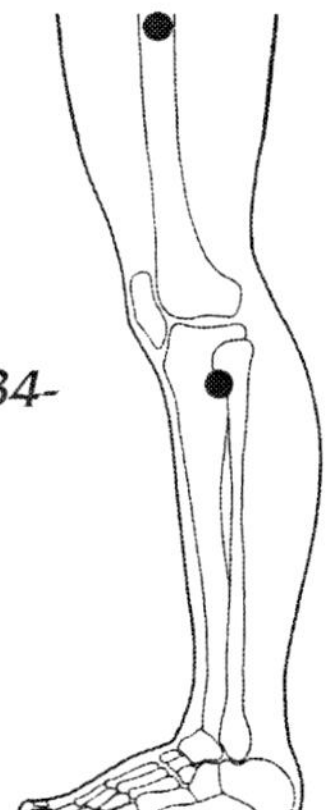

Gb 34-

Fig. 3

TMD/TMJ

Sedate the following points along with any tender points found in the neck and test for improvement. For additional points, see local points next page.

Gb 20 Below the base of the skull, in the hollow just outside the main spinal muscles of neck. *Fig. 1*

B 10 Located 2 fingers width from the middle of the spine at the level of the natural hairline at the back of the neck. ***In the middle of the ropy muscles on each side of the spine.*** *Fig. 1*

Gb 21 This lies halfway between the bone at the base of the neck and the tip of the shoulder, directly on top of the trapezius (shoulder) muscle. *Fig. 1*

Tw 15 1 thumbs width ***below GB 21*** *Fig. 1*

Si 13 4 fingers width ***below GB 21*** just on top of the spine of the shoulder blade. *Fig. 1*

Tender Points
Stimulate these tender points located in the tight muscles at the side of the neck. *Fig. 2*

Si 17 Above the prominent neck muscle, ***at the level of the corner of the jaw.*** *Fig. 2*

Li 18 4 fingers width beside the highest point of the Adam's apple in the prominent muscle at the side of the neck ***(below the corner of the jaw).*** *Fig. 2*

Si 3 On the end of the main transverse crease of the hand. ***Best located with the fist clenched.*** *Fig. 3*

Fig. 1

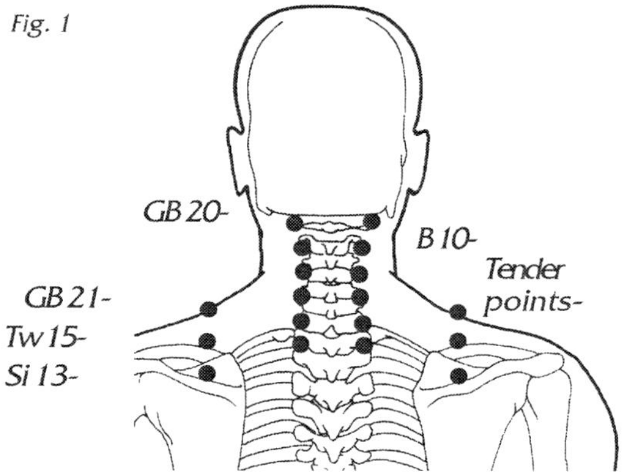

Fig. 2

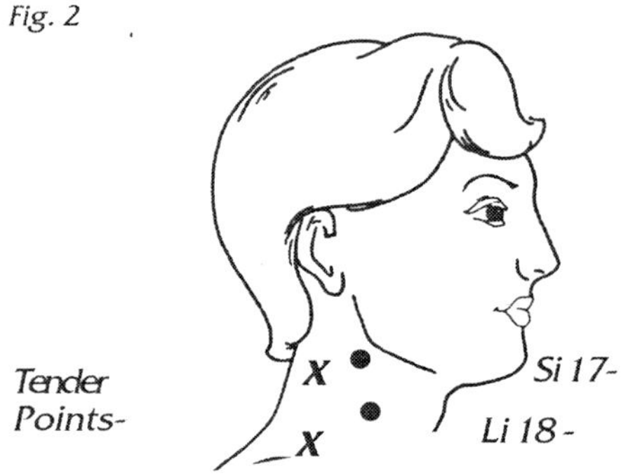

Fig. 3

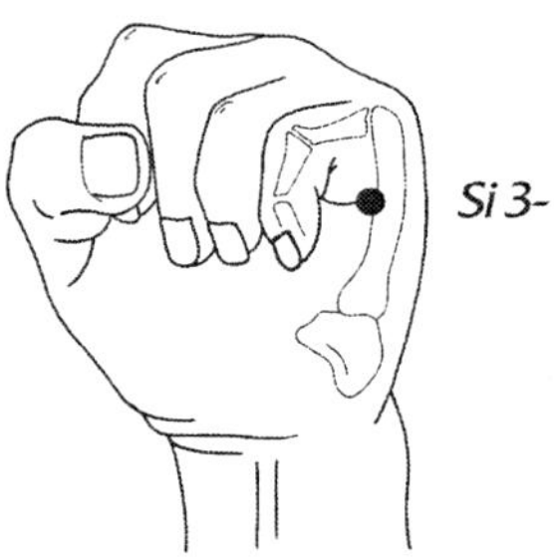

Temporo-Mandibular Pain

***S**edate the following points along with any tender points found in the jaw muscles and test for improvement. Additional points, call 1-800-567-PAIN.*

Tw 21 In front of the midpoint of the ear in the hollow felt when the ***mouth is opened***. *Fig. 1*

Si 19 Just in front of the upper end of the ear lobe in a hollow formed when the ***mouth is opened***. *Fig. 1*

Gb 2 Just in front of lobe of the ear. *Fig. 1*

St 7 2 fingers width in front of the ear, in the hollow ***with the jaw opened.*** *Fig. 2*

Si 18 Below the outer corner of the eye socket, ***directly under the cheek bone***. *Fig. 2*

St 6 Over the highest point of the bulge of the muscle at the angle of the jaw ***when the jaw is clenched***. *Fig. 2*

Tw 5 On the back of the wrist, 2 thumbs width above the wrist crease in between the 2 forearm bones. *Fig. 3*

Li 4 In the centre of the fleshy mass between the thumb and index finger, slightly towards the index finger bone. *Fig. 3*

Fig. 1

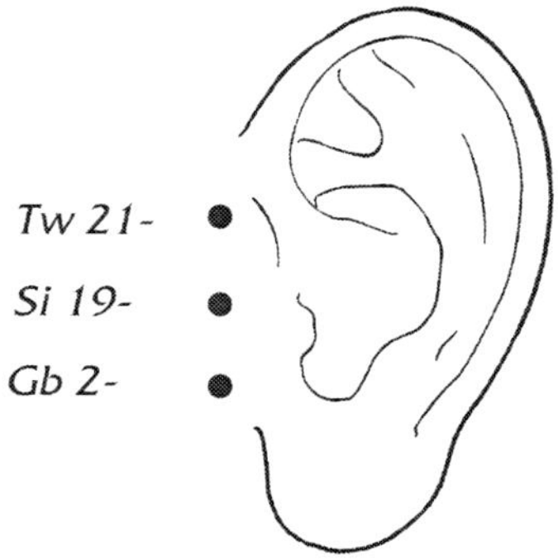

Fig. 2

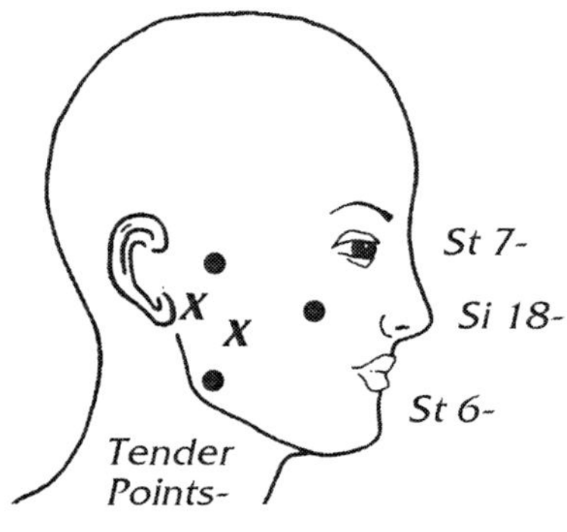

Fig. 3

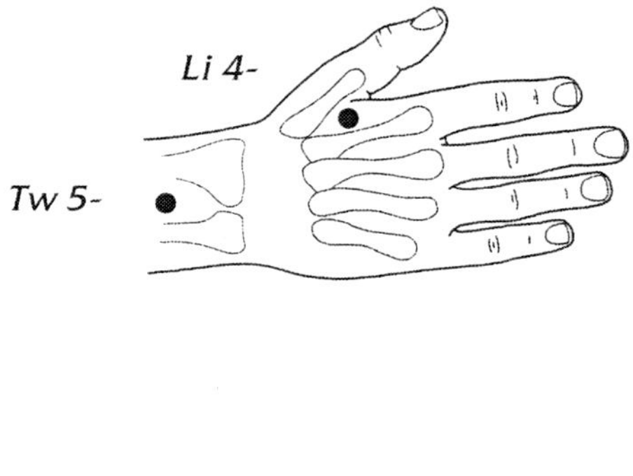

Thigh Pain

Consult a Doctor before treating any points. For chronic conditions, the lower back region should be treated first, follwoed by the jing points. For additional relief, sedate the local on the following page.

Back Shu Points:

Located 2 fingers width to each side of the spinal bones. ***Sedate these points from the lower back to the sacrum. Above points innervate the affected region(s) and often provide substantial relief to the patient.*** *Fig. 1*

Fig. 1

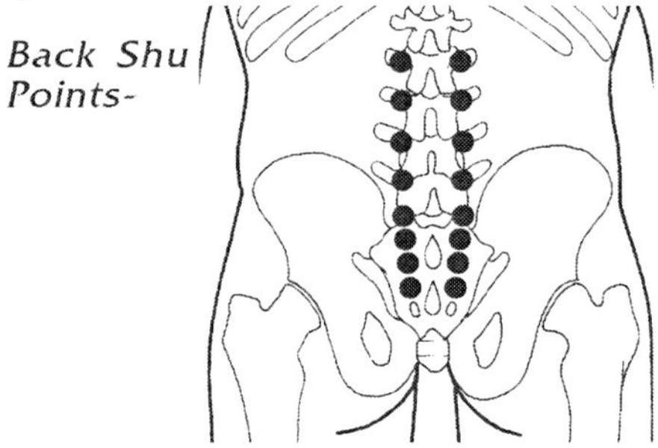

Piriformis Trigger Points:

Approximately half way between the sacrum (the triangular bone at the base of the spine) and the hip joint, or one hands width above GB 30. *Fig. 2*

Fig. 2

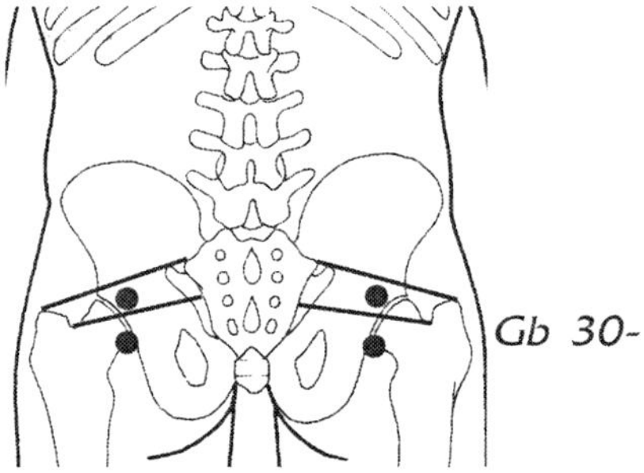

Gb 30 This point is directly in the middle of the each buttocks half, equal distance from all sides. *Fig. 2*

Gb 31 Standing erect with your hands laying the side of the thigh.This point is at the ***tip of the middle finger***. *Fig. 3*

Fig. 3

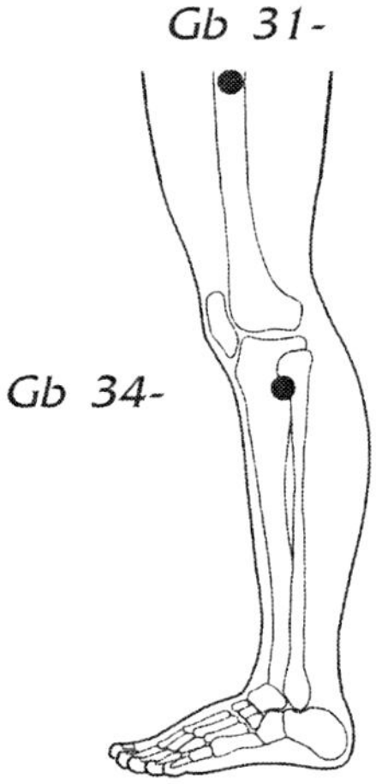

Gb 34 4 fingers width below the outside of the kneecap, and just in front of and below the knobby head of the fibula bone. *Fig. 3*

Fig. 4

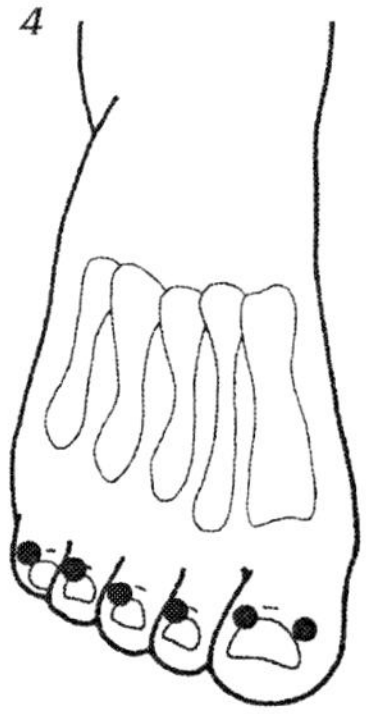

Jing Well Points-

Jing Well Points

Located on each side of the toenails at the base of the nail. *Fig. 4*

Thigh Pain

***S**edate the following points combined with low back pain points on the previous page.*

Gb 31 Stand erect, with hands flat along the side of the thigh. ***This point is at the tip of the middle finger.*** *Fig. 1*

Gb 34 4 fingers width below the outside of the knee and just in front of and below the knobby head of the fibula bone. *Fig. 1*

GB 39 4 fingers width above the tip of the outer ankle bone and just behind the outside leg bone. *Fig. 1*

B 60 In the hollow midway between the tip of the outer ankle bone and the Achilles tendon. *Fig. 1*

St 32 8 fingers width above the outer/upper border of the kneecap. *Fig. 2*

St 38 8 fingers width below the kneecap, and 1 fingers width to the outside of the shinbone. *Fig. 2*

Sp 10 2 thumbs width from the upper/inner border of the kneecap. *Fig. 2*

B 37 On the midpoint in the back of the thigh. *Fig. 3*

B 40 On the middle of the crease behind the knee. *Fig. 3*

B 57 On the mid point of the calf where the calf muscle narrows to form the tendon, between the 2 muscles. *Fig. 3*

Fig. 1

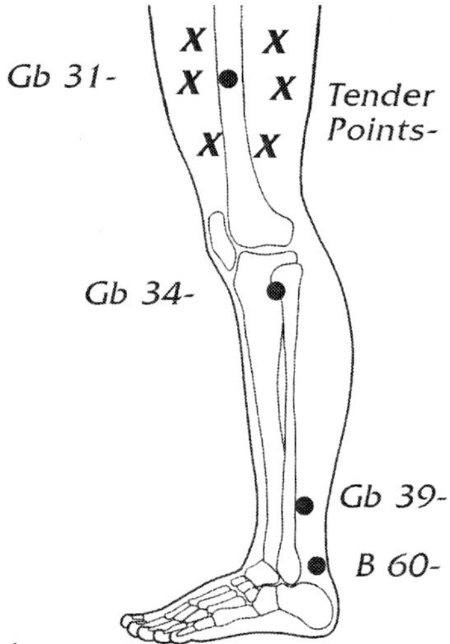

Fig. 2

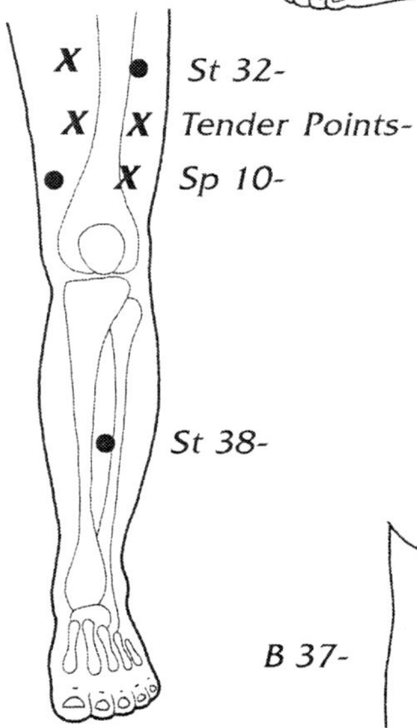

Fig. 3

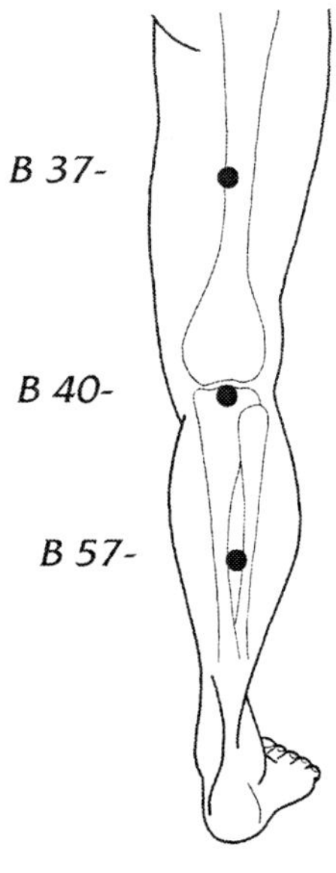

Tendonitis - Elbow

***S**ymptoms of tendonitis include pain and tenderness just outside or surrounding a joint. For chronic conditions, sedate the points in the lower back first and test for improvement. For additional points, see local points next page.*

Back Shu Points:
Located 2 fingers width to each side of the spinal bones. ***Sedate these points from the middle to the lower back. Above points innervate the affected region and often provide substantial relief.*** *Fig. 1*

Piriformis Trigger Points:
Approximately half way between the sacrum (the triangular bone at the base of the spine) and the outside hip joint. Or, one hands width above GB 30. Press and rub (palpate) the general area until tenderness is detected. *Fig. 2*

Gb 30 This point is directly in the middle of the each "cheek" equal distance from all sides. *Fig. 2*

Gb 31 Stand erect, hands flat along the side of the thigh. This point is at the ***tip of the middle finger***. *Fig. 3*

Gb 34 4 fingers width below the outside of the kneecap, and just in front of and below the knobby head of the fibula bone. *Fig. 3*

Fig. 1

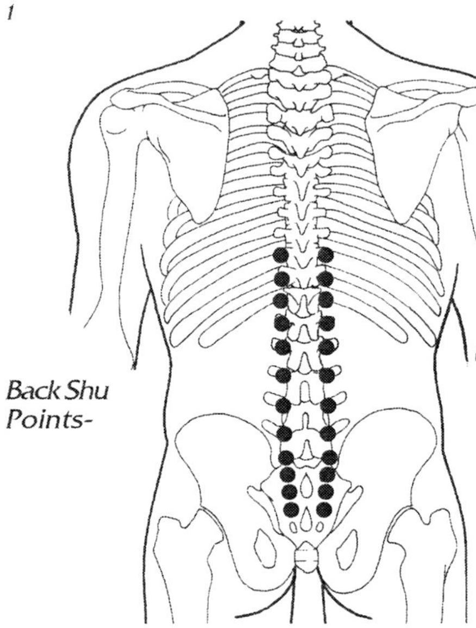

Fig. 2

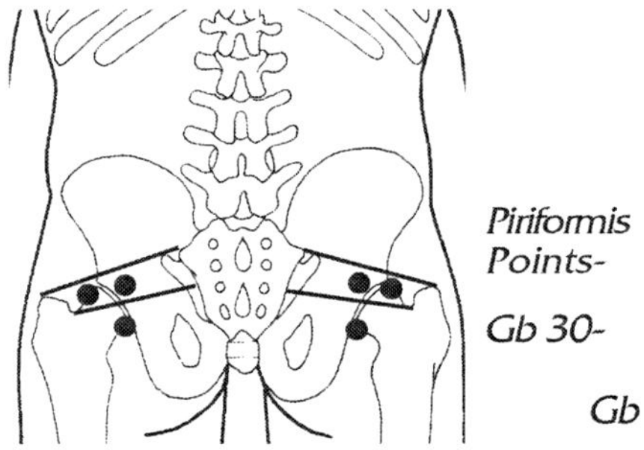

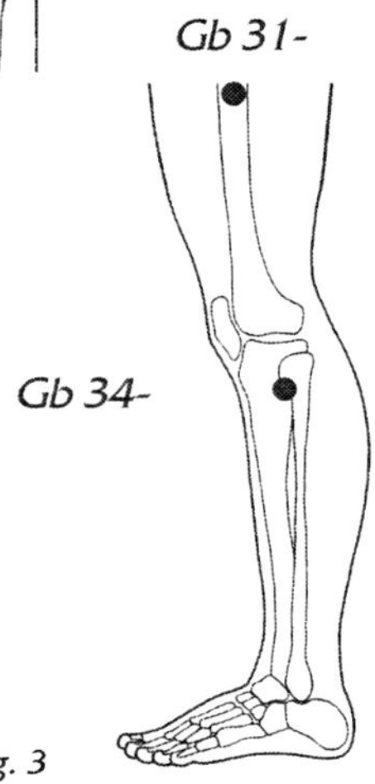

Fig. 3

Tendonitis - Elbow - continued

***S**edate the following points along with any tender points found in the neck and test for improvement. For additional points, see local points next page.*

Gb 20 Below the base of the skull, in the hollow just outside the main spinal muscles of neck. *Fig. 1*

B 10 Located 2 fingers width from the middle of the spine at the level of the natural hairline at the back of the neck. ***In the middle of the ropy muscles on each side of the spine.*** *Fig. 1*

Gb 21 This lies halfway between the bone at the base of the neck and the tip of the shoulder, directly on top of the trapezius (shoulder) muscle. *Fig. 1*

Tw 15 1 thumbs width ***below Gb 21.*** *Fig. 1*

Si 13 4 fingers width ***below GB 21*** just on top of the spine of the shoulder blade. *Fig. 1*

Tender Points
Stimulate these tender points located in the tight muscles at the side of the neck. *Fig. 2*

Si 17 Above the prominent neck muscle, ***at the level of the corner of the jaw.*** *Fig. 2*

Li 18 4 fingers width beside the highest point of the Adam's apple in the prominent muscle at the side of the neck ***(below the corner of the jaw).*** *Fig. 2*

Si 3 On the end of the main transverse crease of the hand. ***Best located with the fist clenched.*** *Fig. 3*

Fig. 1

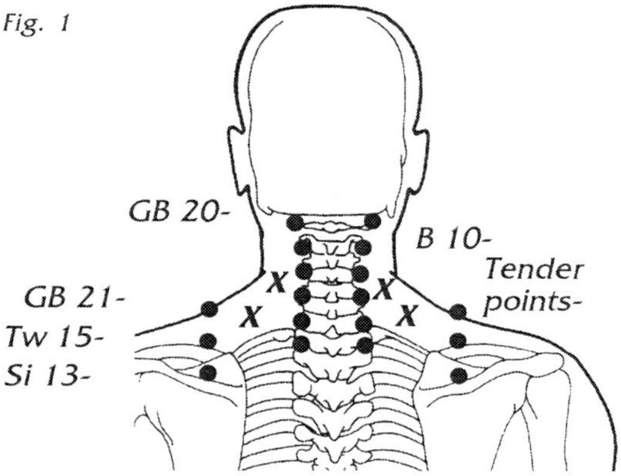

Fig. 2

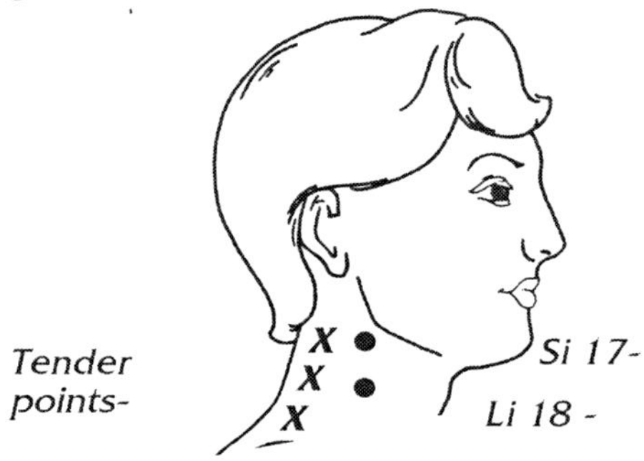

Fig. 3

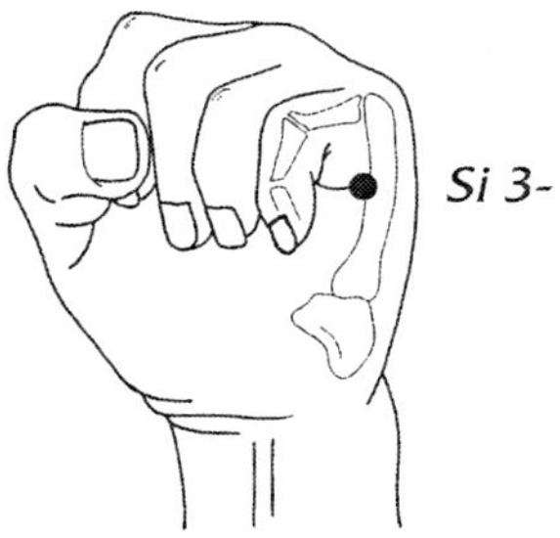

Tendonitis Elbow

I**f additional relief to tendonitis is required after treating the lower back and neck regions, sedate the following points along with any tender points found in the jaw muscles and test for improvement. Additional points, call **toll-free 1-800-567-PAIN.

Li 12 2 fingers width above ***Li 11.*** *Fig. 1*

Li 11 At the end of the outer elbow crease ***with the arm slightly bent.*** *Fig. 1*

Li 10 2 fingers width ***below Li 11***, towards the thumb. ***This point should be tender when pressed.*** *Fig. 1*

Lu 5 On the inner elbow crease, to the outside of the biceps tendon ***(the prominent tendon on the elbow).*** *Fig. 2*

P 3 On the transverse elbow crease, to the ***inside*** of the biceps tendon. *Fig. 2*

H 3 With the elbow flexed, midway ***between*** the inner elbow crease and the inner elbow bone. *Fig. 2*

Si 8 It is located in the hollow ***between*** the 2 heads of the elbow bones. *Fig. 2*

Tender Points

Stimulate any tender trigger points found within the tight muscles. ***The likely areas of location are marked with an "X".*** *Figs. 1 & 2*

Fig. 1

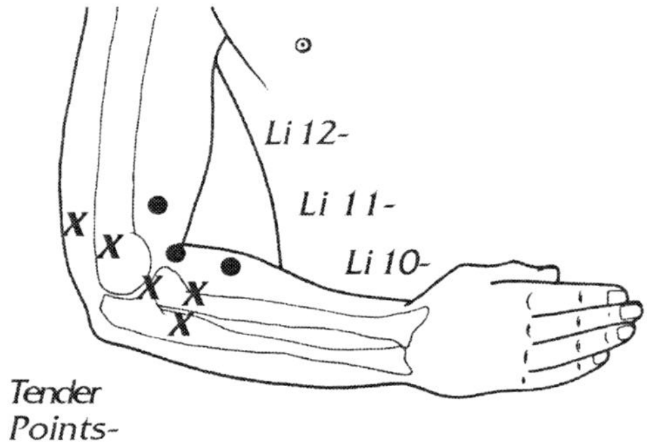

Fig. 2

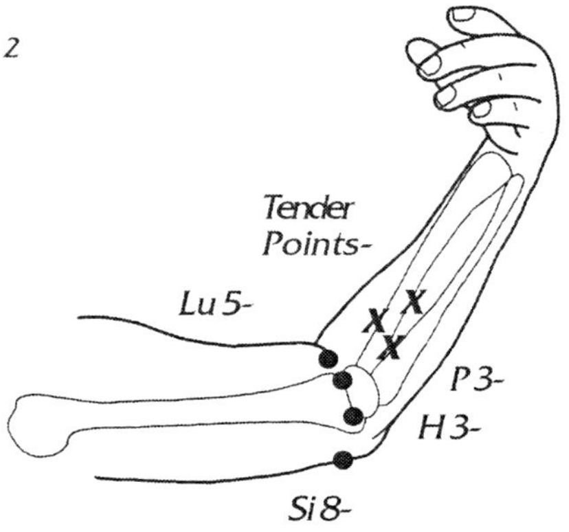

Thyroid - Hyper

***H**yperthyroidism is a condition where the thyroid is overactive. It is characterised by an increase in the metabolic rate of the body. The following points should help reduce that rate and relieve the unpleasant symptoms that are associated with this condition.*

Si 17 Above the prominent neck muscle, ***at the level of the corner of the jaw.*** *Fig. 1*

Li 18 4 fingers width beside the highest point of the Adam's apple, in the middle of the muscle at the side of the neck ***(below the corner of the jaw).*** *Fig. 1*

Cv 22 In the hollow just above the upper border of the breast bone. *Fig. 2*

Cv 17 In the slight depression midway down the breast bone, at the level of the nipples. *Fig. 2*

Li 4 In the middle of the fleshy mass of muscle between the thumb and index finger, and slightly towards the index finger bone. *Fig. 3*

St 36 4 fingers width below the kneecap, and 1 fingers width to the outside of the shin bone. *Fig. 4*

Sp 6 3 fingers width above the inner ankle and just behind the prominent shin bone. ***This tender point may be easily located by pressing and rubbing in the area.*** *Fig. 4*

Fig. 1

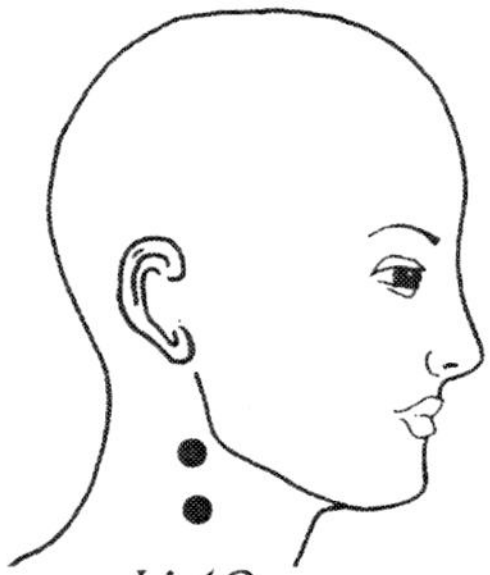

Fig. 2

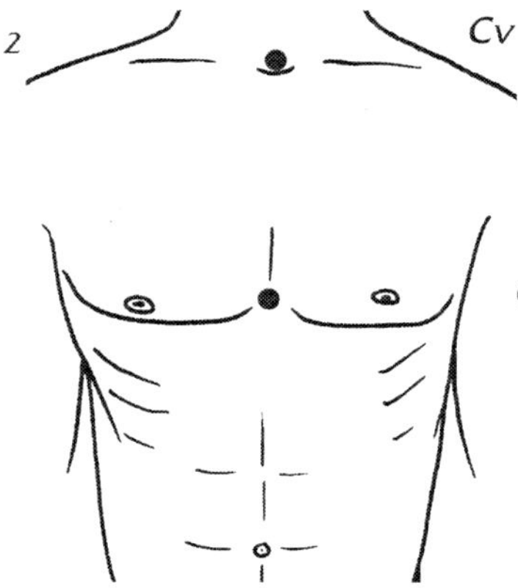

Fig. 3

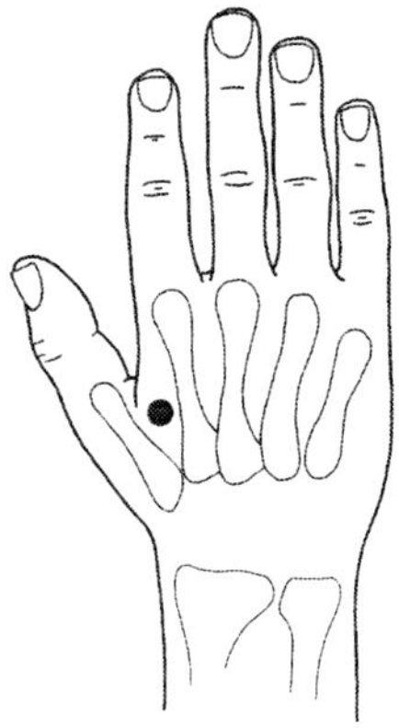

Fig. 4

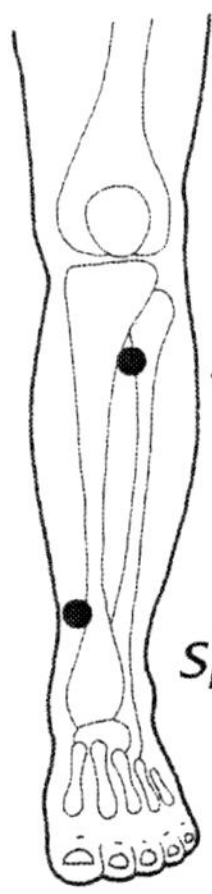

Thyroid - Hypo

***H**ypothyroidism is a condition where the thyroid is underactive. It is characterised by a decrease in the metabolic rate of the body, weight gain and lethargy. The following points should help increase the metabolic rate, increase energy and help reduce the unpleasant symptoms.*

Si 17 Above the prominent neck muscle, ***at the level of the corner of the jaw.*** *Fig. 1*

Li 18 4 fingers width beside the highest point of the Adam's apple, in the middle of the muscle at the side of the neck ***(below the corner of the jaw).*** *Fig. 1*

Fig. 1

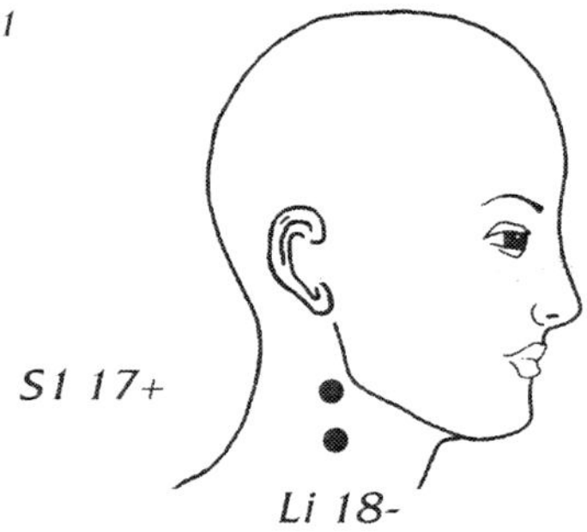

Cv 22 In the hollow just above the upper border of the breast bone. *Fig. 2*

Cv 17 In the slight depression midway down the breast bone, at the level of the nipples. *Fig. 2*

Fig. 2

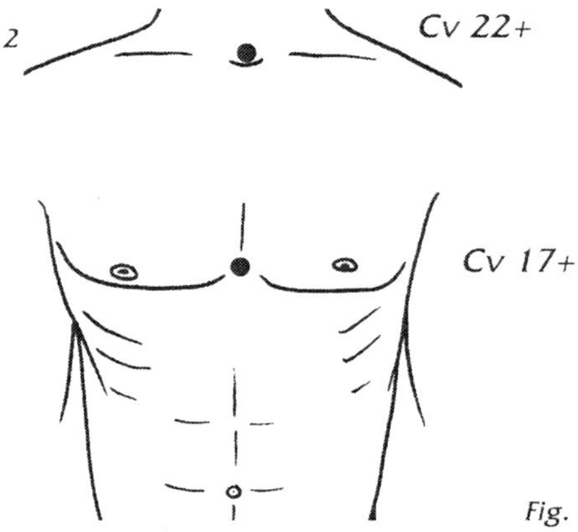

Li 4 In the middle of the fleshy mass of muscle between the thumb and index finger, and slightly towards the index finger bone. *Fig. 3*

Fig. 3

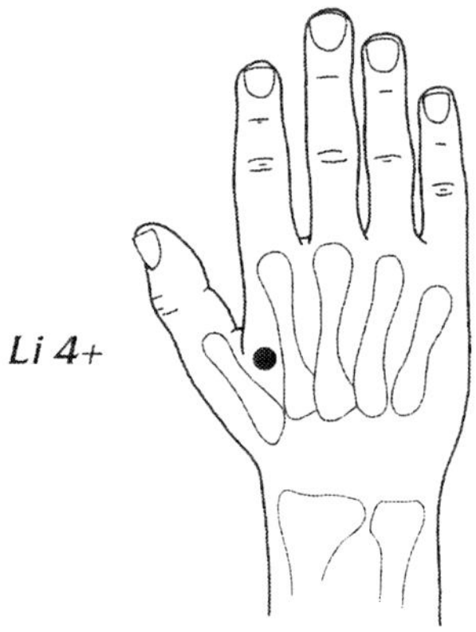

St 36 4 fingers width below the kneecap, and 1 fingers width to the outside of the shin bone. *Fig. 4*

Sp 6 3 fingers width above the inner ankle and just behind the prominent shin bone. ***This tender point may be easily located by pressing and rubbing in the area.*** *Fig. 4*

Fig. 4

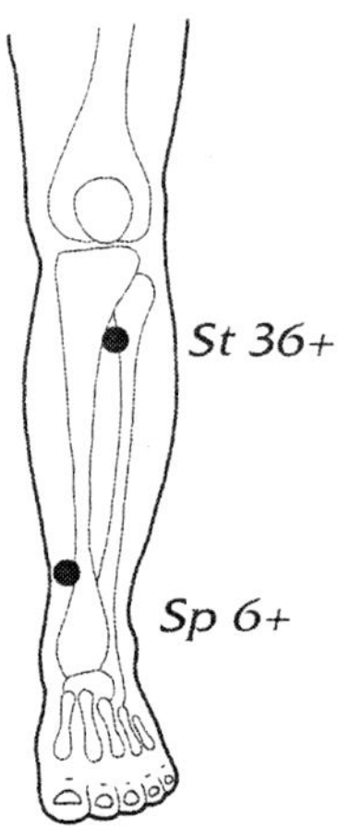

Thumb Pain

T**humb disorders usually arise due to tramatic injuries or repetitive use. For additional relief, sedate the neck pain points **found on pages 112-113.

Li 1 On the thumb side inner corner of the index finger. *Fig. 1*

Li 3 Just proximal to the knuckle at the base of the index finger. *Fig. 1*

Li 4 In the middle of the fleshy mass between the thumb and the index finger (closer to the index finger). *Figs. 1*

Li 5 In the anatomical snuff box, located at the base of the thumb in between the 2 thumb tendons. ***Easily identified when thumb is pulled away from index finger.*** *Fig. 1*

Lu 11 At the base of the inner/outer thumb nail. *Fig. 2*

Lu 9 On the inside of the tendon at the base of the thumb, on the transverse wrist crease. *Fig. 3*

Lu 10 On the palm side, located in the middle of the muscle at the base of the thumb. *Fig. 3*

Lu 6 6½ fingers width **away from** the elbow crease on a line drawn from the biceps tendon to the base of the thumb. *Fig. 3*

P 4 6½ fingers width **above** the midpoint of the inner wrist crease, between the 2 wrist tendons. *Fig. 3*

Fig. 1

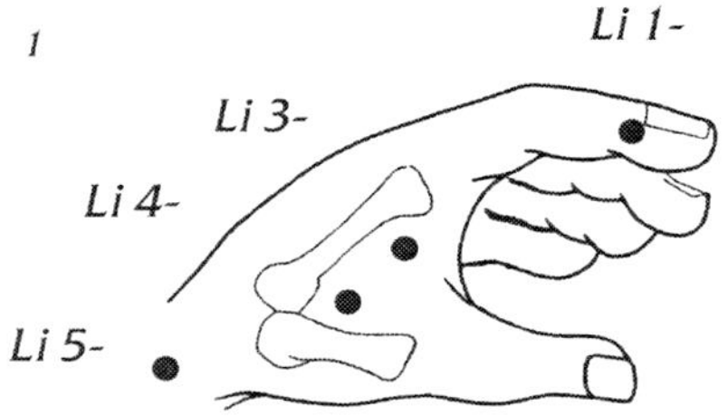

Fig. 2

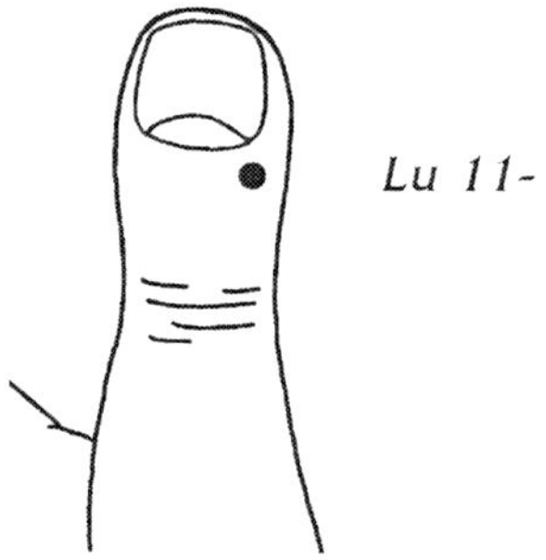

Fig. 3

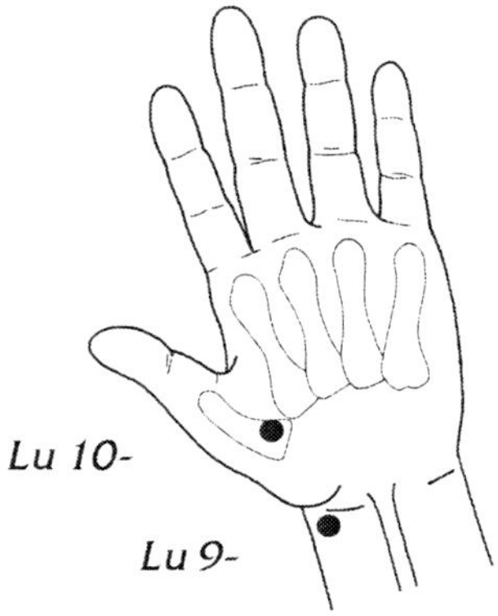

Fig. 4

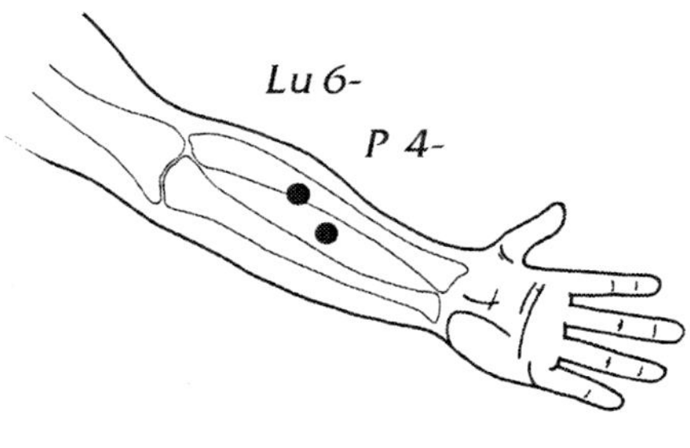

Tinnitus

***T**innitus is the perception of sound without external stimulus. Sedate the following points relating to the neck and test for improvement. For additional points, see next page.*

Gb 20 Below the base of the skull, in the hollow just outside the main spinal muscles of neck. *Fig. 1*

Back Shu Points
These lie 2 fingers width to each side of the spinal bones. *Fig. 1*

Gv 14 This lies just below the most prominent bone at the base of the neck on the midline. *Fig. 1*

Gb 21 This lies halfway between the bone at the base of the neck and the tip of the shoulder, directly on top of the trapezius (shoulder) muscle. *Fig. 1*

Si 13 4 fingers width ***below GB 21*** just on top of the spine of the shoulder blade. *Fig. 1*

Si 17 Above the prominent neck muscle, ***at the level of the corner of the jaw***. *Fig. 2*

Si 3 On the end of the main transverse crease of the hand. ***Best located with the fist clenched***. *Fig. 3*

Li 4 This point is located in the centre of the webbing between the thumb and index finger. *Fig. 4*

Tw 5 On the back of the wrist 2 thumbs width above the wrist crease in between the 2 forearm bones. *Fig. 4*

Fig. 1

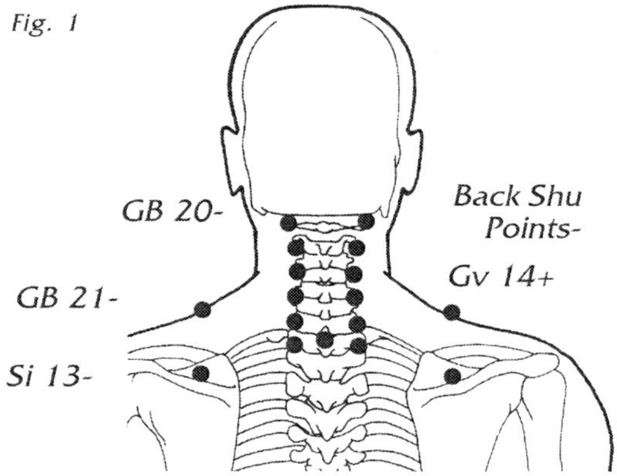

Fig. 2

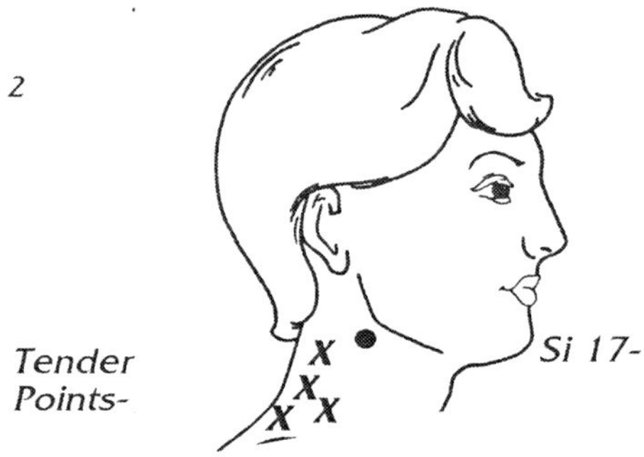

Fig. 3

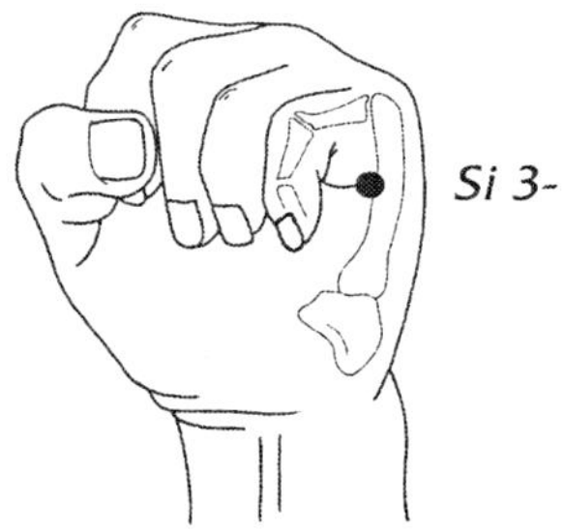

Fig. 4

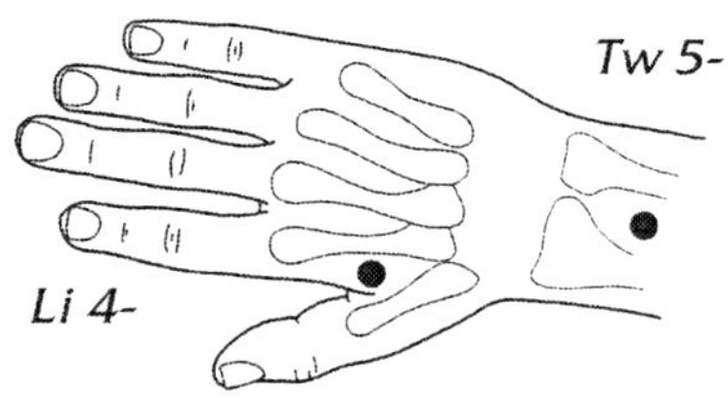

Tinnitus

S**edate the following points along with any tender points found belwo the ear and test for improvement. Additional points, call **1-800-567-PAIN.

Gb 41 In the depression, where the 4th & 5th toe bones meet. *Fig. 1*

B 67 At the outer base of the baby toe nail. *Fig. 1*

Gb 44 At the outer base of the 4th toe nail. *Fig. 1*

Li 11 This lies on the end of the outer elbow crease ***with the arm bent. Tonify.*** *Fig. 2*

Tw 21 In front of the midpoint of the ear in the hollow felt when the ***mouth is opened***. *Fig. 3*

Si 19 Just in front of the upper end of the ear lobe in a hollow formed ***when the mouth is opened***. *Fig. 3*

Gb 2 Just in front of lobe of ear. *Fig. 3*

Tw 17 On the indentation directly ***behind*** the ear lobe. *Fig. 3*

H 7 On the little finger side of the wrist crease, to the inside of the tendon. *Fig. 4*

P 6 3 fingers width from the most distal wrist crease, in between the tendons. *Fig. 4*

Fig. 1

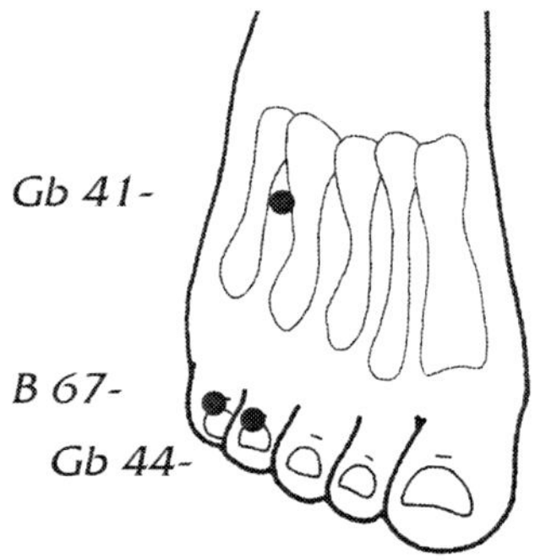

Fig. 2

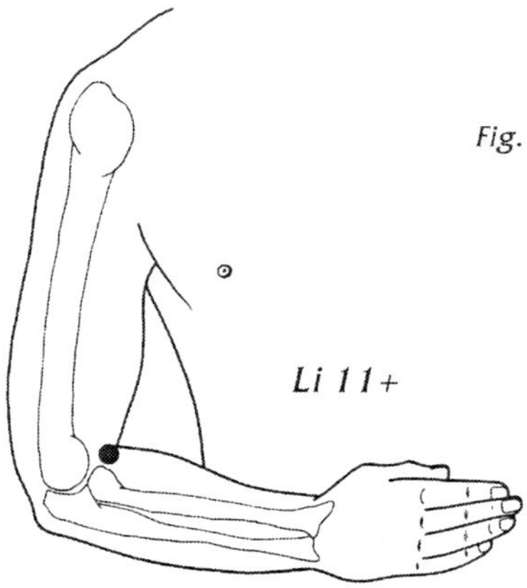

Fig. 3

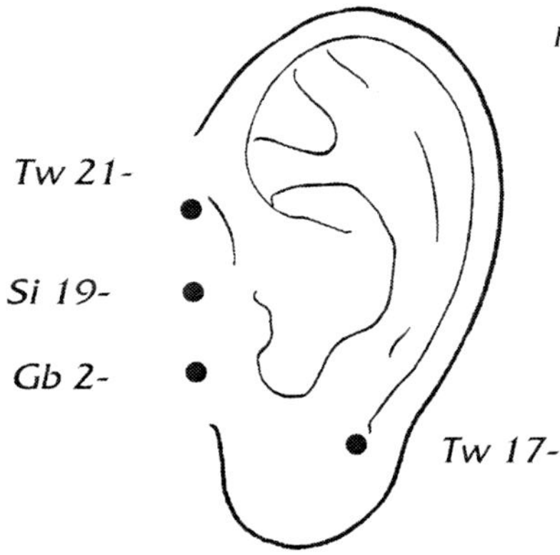

Fig. 4

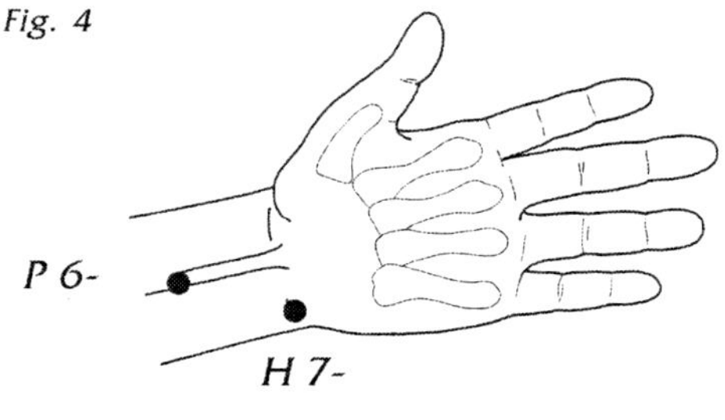

Wrist Pain

***P**ain may be caused by tendon inflammation, arthritis or acute injury. Sedate the following points for relief of symptoms.* **For chronic wrist conditions sedate the neck pain points illustrated on page 112-113.**

P 8 ***While clenching the fist*, the tip of the middle finger touches this point.** *Fig. 1*

Lu 9 In the groove at the thumb side of the wrist crease, and inside of the tendon. *Fig. 1*

P 7 On the wrist crease, in between the 2 wrist tendons. *Fig. 1*

H 7 On the little finger side of the wrist crease, to the inside of the bone. *Fig. 1*

P 6 3 fingers width from the most distal wrist crease, in between the tendons. *Fig. 1*

Li 4 This lies in the fleshy mass between the thumb and index finger, and slightly towards the index finger bone. *Fig. 2*

Li 5 In the snuff box hollow formed between the 2 tendons at the base of the thumb. ***Easily identified when the thumb is pulled away from the index finger.*** *Fig. 2*

Tw 4 On the midpoint of the crease on the back of the wrist. *Fig. 2*

Si 4 On the outside of the wrist crease. *Fig. 2*

Tw 5 On the back of the wrist 2 thumb widths above the wrist crease in between the 2 forearm bones. *Fig. 2*

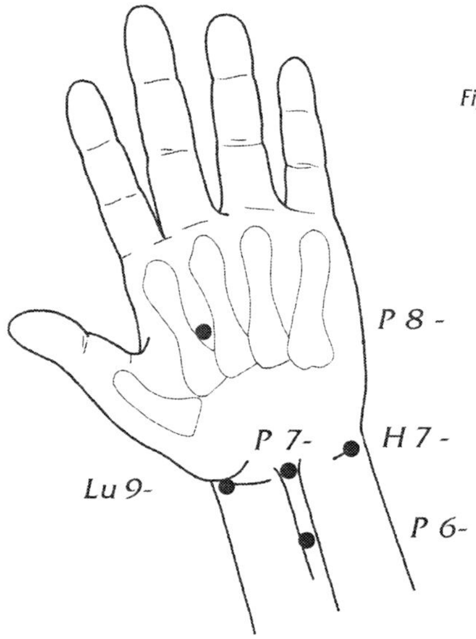

Fig. 1

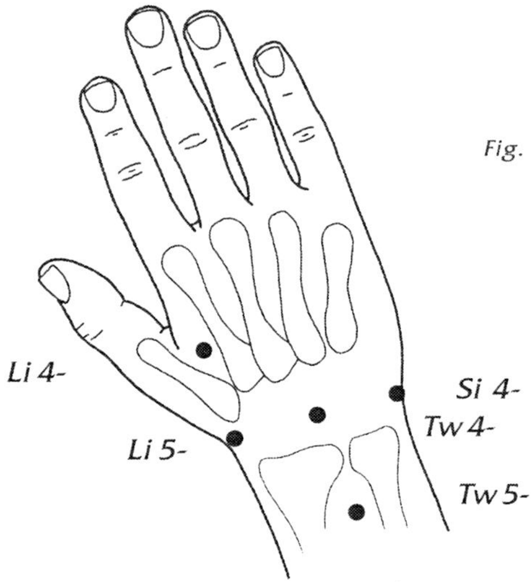

Fig. 2

World Health Organization

The World Health Organization (WHO) has listed a series of disorders for which Acupuncture has proven clinically effective throughout the world.

Neurological and Orthopaedic Disorders

Headaches
Migraines
Trigeminal Neuralgia
Bell's Palsy (Facial paralysis)
Paralysis after apoplectic fit
Peripheral neuropathy
Polio Paralysis
Ménière's syndrome
Neurogenic bladder dysfunction
Bed wetting (nocturnal enuresis)
Intercostal neuralgia
Periarthritis numeroscapularis
Tennis elbow
Sciatica
Back pain
Rheumatoid arthritis

Gastrointestinal Disorders

Spasm of esophagus and cardia
Hiccups
Gastroptosis
Acute and Chronic gastritis
Gastric hyperacidity
Chronic duodenal ulcer
Acute & chronic colitis
Acute bacterial dysentery
Constipation
Diarrhoea
Paralytic ileus

Respiratory Tract

Acute sinusitis
Acute rhinitis
Common cold
Acute tonsilitis

Bronchopulmonary Disorders

Acute bronchitis
Bronchial asthma

Disorders of the eye

Acute conjunctivitis
Central retinitis
Myopia (in children)
Cataract (without complications)

Disorders of the Mouth Cavity

Toothache
Pain after tooth extraction
Gingivitis
Acute and chronic pharyngitis

Index

ETPS Therapy Introduction .... 1 - 15
Quick Reference Guide .... 16 - 17
Dermatome Chart 18
Finger Measurements (How to Find Treatment Points) 19
ETPS Pain Therapy Introduction .... 20 - 49
Parasympathetic Points .... 21 - 22
Standard Protocol - Back & Lower Limb .... 23 - 27
Standard Protocol - Neck & Upper Limb .... 28 - 30
World Health Organization (WHO) 157

Pain Disorders

Abdominal Pain 32
Achilles Tendonitis .... 33 - 34
Ankle Sprain and Strain .... 35 - 36
Ankylosing Spondylitis .... 37 - 38
Back Pain - Lower .... 39 - 40
Back Pain - Upper .... 41 - 42
Anxiety & Stress *(see Parasympathetic Points)* .... 21 - 22
Bell's Palsy .... 42 - 43
Bursitis of the Shoulder .... 44 - 45
Calf Pain - General .... 46 - 47
Carpal Tunnel Syndrome .... 48 - 49
Cervical Spondylosis .... 50 - 51
Chronic Fatigue Syndrome .... 52 - 53
Coccyx Injury 54
Constipation 55
Costochondritis .... 56 - 57
Digestive Problems .... 58 - 59
Dupuytren's Contracture .... 60 - 61
Earache .... 62 - 63
Elbow Problems - Golfer's .... 64 - 66
Facial Pain & Neuralgia (toothache) .... 67 - 68
Fibromylgia .... 69 - 70
Finger Pain - Arthritis 73
Foot Pain 74
Ganglion 75
Gout .... 76 - 77
Groin Injury .... 78 - 79
Hand Pain & Stiffness 80
Hamstring Injuries 81

Heel Pain 82
Hernia ..... 83 - 84
Herpes Zoster *(see shingles)* ..... 130 - 133
Hip Pain ..... 85 - 86
Immunity - To Enhance 87
Impotence - Male 88
Insomnia - Stress - Apnea *(also see Parasymapthetic Points)* 89
Intercostal Neuralgia ..... 90 - 91
Irritable Bowel Syndrome ..... 92 - 93
Kidney Disorders *(see Renal Disorders)* 122
Knee - Runner's Knee ..... 94 - 95
Mandibular Arthritis ..... 96 - 97
Menstrual Cramps - PMS ..... 98 - 99
Metatarsalgia ..... 100 - 101
Migraine ..... 102 - 103
Multiple Sclerosis ..... 104 - 105
Muscle Cramps ..... 106 - 107
Muscle - Pulled or Strained ..... 108 - 109
Muscle - Sports Injuires *(see Muscles Pulled)* ..... 108 - 109
Nausea ..... 110 - 111
Neck Pain ..... 112 - 113
Osteoarthritis - Knee ..... 114 - 115
Parasympathetic - Calming 116
Pelvic Pain 117
Peripheral Neuropathy *(feet)* 118
Peripheral Neuropathy *(hands)* 119
Post Operative Pain 120
Plantar Fasciitis *(see Foot Pain)* 74
Prolapsed Disc (Low Back) 121
Renal (Kidney) Disorders 122
Rheumatoid Arthritis ..... 123 - 124
Sciatica ..... 125 - 126
Scoliosis 127
Shin Splints ..... 128 - 129
Shingles (Herpes Zoster) ..... 130 - 133
Shingles - Post for Immuniity 134
Shoulder Pain - Frozen ..... 135 - 136
Sinus Problems & Immunity ..... 137 - 138
Sleep Apnea *(see Insomnia)* 139
Snoring *(see Sleep Apnea/Insomnia)* 139
Spondylosis 140
Stress *(also see Parasympathetic Points)* 116
Temporomandibular Pain (TMD/TMJ) ..... 141 - 142
Thigh Pain ..... 144 - 145

Tendonitis - Elbow Pain ..... 146 - 148
Tenosynovitis - *(see Elbow Pain)* ..... 147 - 148
Thyroid - Hyper 149
Thyroid - Hypo 150
Thumb Pain 151
Tinnitus ..... 152 - 153
Toothache *(also see Facial Pain)* ..... 67 - 68
Whiplash *(also see Neck Pain)* ..... 28 - 30
Wrist Pain 156
World Health Organization 157

Happy Healing from Acumed